LE3 0QU

G000114846

Risks and outcomes in developmental psychopathology

Risks and outcomes in developmental psychopathology

Edited by

Hans-Christoph Steinhausen

Department of Child and Adolescent Psychiatry, University of Zürich

and

Frank C. Verhulst

University Hospital Rotterdam, Sophia Children's Hospital

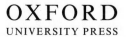

OXFORD
UNIVERSITY PRESS

OXFORD
UNIVERSITY PRESS

Great Clarendon Street, Oxford OX2 6DP

Oxford University Press is a department of the University of Oxford.
It furthers the University's objective of excellence in research, scholarship,
and education by publishing worldwide in

Oxford New York

Athens Auckland Bangkok Bogotá Buenos Aires Calcutta
Cape Town
Chennai Dar es Salaam Delhi Florence Hong Kong
Istanbul Karachi Kuala Lumpur Madrid Melbourne
Mexico City Mumbai Nairobi Paris São Paulo Singapore
Taipei Tokyo Toronto Warsaw

with associated companies in Berlin Ibadan

Oxford is a registered trade mark of Oxford University Press
in the UK and in certain other countries

Published in the United States
by Oxford University Press, Inc., New York

A catalogue record for this book is available from the British Library

Library of Congress Cataloging in Publication Data

Risks and outcomes in developmental psychopathology / edited by
H. -C. Steinhausen and Frank C. Verhulst.
Includes bibliographical references and index.
Running title: Risks and outcomes in adolescent psychopathology.
1. Child psychopathology. 2. Adolescent psychopathology. 3. Outcome
assessment (Medical care) I. Steinhausen, Hans-Christoph. II. Verhulst,
Frank C. III. Title: Risks and outcomes in adolescent psychopathology.
[DNLM: 1. Mental Disorders–in infancy & childhood. 2. Mental
Disorders–diagnosis. 3. Mental Disorders–therapy. 4. Risk
Factors. 5. Outcome Assessment (Health Care). 6. Psychopathology
in infancy & childhood. WS 350 R595 1999]
RJ499.R566   1999   618.92'89–dc21   98-52302

ISBN 0 19 262799 6

Typeset by Bibliocraft Ltd, Dundee

Printed and Bound by Thomson Press (India) Ltd.

Contributors

Dr Tyrone D. Cannon   Department of Psychology, University of Pennsylvania, 3815 Walnut Street, Philadelphia, Pennsylvania 19104, USA

Professor David P. Farrington   Institute of Criminology, Cambridge University, 7 West Road, Cambridge CB3 9DT, UK

Dr Robert F. Ferdinand   Department of Child and Adolescent Psychiatry, Sophia Children's Hospital, Erasmus University Rotterdam, Dr Molewaterplein 60, PO Box 700 29, NL–3015 GJ Rotterdam, The Netherlands

Dr Martine F. Flament   Pavillon Clerambault, INSERM, CNRS, UMR 7593, Hôpital La Salpêtrière, 47 Boulevard de L'Hôpital, 75651 Paris, France

Professor M. Elena Garralda   Imperial College School of Medicine, St. Mary's Campus, Academic Unit of Child and Adolescent Psychiatry, Norfolk Place, London W2 1PG, UK.

Professor Christopher Gillberg   University of Göteborg, Department of Child and Adolescent Psychiatry, Child Neuropsychiatry Centre, Annedal Clinics, Box 17113, S–413 45 Göteborg, Sweden

Professor Constance Hammen   Department of Psychology, University of California, 405 Hilgard Avenue, Los Angeles, California 90095, USA

Professor Richard C. Harrington   University of Manchester, Royal Manchester Children's Hospital, Hospital Road, Pendlebury, Manchester M27 4HA, UK

Professor Yifrah Kaminer   Alcohol Research Center, Department of Psychiatry, University of Connecticut Health Center, 263 Farmington Avenue, Farmington, Connecticut 06030–2103, USA

Dr Youngshin Kim   Child Study Center, Yale University School of Medicine, PO Box 3333, New Haven, Connecticut 06510, USA

Professor James F. Leckman   Child Study Center, Yale University School of Medicine, PO Box 3333, New Haven, Connecticut 06510, USA

Dr Jon M. McClellan   Child Study and Treatment Center, W27–25, 8805 Steilacoom Blvd SW, Lakewood, Washington 98498–4771, USA

Professor Sarnoff A. Mednick   Social Science Research Institute, University of Southern California, University Park MC 1111, Los Angeles, California 90089–1111, USA

Professor Heino F.L. Meyer-Bahlburg Department of Psychiatry, Columbia University, 1051 Riverside Drive, New York, New York 10032–2659, USA

Dr Michelle New Department of Psychiatry & Behavioral Sciences, Children's National Medical Centre, 111 Michigan Avenue NW, Washington DC, 20010–1970, USA

Dr Su-chin Serene Olin Social Science Research Institute, University of Southern California, University Park AHF B51, Los Angeles, California 90089–0375, USA

Professor Thomas Ollendick Department of Psychology, Virginia Polytechnic Institute and State University, Blacksburg, Virginia 24061–0436, USA

Professor Josef Parnas Institute of Preventive Medicine, Copenhagen Hospital Corporation, 1399 Copenhagen, Denmark

Dr Luiza A.D. Rangel Imperial College School of Medicine, St. Mary's Campus, Academic Unit of Child and Adolescent Psychiatry, Norfolk Place, London W2 1PG, UK

Professor Fini Schulsinger Hvidovre Hospital, Psychiatric Department, Brondbyostervej 160, 2650 Hvidovre, Denmark

Dr Laura Seligman Department of Psychology, Virginia Polytechnic Institute and State University, Blacksburg, Virginia 24061–0436, USA

Professor David Skuse Behavioral Sciences Unit, Institute of Child Health, 30 Guilford Street, London WC1N 1EH, UK

Professor Hans-Christoph Steinhausen Department of Child and Adolescent Psychiatry, University of Zürich, Neumünsterallee 9, Postfach, CH–8032 Zürich, Switzerland

Professor Ralph E. Tarter Western Psychiatric Institute and Clinic, 3811 O'Hara Street, Pittsburgh, Pennsylvania 15213, USA

Professor Eric Taylor Department of Child and Adolescent Psychiatry, Institute of Psychiatry, Denmark Hill, London SE5 8AF, UK

Dr Anneloes L. van Baar Emma Kinderziekenhuis, University of Amsterdam, Department of Neonatology, Meibergdreef 9, Postbus22660 NL–1100 Amsterdam Zuidoost, The Netherlands

Professor Frank C. Verhulst Department of Child and Adolescent Psychiatry, Sophia Children's Hospital, Erasmus University Rotterdam, Dr Molewaterplein 60, PO Box 700 29, NL–3015 GJ Rotterdam, The Netherlands

Dr Herma J.M. Versluis-den Bieman Department of Child and Adolescent Psychiatry, University Hospital Rotterdam, Sophia Children's Hospital, Dr Molewaterplein 60, PO Box 700 29, NL–3015 GJ Rotterdam, The Netherlands

Jennifer B. Watson Social Science Research Institute, University of Southern California, University Park AHF B51, Los Angeles, California 90089–0375, USA

Professor John S. Werry Department of Psychiatry, University of Auckland, Private Bag, Auckland, New Zealand

Abbreviations

ADHD	attention deficit hyperactivity disorder
APD	antisocial personality disorder
CAH	congenital adrenal hyperplasia
CAIS	complete androgen insensitivity
CBCL	Child Behavior Checklist
CBT	cognitive-behavioural therapy
CD	conduct disorder
CDAP	children of drug-addicted parents
CGAS	Children's Global Assessment Scale
CNS	central nervous system
CTD	chronic tic disorder
DIS	Diagnostic Interview Schedule
DISC	Diagnostic Interview Schedule for Children
DISC-C	Child version of the Diagnostic Interview Schedule for Children;
DISC-P	Parent version of the Diagnostic Interview Schedule for Children;
DSM	Diagnostic and Statistical Manual of Mental Disorders
EEG	electroencephalogram
EOS	early onset schizophrenia
ESCRF	end-stage chronic renal failure
GAF	Global Assessment of Functioning
GID	gender identity disorder
HIA	hyperactivity–impulsivity–attention deficit
HOME	Home Observation and Measurement of the Environment
HR	high risk
IBQ	Infant Behavior Questionnaire
IT	interactional therapy
MST	multi-systemic therapy
NAS	neonatal abstinence syndrome
NBAS	Neonatal Behavioral assessment Scale
NMI	no mental illness
NIMH	National Institute of Mental Health
ODD	oppositional defiant disorder
OCD	obsessive–compulsive disorder
PRF	Pupil Rating Form
RCT	randomized clinical trials
ROC	receiver operating characteristic

SPD	schizotypal personality disorder
SSRI	serotonin-selective re-uptake inhibitors
SUD	substance use disorder
T-ASI	Teen-Addiction Severity Index
TCA	tricyclic antidepressant
TEACCH	The Education of Autistic and Communication handicapped Children
TRF	Teacher Report Form
TS	Tourette syndrome
VEOS	very early onset schizophrenia
YABCL	Young Adult Behavior Checklist
YASR	Young Adult Self Report
YSR	Youth Self Report

Contents

Introduction

H.-C. Steinhausen and F.C. Verhulst

Since the early 1980s, interest in the concepts and findings of developmental psychopathology has increased considerably. The understanding that all psychopathology must be regarded in the framework of development is one of the cornerstones of modern child and adolescent psychiatry. Based on this core identity, the more recent research discipline of developmental psychopathology has raised various questions about continuities and discontinuities over time and over the various manifestations of behavior.

With this perspective, questions about causal mechanisms and processes have been the subjects of research. In order to tackle these questions, adequate research tools had to be developed or used. Epidemiological studies based on both cross-sectional and longitudinal designs have become a primary tool that has considerably increased our understanding of processes within the framework of developmental psychopathology. To study the natural course of childhood psychopathology and the factors that influence this course, we particularly need longitudinal assessments both of general population samples and of specific cohorts. The advantage of general population samples over clinical samples is that conclusions drawn from representative general population samples can be generalized, whereas conclusions drawn from the study of clinical samples are limited owing to selection factors connected with the referral process. Few studies exist that investigated the long-term longitudinal course of psychopathology in the general population from childhood into adulthood with measures of psychopathology that can be compared across time. Accordingly, the first section of this monograph, on high risk groups, starts with a chapter on community studies.

The topic on high risk groups continues with chapters on the offspring of parents who have a psychiatric illness. There is overwhelming evidence that these children have an increased risk of later developing the same disorder in a homotypic fashion, or of developing other forms of maladjustment or some other psychiatric disorder in a heterotypic fashion. The process involved in these outcomes include both genetic and environmental risk factors and their interaction. So far, various projects have studied these processes in the offspring of schizophrenic, affectively ill, alcoholic, or drug-addicted parents. In these studies the status of children who have been adopted away has often served as a means of investigating whether or not genetic liabilities are ultimately stronger than a protecting environment for the manifestation of certain disorders. However, the status of adoption may itself represent a risk factor for development because of the strain of environmental re-adaptation for the exposed infant or child. Because of this very nature of adoption as a potential risk factor, it is also reviewed in this monograph.

The clinical interest in developmental psychopathology focuses very strongly on the question of the outcome of the various psychiatric disorders originating in childhood. To what extent do certain disorders remit, how do they transform into adult psychiatric disorders, what are the risk factors for persistent disorder, are the relations between child and adult psychiatric disorder more of a continuity or a discontinuity type—these are just some of the many intriguing questions that are dealt with in the second section of the monograph. These questions are addressed in a series of chapters in which the various child and adolescent psychiatric disorders are described with regard to their clinical characteristics, their course, and their outcome. In addition, these chapters tackle the issue concerning the extent to which intervention has effects on the outcome and the development of the affected children.

Various conclusions can be drawn from the first chapter on children from the community at risk for psychopathology in adulthood. The first is that the continuity from adolescence to adulthood is considerable. In addition, it becomes clear that the study of community samples in contrast to clinical samples leads to different insights. In clinical samples selection factors including comorbidity and associated risk factors usually contribute to a poor outcome. Community studies make it possible to disentangle the effects of psychopathology as such on outcome from the effects of associated risk factors.

However, a disadvantage of community studies is the fact that very large samples are needed to study rare disorders and risk factors. One way of overcoming these problems is the use of the high risk study paradigm in which the offspring of psychiatrically ill parents are studied. These children are exposed to high genetic and environmental risks. The fruitfulness of this approach is shown in the chapter on children of schizophrenic parents. The authors give an authoritative review of the various eminent projects in this field. There is overwhelming evidence stemming from these projects that schizophrenia is a developmental disorder. These studies also identified a number of premorbid behaviors that later distinguished schizophrenics from normal children. However, more research is needed to discern whether or not a combination of these behaviors with other risk indicators such as perinatal complications, motor abnormalities, and positive family history of schizophrenia will improve the early identification of individuals who will later develop schizophrenia. The hope is that this could also lead to effective early intervention.

The enormous progress that has been made in studies on the offspring of affectively ill parents is also evident. After a first generation of studies on affective and other disorders in children, the mechanisms and modifiers of risk have been analyzed in more recent studies. They include parent–child interactions in younger and in older children, biological mechanisms, and multiple risk factor models. Among the modifiers, chronicity and severity of the parental disorder, the timing of exposure to maternal depression, and the role of the unaffected father are under discussion. This chapter also highlights methodological gaps in high risk research and reflects on future avenues for conceptual and empirical issues, e.g. the specificity of depression versus other indicators of malfunctioning.

Because of the high prevalence of alcoholism in adults, many children also suffer from maladaptation. The three major risk factors that affect their development are genetic, teratogenic, and family environmental factors. Although it is clear that a considerable proportion of the familial aggregation of alcoholism can be attributed to genetic factors, the specific inherited components of alcoholism are still unknown. Furthermore, owing to prenatal alcohol exposure, a considerable proportion of children suffer from long-standing physical, mental, and behavioral symptoms. There is a clear dose–response relationship between the amount and duration of exposure to alcohol during pregnancy and developmental outcome. In addition, the family environment, especially in the period of active alcoholism, is crucial to the development of the child. This has been shown for various disorders in the offspring, including conduct disorders and delinquency, hyperkinetic disorders, substance abuse, emotional disorders, somatic problems, and even cognitive and neuropsychological functioning. In conclusion, this chapter gives a broad account of the various factors that need to be considered in public health discussion of parental alcohol use and its consequences for the developing child.

It has also been shown that various developmental domains are affected in the offspring of drug-addicted parents. Again, in these children, the threefold risk factor model is applicable. Studies on the development of children who had been exposed to drugs prenatally clearly show that parental use of cocaine, heroin, and methadone lead to a variety of problems, which become more and more evident with increasing age. Beyond the subtle effects on growth and neuromotor development there are more serious delays in cognitive and socioemotional development. The most probable adverse outcomes include language impairment, conduct disorder, hyperkinetic disorders, and substance abuse. Among the various unresolved research issues are the interactions of the various main risk factors and the delineation of effective intervention programs from this research, including the prevention of the intergenerational cycle of addiction and psychiatric disorders.

Adoption is usually thought of as a means of reducing environmental risks by placing children exposed to unfavorable environmental influences into a more favórable environment. Indeed, many studies do confirm the beneficial effects of adoption. However, these studies are mainly restricted to white and intraracially adopted children. The Dutch international adoption study has shown that the adoption of children from developing countries by white parents challenges these previous findings. Internationally adopted children are at increased risks for later malfunctioning, especially as they move into adolescence. This is demonstrated not only with cross-sectional data but also using a longitudinal approach. An issue that still needs to be resolved is the reason why adopted children are more vulnerable to psychopathology in adolescence than non-adopted children.

The second section of the monograph covers the various child and adolescent psychiatric disorders. Each chapter is structured in the same way. After a brief introduction of the clinical picture of the respective disorder, studies of natural course are reviewed as far as they are available. In addition, the effects of intervention studies are highlighted. This is followed by a description of short-term and long-term outcomes. A further section deals with the question of continuity or discontinuity of the respective disorder over time. The penultimate section of each chapter deals with the discussion of risks and prognostic factors and, finally, some conclusions are drawn.

The first chapter in this second section deals with anxiety disorders. Regrettably, there is little research on the effects of intervention except for the positive effects of cognitive-behavioral treatment (CBT). There is also a substantial lack of controlled pharmacological studies. Contrary to what is often assumed, anxiety disorders do have negative consequences on later development in untreated samples. Although the outcome is better in treated samples, there are a number of open questions. The latter deal, for instance, with effects beyond diagnosis, including specific treatment factors. Although there is some evidence for a homotypic continuity of anxiety in childhood and adolescence, little is known about the course into adulthood. This also applies to the risks and prognostic factors related to outcome.

From the few intervention studies on depression, no clear answer as to the best treatment can be generated. As with the anxiety disorders, there are only a few controlled studies on psychological treatment. Again, CBT has been shown to be effective. Controlled trials with tricyclic antidepressants have shown no significant benefits over placebo in adolescents, in contrast to adults; there is also some concern over the side-effects of these compounds, especially in children. The greater effectiveness and lower rate of side-effects of the serotonin selective reuptake inhibitors (SSRIs) have led to some clinical optimism. However, carefully controlled studies are still lacking in the age range of childhood and adolescence. Despite a high recovery rate from the index episode, there is an increased short-term risk of subsequent episodes of depression. The long-term outcome is marked by a strong child-to-adult continuity of depression. Among the risk and prognostic factors that have been identified so far are those of older age at onset of depression, family stress, and extra-familial adversities.

As with the anxiety and affective disorders, positive intervention effects of CBT have been shown in some studies—predominantly in open studies—on patients suffering from obsessive–compulsive disorders. Furthermore, a substantial reduction of obsessive–compulsive symptoms has been documented in pharmacological studies using SSRIs. Both retrospective and prospective studies after treatment underline the severity of the disorder which, once established, most frequently takes a chronic, fluctuating course. Surprisingly few demographic and clinical features predict the long-term outcome of this disorder.

In the hyperkinetic disorders there is solid evidence based on controlled trials for the effects of various treatments. This is strongest for the stimulants, especially methylphenidate. However, the long-term effects of this medication are less clear. Some forms of behavior modification at school and at home are also effective. So far, direct comparisons between interventions and combinations of interventions have received little attention. Although some children may benefit from a specified diet, the question is open as to how many and which children can be helped in this way and whether diets are superior to other interventions. Although the short-term outcome can be inferred from the sizable treatment effects, the long-term outcome shows a remarkable proportion of persistent hyperactivity and other adverse outcome, even when treatment is provided. The adverse outcomes include aggressive and antisocial behavior, substance abuse, and poor educational careers. Among the various risk factors for continuity, the combination with conduct disorders is specifically worrisome.

For conduct disorder and delinquency there is long-standing accumulated knowledge that these disorders are associated with a poor outcome in a sizable proportion of the affected children and youngsters. However, intervention studies have proved that both early prevention and effective intervention are possible. Parent training, skills training, certain school programs, and multimodal programs have been shown to be helpful interventions. The outcome of conduct disorders is disproportionately followed by antisocial personality disorder in adulthood, and delinquency again is associated with many antisocial careers. Furthermore, there is considerable homotypic stability for both disorders. The main risk factors include low IQ and attainment, certain temperament and personality features, deficits in parental child-rearing behavior, parental disharmony and separation, antisocial behavior in the parents and large families, low socioeconomic status, and school influences.

Although there is a large number of treatment outcome studies of adolescents with substance use disorders, the outcome is highly variable. Relapse rates are high, according to short-term follow-up studies, and long-term outcome studies are lacking. However, drug use in most adolescents subsides or ceases by adulthood. Substance dependence in adulthood is predicted by behavioral or affective dysregulation, poor social skills, a limited social network, and substance use during late adolescence. Despite the mounting public concern regarding the physical and mental health outcomes among adolescents who use psychoactive drugs, it appears that modest experimental exposure to drugs may be a component of normative socialization and may not necessarily imply a poor prognosis.

For anorexia nervosa, one of the major eating disorders, there is some limited evidence from studies of natural course that a substantial proportion of subjects at risk and untreated cases remain stable with regard to their condition. Among the few controlled studies, only family therapy and some behavioral interventions have been shown to be effective. There is a substantial mortality rate (5%); full recovery has been found in only 43% of the patients, although 33% improve, and close to 20% develop a chronic course. There is a long and heterogeneous list of risks and prognostic factors related to the outcome.

In bulimia nervosa there is also remarkable stability of symptoms and diagnoses across time. CBT reduces target behavior and improves the accompanying psychopathology. Various antidepressants have been shown to be effective. However, little is known about matching patients to treatments. Furthermore, the majority of treated patients remains symptomatic at the end of treatment. Mortality rates are lower than in pure anorexia nervosa, and the recovery rate is slightly higher. Little is known about prognostic factors.

Children with various manifestations of somatoform disorders show up rather frequently in various clinical settings. Most of our clinical knowledge on treatment is based on case reports and uncontrolled studies, except recurrent abdominal pain, migraine, and functional headache. Obviously, more work is needed to identify the most efficient treatments for the various functional symptoms. Although approximately two-thirds of the children with these symptoms recover in the short term, the little that is known about the long-term outcome indicates a less favorable outcome, especially for abdominal pain, which tends to continue into gastrointestinal symptoms. In addition, there is insufficient evidence of any links between childhood somatoform disorders and other types of psychiatric disorders in adulthood. Unfortunately, very little is also known about the contribution of risk factors to the continuation of symptoms.

Despite the enormous psychological burdens on children with chronic physical illness, e.g. asthma, epilepsy, chronic renal failure, diabetes mellitus, cystic fibrosis, or congenital heart disease, the adult adjustment of children surviving these conditions is not compromised. If psychiatric disorders—i.e. mainly emotional disorders such as depression and anxiety disorders—are present in childhood, there is continuity more in the type than in the level of psychiatric disturbance. Severity of the physical condition and brain involvement seem to be the major risk factors for adult psychiatric disorder. Self-esteem might be an important protective factor.

Both studies of natural course and intervention studies in children with autism spectrum disorders reveal that the majority of these children will show deviance throughout life. Others will improve enough to make it possible to lead an almost independent life. Despite the short-term benefits of some specific forms of treatment, the extent to which these interventions have a long-term beneficial effect is still unknown. The level of intelligence and communications skills, together with neuropsychological functioning, i.e. flexibility and cognitive shifting abilities, are the predictors of long-term outcome.

Because of the very low incidence of early onset schizophrenia, there is very little systematic research on its natural course. For instance, it is not known whether or not it follows a longitudinal pattern as in adult schizophrenia. In 80% of the young patients with more than one episode, recovery is incomplete. Although clinical practice clearly shows that an array of therapeutic resources are needed and should take into account the specific developmental needs of children and adolescents, more needs to be known about the differential contribution of the various components to treatment and outcome. The long-term outcome of early onset schizophrenia is consistent with the adult finding that approximately 50% suffer from chronic impairment. However, more recent studies show that the prognosis might be even worse in very young people. Among the known prognostic factors are age at onset, premorbid functioning, intellectual functioning, and degree of recovery from the first episode.

Various pharmacological agents have been studied in children and adolescents suffering from tic disorders, so there is sufficient knowledge about the beneficial effects and the side-effects of these substances in clinical practice. In addition, controlled studies indicate that among various behavior modification procedures, habit reversal is superior to other modes in reducing tic symptoms. The long-term prognosis of tic disorders is characterized by a marked reduction of symptoms in late adolescence and early adulthood. The psychosocial outcomes might be less favorable in patients suffering from Tourette's syndrome, owing to restricted educational and vocational opportunities. The findings on prognostic factors are inconclusive across studies.

Two variants of gender differentiation are considered among the psychosexual disorders, i.e. gender identity disorder (GID) and gender identity problems in intersexuality. Because of the relatively rare occurrence of these problems, only few studies based on larger samples have been performed. In males, the GID appears to fade away during the years of middle childhood with a substantial proportion of boys with GID showing homosexuality as adults. Research on the development of children with intersexuality is important with respect to our understanding of gender differentiation. No well-established standard treatment regimes for childhood GID or for gender problems in intersexuality are currently available. Given the magnitude of psychosocial factors influencing gender differentiation, there is no clear picture of the most influential prognostic factors for both the development of GID and gender problems in intersex children.

The final chapter on child maltreatment deals with neglect and physical abuse, including sexual abuse. Although intervention can result in improvement, more systematic research is needed to determine which factors influence treatment outcome. However, it is well established that both physical and sexual abuse have far-reaching consequences on later functioning in important areas of adult life such as interpersonal relationships, sexual functioning, cognitive functioning, and socioemotional functioning. There is also a special concern about potential intergenerational effects on parenting practices.

In conclusion, this monograph provides a rich source of information on the risks and outcomes in developmental psychopathology. Because of the individual and the societal burdens that are inherent in the less favorable courses of many child and adolescent psychiatric disorders, it is vital that we proceed to gain more empirical knowledge of these developmental processes. In contrast to the more widely prevalent disorders, e.g. hyperkinetic or conduct disorders, there are much wider gaps in our knowledge of the rarer conditions such as schizophrenia, obsessive–compulsive disorders, or gender identity problems. This poses a challenge to setting up international collaborative studies. Projects of this kind would certainly profit from the growing awareness of using standardized diagnostic procedures and common methodologies that have been successfully implemented in child and adolescent psychiatric research in the recent past. Hopefully, the unraveling of developmental mechanisms will also stimulate the design of more effective interventions and prevention in order to help troubled youth.

High risk groups

1 Children from the community at risk for psychopathology in adulthood

Robert F. Ferdinand and Frank C. Verhulst

To assess the outcome of child and adolescent psychopathology, and to identify children and adolescents from the community who are at risk for psychopathology or maladjustment in adulthood, longitudinal studies are indispensable. Knowledge of longitudinal pathways of problems in unselected samples is needed to understand causal mechanisms, to determine the necessity of intervention, and to test and improve appropriate intervention strategies. During the past decade various community studies have investigated the course of child and adolescent psychopathology into young adulthood. These studies have provided valuable information on the course of psychopathology across an important developmental phase: the transition from childhood into adulthood.

In this chapter, results of existing longitudinal community studies, spanning the transition from childhood or adolescence into adulthood, are presented. Furthermore, a number of methodological issues, including possible longitudinal designs, diagnostic paradigms, assessment procedures, and data analyses are discussed. The characteristics of the epidemiological studies spanning the transition from adolescence to adulthood that are reviewed in this chapter are summarized in Table 1.1. We have included only prospective studies that used reliable and valid assessment procedures in representative community samples. The main information provided by these studies concerns associations between psychopathology in adolescence and psychopathology or maladjustment in young adulthood. These associations therefore constitute the main topic of the present chapter; risk factors for maladjustment in adulthood, other than psychopathology in childhood or adolescence, are not reviewed here.

Paradigms of the studies

Two main paradigms

The lack of a gold standard to determine morbidity is a major problem in psychiatric epidemiology, hampering comparability across studies and across time. Two nosological systems are widely used to assess child and adolescent psychopathology:

- the DSM system (APA 1994)
- the empirically derived taxonomic constructs that are associated with the Child Behavior Checklist and its derivatives (Achenbach 1991a–d).

Table 1.1 Studies that have provided information on continuity and change of psychopathology at the transition from adolescence to adulthood in community samples

Country	Sample	Initial age (years)	Diagnostic system	Age at follow-up (years)	Diagnostic system	Main sources
USA	National sample	13–16	Achenbach's taxonomy	19–22	Achenbach's taxonomy	Achenbach et al. (1995) McDonald and Achenbach (1996)
USA	Nine Western Oregon high schools	14–18	DSM-III-R	15–19	DSM-III-R	Orvaschel et al. (1995)
New Zealand	Birth cohort from Dunedin hospital	0	DSM-III behavior observations	21	DSM-III-R	Schaughency et al. (1994) Feehan et al. (1995) Caspi et al. (1996) Bardone et al. (1996)
The Netherlands	Province of Zuid Holland	11–16	Achenbach's taxonomy	19–24	Achenbach's taxonomy DSM-III-R	Ferdinand & Verhulst (1995) Ferdinand et al. (1995a, b) Ferdinand et al. (1998)

The DSM system has greatly influenced research on psychopathology. However, most of its childhood categories are not based on empirical findings. Furthermore, major shifts have been introduced in definitions of childhood disorders from DSM-III to DSM-III-R, and from DSM-III-R to DSM-IV. This is an especially serious handicap to longitudinal studies, because diagnostic criteria used at the time of the initial assessment may be obsolete by the time of the next measurement.

In contrast to the DSM classification system, the taxonomic constructs derived by Achenbach (1991a–d) are easily applicable to longitudinal data. Achenbach (1991a) constructed eight syndromes:

- Withdrawn
- Somatic Complaints
- Anxious/Depressed
- Thought Problems
- Social Problems
- Attention Problems
- Aggressive Behavior
- Delinquent Behavior.

These syndromes were derived from multivariate analyses of parent, teacher, and self-report data on large clinical samples. Data were obtained via the Child Behavior Checklist (CBCL), its teacher version (Teacher's Report Form; TRF) and its self-report (Youth Self Report; YSR) version (Achenbach 1991b–d). Although the 1991 CBCL syndromes differ from earlier versions, this did not complicate longitudinal comparisons, since the 1991 version of the CBCL is almost identical to the 1983 version. Hence, new scoring methods can be applied to longitudinal data that were obtained prior to 1991, which facilitates the application of the CBCL and its derivatives in longitudinal research.

Outcome measures as external validators

The outcome of psychopathology across time can also be investigated by testing the power of psychopathology measures to predict measures of later malfunctioning that can be regarded a consequence of psychopathology. Associations between initial psychopathology and later indices of psychopathology that are external to initial assessment procedures can be used to test the validity of associations between longitudinal data that rely on similar assessment procedures across time. For instance, in their 8 year follow-up of initially 13–16 year olds, Ferdinand and Verhulst (1995) assessed several signs of malfunctioning at follow-up, including expulsion from school or work, police or judicial contacts, and referral to mental health services.

The need for different informants

Reliable standardized information on behavioral and emotional problems in children can be provided by parents and teachers. As children grow older, they themselves become a reliable source of information.

Agreement between parent, teacher, and self-report data is usually moderate or low, irrespective of the diagnostic procedures used (McConaughy *et al.* 1992, Verhulst and van der Ende 1992, Verhulst and Koot 1992, Verhulst *et al.* 1997a). A number of studies have tried to ascertain which informant is best for assessing certain disorders (Reich and Earls 1987, Loeber *et al.* 1990, Bird *et al.* 1992) but encountered the problem of which criterion to use in determining the validity of information from different sources.

Longitudinal research can be of use to compare the validity of information from different informants, by comparing the differential predictive value of different informants' ratings of problem behavior for indices of malfunctioning over time. A comparison of the ability of parents', teachers', and adolescents'self-reports of problem behaviors to predict signs of maladjustment across time was carried out by Verhulst *et al.* (1997b). This study tested the ability to predict referral for mental health services, and need for professional help without actually being referred, of parent ratings on the CBCL, teacher ratings on the TRF, and adolescents' ratings on the YSR. Subjects from the Dutch general population were initially assessed at ages 11–14, and were reassessed 4 years later.

It was found that deviant scores on the CBCL scale Delinquent Behavior and on the TRF scales Withdrawn and Thought Problems at initial assessment were the best predictors of referral for mental health services. Furthermore, deviant scores on the CBCL scale With-drawn, the TRF scale Social problems, and the YSR scale Aggressive Behavior were the best predictors of the youths indication of need for professional help, without actually being referred. Hence, each of the three types of informants had a unique contribution to the prediction of maladjustment across time. It is especially important to note that teachers evaluations of adolescents problems were important predictors of later problems, although many mental health professionals perceive that teachers are less valuable for assessing internalizing problems than are parents and children themselves (Achenbach 1991c). Apparently the evaluations of multiple informants are needed in order to obtain comprehensive information on psychopathology in adolescents.

Impairment measures

Subjects who meet the criteria for a DSM diagnosis are not necessarily impaired in daily functioning. This was indicated by findings of Bird *et al.* (1990) who assessed the prevalence of psychiatric disorder in 4–16 year olds from the general population of Puerto Rico. Subjects were assessed with the 1985 version of the Diagnostic Interview Schedule for Children (DISC) and with the Childrens Global Assessment Scale (CGAS; Shaffer *et al.* 1983). They found that 63.8% of subjects who fulfilled criteria for a DSM-III diagnosis, were only mildly impaired, if at all, when assessed via the DISC. Similarly, Ferdinand *et al.* (1995b) assessed 19–25 year olds from the Dutch general population with the Young Adult Self Report (YASR; Achenbach 1990) and with the Global Assessment of Functioning scale (GAF; APA 1987), which indicates general functioning in adults. They found that many subjects with deviant YASR total problem scores, exceeding the 90th percentile of the cumulative frequency distribution of the general population, were only mildly impaired (27.3%), or not impaired at all (25.0%). Apparently, to obtain a valid judgment on the severity of psychopathology, instruments that assess impairment in daily functioning can provide valuable information, in addition to psychopathology measures.

Methods and designs

The need for comparable measures across time

In New Zealand, Feehan *et al.* (1995) assessed a general population sample of 15 year olds with the Diagnostic Interview Schedule for Children (DISC; Shaffer *et al.* 1993). At age 18, subjects were reassessed with the Diagnostic Interview Schedule (DIS; Robins *et al.* 1981). It was found that the presence of a DISC/DSM-III diagnosis at age 15 was predictive of a DIS/DSM-III-R diagnosis in 18 year old females (odds ratio = 3.6) and males (odds ratio = 5.0).

This finding suggested moderate stability of psychopathology. However, different assessment procedures (DISC versus DIS) and different nosological systems (DSM-III versus DSM-III-R) were used for 15 year olds versus 18 year olds. A stronger connection in psychopathology across time might have been found if similar assessment procedures had been applied across time. Now, it is unclear whether changes in the level of psychopathology reflected developmental changes, or merely differences between diagnostic constructs.

To enable assessment of psychopathology which will reveal results that are comparable from childhood to adulthood, Achenbach (1990) constructed the Young Adult Self-Report (YASR), a self-report questionnaire, and the Young Adult Behavior Checklist (YABCL; Achenbach *et al.* 1995), a parent questionnaire, to assess psychopathology in 18–30 year olds. The YASR and the YABCL have the same format as the Youth Self-Report (YSR; Achenbach 1991d), a self-report questionnaire for ages 11–18, and the Child Behavior Checklist

(Achenbach 1991b), a parent questionnaire for ages 4–18. By using these instruments in longitudinal research, comparable information can be obtained on the course of psychopathology, across the transition from adolescence to young adulthood.

Dimensional versus categorical data

Two main approaches can be applied to psychopathology in children and adolescents: a categorical approach and a dimensional approach.

- Following a *categorical approach*, subjects are considered abnormal if they fulfill criteria for a diagnosis, or normal if they do not fulfill diagnostic criteria. The DSM system is an example of a categorical approach.
- Following a *dimensional approach*, psychiatric problems are not rated as present or absent. Instead, to derive information on psychiatric problems, subjects are rated on symptom scales. Psychiatric problems are regarded as quantitative deviations from normative data. The application of a dimensional instead of a categorical approach to describe psychopathology in children and adolescents was supported by Achenbach (1991 a–d). In subjects from the general population of the USA, he found that all CBCL, TRF, and YSR scale scores followed a continuous distribution, instead of being divided into categories.

Analyses of categorical data

To obtain information on subjects with deviant scores on psychopathology measures, it can be useful to divide ratings on symptom scales into categories. The division of information into categories may also help to enhance the translation of research findings into a language that can easily be interpreted. Logistic regression analysis, a method of categorical data analysis that is often used in longitudinal studies, is explained here.

Logistic regression analysis

To identify connections between syndrome scores across time at a categorical level, logistic regression analyses can be used. Logistic regression analyses produce odds ratios for specific outcomes in relation to predictor variables. Odds ratios are computed by dividing two probabilities:

- the probability that an outcome will occur if a certain condition *is* present
- the probability that the same outcome will occur if the condition *is not* present.

Values greater than 1 indicate a positive association between predictor and outcome, values less than 1 a negative association.

By performing stepwise analyses, it is possible to determine the best set of predictors for a certain outcome variable. In this way, only variables contributing independently of other variables to the prediction of an outcome variable are identified. In other words, it is possible to correct for comorbidity between possible predictor variables.

Analysis of dimensional data

The two most important methods of analysis of dimensional data that have been used in longitudinal community studies are computation of correlation coefficients and application of path models.

Correlation coefficients

Correlation coefficients provide information on the extent to which subjects retain their rank order on the cumulative frequency distribution of scores. They can therefore be regarded as stability coefficients. According to Cohen (1988), correlation coefficients < 0.30 are small, between 0.30 and 0.50 medium, and > 0.50 large.

Correlations provide information on the stability of problems. However, stability coefficients do not give information on differences in mean scores across time. In other words, even if the stability of problem scores may be very high, the level of problems may increase or decrease significantly. Hence, in addition to stability coefficients, information on differences in mean scores is necessary to obtain a comprehensive picture of the development of psychopathology across time.

Path analyses

Achenbach *et al.* (1995) used path analyses to assess associations between dimensional scores across time. The advantage of path analyses over correlation/stability coefficients is that path analyses correct for dependency between possible predictors. Achenbach *et al.* (1995) assessed 13–16 year olds (Time 1) with the ACQ, which covers similar problems to the CBCL. The CBCL and the YSR were completed at 3 year follow-up (Time 2), and the YABCL and the YASR at 6 year follow-up (Time 3).

To identify the ability of Time 1 ACQ syndrome scores and Time 2 CBCL/YSR syndrome scores to predict Time 3 YASR/YABCL scores, path analyses were performed. Scores on each YASR/YABCL syndrome served as an outcome in a multiple regression, where the candidate predictors were Time 1, Time 2 and Time 3 family variables; Time 1 ACQ syndrome scores and Time 2 CBCL and YSR scores; and stressful experiences occurring between Time 1 and Time 2 or between Time 2 and Time 3.

Three groups of path analyses were conducted for each sex, with YASR syndrome scores, YABCL syndrome scores, and composite YASR/YABCL syndrome scores as outcome variables respectively (see Achenbach *et al.* 1995 for details). Predictors that were significant in two groups of analyses were considered to be robust.

Findings

In this section, data on continuity and change of psychopathology across the transition from adolescence to young adulthood will be summarized at the following levels:

- psychopathology in general
- internalizing versus externalizing problems
- specific syndromes.

Continuity of psychopathology in general

At the transition from adolescence to young adulthood, problems are rather stable. In initially 16–19-year-olds from the American general population, Achenbach *et al.* (1995) found 3-year stability coefficients of 0.69 and 0.55 for CBCL/YABCL Total Problem scores and YSR/YASR Total Problem scores respectively, and Ferdinand *et al.* (1995a) found a 4-year stability coefficient of 0.49 for YSR/YASR Total Problem scores in initially 15–18 year old Dutch adolescents.

To obtain information on subjects with deviant Total Problem scores, Ferdinand *et al.* (1995a) tracked subjects across time according to their YSR/YASR Total Problem scores, which were divided into categories. Initially 15–18 year-olds were followed up at intervals of 2 years (17–20 years of age) and 4 years (19–22 years of age). At each assessment, 18 year old subjects completed the YSR, and older subjects completed the YASR. (The YSR and the YASR yield comparable syndrome scores.)

To assess the continuity of problems, YSR and YASR Total Problem scores were recoded. To identify deviant subjects, cutoffs were applied at the 90th percentile (P90) of the cumulative frequency distribution of YSR and YASR Total Problem scores, separately for each sex. An important aim of the study was to assess meaningful changes in problem behavior across time. Changes from above P90 to just below the clinical cutoff can hardly be regarded as meaningful. Therefore, the 50th percentile (P50) of the cumulative frequency distribution was chosen as the border below which individuals are considered to function well. Hence, the use of P50 and P90 enabled the authors to identify individuals whose functioning improved or worsened significantly over time.

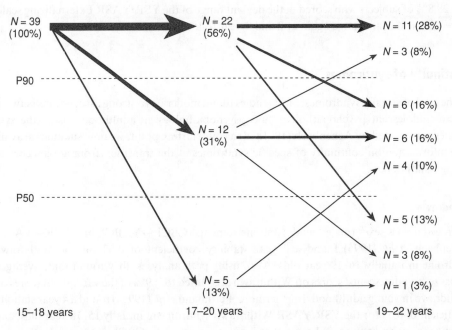

Fig. 1.1 Developmental pathways of 15–18 year olds who scored above P90 on the Total Problem score of the YSR in the Dutch sample. Source: Ferdinand *et al.* (1995a).

At initial assessment, 39 15–18 year olds were classified as deviant. Figure 1.1 shows the developmental course of these subjects across the 4 year follow-up. Subjects with high problem levels (> P90) in adolescence often remained above P90 (36%) or scored between P50 and P90 (42%) in young adulthood.

Findings from the American and Dutch follow-up studies seem to be confirmed by Feehan *et al.* (1995) who performed logistic regression analyses. They found odds ratios of 3.6 (in males) and 5.0 (in females) for a DSM-III-R Axis 1 diagnosis at age 18, when there had been a DSM-III Axis 1 diagnosis at age 15. This indicated that the problems might be moderately stable. However, different assessment methods were used across time, which hampers exact interpretation of those findings.

Continuity of internalizing and externalizing problems

The stability of internalizing problems is similar to that of externalizing problems. Averaged across sex, Achenbach *et al.* (1995) found stability coefficients of 0.64 and 0.69 for the CBCL/YABCL scales Internalizing problems and Externalizing problems respectively; stability coefficients for the YSR/YASR Internalizing problems and Externalizing problems scales were 0.53 and 0.55 respectively. Similarly, Ferdinand *et al.* (1995a) found YSR/YASR 4 year stability coefficients of 0.47 for Internalizing problems and 0.56 for Externalizing problems in initially 15–18 year olds.

Continuity of internalizing and externalizing problems is also similar at a categorical level. In initially 15–18 year olds from the general population, Ferdinand *et al.* (1995a) found that 28.8% of subjects who scored in the deviant range of the YSR/YASR Internalizing scale, and also 28.8% of subjects who scored in the deviant range of the YSR/YASR Externalizing scale, scored in the deviant range again at 2 and 4 year follow-up.

Continuity of syndromes

At the level of specific syndromes, most studies found moderate to strong associations between child or adolescent psychopathology and psychopathology in adulthood. Using the syndromes constructed by Achenbach (1991a–d) as our starting point, we now summarize available information on continuity of specific syndromes at the transition from adolescence to young adulthood.

Withdrawn

Averaged across sexes (male/female) and instruments (CBCL→YABCL and YSR→YASR) Achenbach *et al.* (1995) found a 3 year stability coefficient of 0.53 for the Withdrawn syndrome in initially 16–19 year olds. Also, using path analyses, they found that, averaged across sexes, adolescents' scores on Withdrawn accounted for 29% of the variance in scores on Withdrawn in young adulthood. Furthermore, Ferdinand *et al.* (1995a) found a 4 year stability coefficient of 0.37 for the YSR/YASR Withdrawn syndrome in initially 15–18 year olds, and logistic regression analyses indicated that deviant scores on the CBCL syndrome Withdrawn in initially 13–16 year olds predicted deviance on the YASR syndrome Withdrawn 8 years later (odds ratio = 3.3; Ferdinand and Verhulst 1995). The significance of the stability of withdrawal from contacts with others was underscored by the finding that deviant scores on the CBCL syndrome Withdrawn in 13–16 year olds from the Dutch sample predicted suicide attempts during young adulthood (odds ratio = 14.5; Ferdinand and Verhulst 1995).

Somatic complaints

Achenbach *et al.* (1995) found an average 3 year stability coefficient of 0.43 for the Somatic Complaints syndrome in initially 16–19 year olds from the American general population, whereas Ferdinand *et al.* (1995a) reported a 4 year YSR/YASR stability coefficient of 0.37 in Dutch initially 15–18 year olds. Furthermore, path analyses in the American sample indicated that adolescents' scores on the Somatic Complaints scale accounted for 13% of the variance in scores on the Somatic Complaints scale in young adulthood. In the Dutch sample, analyses at a categorical level indicated that deviance on the CBCL syndrome Somatic Complaints in 13–16 year olds predicted deviance on the YASR syndrome Somatic Complaints 8 years later (odds ratio = 2.3; Ferdinand and Verhulst 1995).

Ferdinand *et al.* (1998) assessed relations between CBCL scores in initially 11–16 year olds from the Dutch general population and DSM-III-R Axis I diagnoses assessed using the Schedules for Clinical Assessment in Neuropsychiatry (SCAN; World Health Organization 1991) approximately 9 years later. They found that adolescents with deviant scores on the Somatic Complaints scale of the CBCL were at risk for a DSM-III-R diagnosis in young adulthood. However, the predictive value of the Somatic Complaints scale was blotted out when functional impairment in daily life, assessed using the GAF, was added as a morbidity criterion to DSM-III-R diagnoses. Hence, despite the fact that adolescents' somatic complaints with unknown medical origin were linked with later DSM-III-R diagnoses, the addition of an impairment measure to the DSM classification system indicated that somatic complaints probably do not represent a risk factor for later serious maladjustment.

Anxious/Depressed

The average 3 year stability coefficient for the Anxious/Depressed syndrome in 16–19 year olds was 0.57 in the American sample of Achenbach *et al.* (1995); adolescents' scores on Anxious/Depressed accounted for 16% of the variance of scores in young adulthood. In the Dutch sample (Ferdinand *et al.* 1995a), the average 4 year YSR/YASR stability coefficient for Anxious/Depressed in initially 15–18 year olds was 0.43, and logistic regression analyses indicated that deviance on the CBCL scale Anxious/Depressed predicted deviance on the YASR scale Anxious/Depressed (odds ratio = 3.0).

Furthermore, Ferdinand *et al.* (1998) found that deviance on Anxious/Depressed in 11–16 year olds predicted the presence of a DSM-III-R Axis 1 disorder, even when functional impairment in daily life was added as a morbidity criterion.

As the Anxious/Depressed syndrome, DSM diagnoses of major depression and anxiety disorders are also rather stable. In their high school sample in Western Oregon, USA, Orvaschel *et al.* (1995) also assessed the continuity of anxiety and depression in older adolescents. They found that a DSM-III-R diagnosis of major depression in initially 14–18 year olds predicted major depression at 1 year follow-up (relative risk = 1.6), while initial anxiety disorder predicted anxiety disorder (relative risk = 3.3) and dysthymia (relative risk = 4.4) across the 1 year period. In the New Zealand study (Bardone *et al.* 1996) depression at age 15 predicted depression at age 21.

The importance of anxiety and depression as a rather stable condition in adolescents was supported by the finding from logistic regression analyses that deviance on the CBCL scale Anxious/Depressed in 13–16 year olds predicted referral to mental health services in young adulthood (odds ratio = 4.0; Ferdinand and Verhulst 1995). Furthermore, Bardone *et al.* (1996) found that depressed 15 year old girls were at risk for early school leaving, low education attainment and multiple drug use.

Social Problems

In the American national sample, the average 3 year stability coefficient of the Social Problems scale in initially 16–19 year olds was 0.45 (Achenbach *et al.* 1995); the mean 4 year stability coefficient in 15–18 year olds from the Dutch sample was 0.39. Furthermore, in the Dutch and the American samples adolescents' problems with aggression predicted social problems in young adulthood. Ferdinand *et al.* (1995a) found that deviant scores on the CBCL Delinquent Behavior scale in initially 13–16 year olds predicted deviance on the YASR Social Problems scale (odds ratio = 2.6) across an 8 year interval, and Achenbach *et al.* (1995) found that scores on the Aggressive Behavior scale in 16–19 year old males accounted for 15% of the variance in scores on the Social Problems scale 3 years later.

Thought Problems

In the Dutch sample, the 4 year stability coefficient for the YSR/YASR Thought Problems scale was 0.31. Because the Thought Problems scale is a valid measure for psychopathology in American adolescents, but not in young adults, Achenbach *et al.* (1995) computed correlations between adolescents' scores on the YSR syndrome Thought Problems and the YASR syndrome Strange, its closest young adult counterpart. They found an average correlation of 0.40. Furthermore, in the Dutch sample (Ferdinand and Verhulst 1995) deviant scores on the CBCL scale Aggressive Behavior in 13–16 year olds predicted high scores on the YASR scale Thought Problems in young adulthood (odds ratio = 3.0).

Attention Problems

Achenbach *et al.* (1995) found an average 3 year correlation of 0.62 in initially 16–19 year olds between the CBCL Attention Problems scale and its closest young adult counterpart, the YABCL scale Irresponsible; in the Dutch sample the 4 year YSR/YASR stability coefficient for initially 15–18 year olds was 0.44 (Ferdinand *et al.* 1995a). Some studies indicated that adolescents' attention problems might be a risk factor for later conduct problems. Ferdinand and Verhulst (1995) found that 13–16 year olds' deviant CBCL scores on the Attention Problems scale predicted police or judicial contacts in young adulthood (odds ratio = 6.6), and Schaughency *et al.* (1994) found that DSM-III attention deficit disorder (ADD) in 15 year olds from New Zealand was a risk factor for ADD at age 18, but also for later externalizing problems. However, after controlling for comorbid conduct problems at initial assessment and follow-up, MacDonald and Achenbach (1996) found that attention problems in 12–16 year olds made little contribution to later conduct problems in a 6 year follow-up of their American national sample.

Aggressive Behavior

In the American national sample, the average 3 year stability coefficient for the Aggressive Behavior scale in initially 16–19 year olds was 0.55, while the mean percentage of variance in young adults' scores on the Aggressive Behavior scale accounted for by adolescents' scores on the Aggressive behavior scale was 24%. This indicated that the stability of aggressive behaviors at the transition from adolescence to young adulthood was considerable, which was supported by findings in the Dutch sample. Ferdinand *et al.* (1995a) found a 4 year YSR/ YASR stability coefficient of 0.47 in initially 15–18 year olds, and deviance on the CBCL scale Aggressive Behavior in 13–16 year olds predicted deviance on the YASR scale Aggressive Behavior 8 years later (odds ratio = 3.0; Ferdinand and Verhulst 1995). Similarly, in their Oregon high school sample Orvaschel *et al.* (1995) found that DSM-III-R disruptive disorders in 14–18 year olds predicted disruptive disorders across a 1 year period (relative risk = 6.9).

Delinquent Behavior

In the Dutch sample, the 4 year stability coefficient for the Delinquent Behavior scale in 15–18 year olds was 0.41 (Ferdinand *et al.* 1995), which was in the same range as the mean 3 year stability coefficient of 0.49 for 16–19 year olds from the American national sample (Achenbach *et al.* 1995). Furthermore, Achenbach *et al.* (1995) found that 23% of the variance in young males' scores on the Delinquent Behavior scale was accounted for by scores on the Delinquent Behavior scale in adolescence; the percentage of variance in young adult females was lower (7%). The adverse outcome of conduct problems in girls was supported by Bardone *et al.* (1996) who found that DSM-III conduct disorder in 15 year old girls predicted early school leaving, early pregnancy, and violent victimization by a partner at age 21.

Conclusions

Continuity of psychopathology

So far, existing general population studies on the connectedness between problems in childhood, adolescence, and adulthood have yielded important information on the development of psychopathology. Several associations between psychopathology in adolescence and psychopathology and problems of adjustment in young adulthood have been found.

At the transition from adolescence to young adulthood, the stability of problems is considerable. This indicates that intervention programs to prevent psychopathology in adulthood should probably be aimed at children and adolescents. Therefore, long-term studies investigating preventive effects of intervention in children and adolescents from the general population are needed.

Most types of problems in adolescence increase the risk for psychopathology or maladjustment in young adulthood, and therefore could be used as targets for prevention studies

Table 1.2 The possible design of future longitudinal general population studies

	Time 1	Time 2	Time 3	Time 4
Age (yrs)	4–18	8–18	12–18	16–18
Instruments	CBCL	CBCL	CBCL	CBCL
	YSR	YSR	YSR	YSR
	TRF	TRF	TRF	TRF
	DISC-P	DISC-P	DISC-P	DISC-P
	DISC-C	DISC-C	DISC-C	DISC-C
	CGAS	CGAS	CGAS	CGAS
Age (yrs)		19–22	19–26	19–30
Instruments	YABCL	YABCL	YABCL	
	YASR	YASR	YASR	
	DIS	DIS	DIS	
	GAF	GAF	GAF	
All ages	Outcome variables	Outcome variables	Outcome variables	

CBCL, Child Behavior Checklist; DIS, Diagnostic Interview Schedule; DISC-C, Child version of the Diagnostic Interview Schedule for Children; DISC-P, Parent version of the Diagnostic Interview Schedule for Children; TRF, Teachers' Report Form; YABCL, Young Adult Behavior Checklist; YASR, Young Adult Self-Report; YSR, Youth Self-Report.

in adolescents from the general population. Since existing longitudinal community studies indicated to which outcome psychopathology in adolescence is linked, the results of existing studies can be useful to determine which variables can be assessed to determine the effect of intervention programs.

Study designs

Several existing studies have been hampered by methodological difficulties with the assessment of problems. Furthermore, most studies differed with respect to assessment procedures and data analyses, which hampered the comparability of results.

Future studies investigating stability and change of psychopathology, from childhood or adolescence into young adulthood, using similar assessment procedures relying on multiple informants (parents, teachers, subjects themselves) at both initial assessment and follow-up are needed. If similar studies yielding comparable results could be performed in different countries in the future, this would yield valuable information on developmental psychopathology in children and adolescents. In Table 1.2, a possible design of a longitudinal study using multiple informants at different times of assessment is shown.

To assess psychopathology, the CBCL, YSR, and TRF, and their adult counterparts, could be used to obtain data that are comparable across informants, across ages, and across time. At each assessment, instruments that yield DSM diagnoses could be added, to facilitate comparisons with clinical data. However, DSM criteria are liable to change across time. Also, child and adult diagnostic criteria may not be comparable. Besides psychopathology, it is also important to assess impairment in functioning at consecutive times of assessment. To achieve this, the CGAS could be used, especially because CGAS scores for children and adolescents can easily be compared to GAF scores for adults, since the CGAS and the GAF have a similar scoring format. At follow-up assessments outcome variables such as referral to mental health service, police or judicial contacts, suicide attempts, alcohol abuse, and expulsion from school or job can be important indices of a person's functioning.

References

Achenbach, T.M. (1990). *The Young Adult Self-Report*. University of Vermont Department of Psychiatry, Burlington, VT.

Achenbach, T.M. (1991a). *Integrative Guide to the 1991 CBCL/4–18, YSR, and TRF Profiles*. University of Vermont Department of Psychiatry, Burlington, VT.

Achenbach, T.M. (1991b). *Manual for the Child Behavior Checklist/4 18 and 1991 Profile*. University of Vermont Department of Psychiatry, Burlington, VT.

Achenbach, T.M. (1991c). *Manual for the Teachers Report Form and 1991 Profile*. University of Vermont Department of Psychiatry, Burlington, VT.

Achenbach, T.M. (1991d). *Manual for the Youth Self Report and 1991 Profile*. University of Vermont Department of Psychiatry, Burlington, VT.

Achenbach, T.M., Howell, C.T., McConaughy, S.H., and Stanger, C. (1995). Six-year predictors of problems in a national sample: III. Transitions to early adult syndromes. *Journal of the American Academy of Child and Adolescent Psychiatry*, **34**, 658–669.

APA (1987). *Diagnostic and statistical manual of mental disorders*, 3rd edn, revised. American Psychiatric Association, Washington, DC

APA (1994). *Diagnostic and statistical manual of mental disorders*, 4th edn. American Psychiatric Association Washington, D.C.

Bardone, A.M., Moffitt, T.E., Caspi, A., Dickson, N., and Silva, P.A. (1996). Adult mental health and social outcomes of adolescent girls with depression and conduct disorder. *Development and Psychopathology*, **8**, 811–829.

Bird, H.R., Yager, T.J., Staghezza, B., Gould, M.S., Canino, G., and Rubio-Stipec, M. (1990). Impairment in the epidemiological measurement of childhood psychopathology in the community. *Journal of the American Academy of Child and Adolescent Psychiatry*, **29**, 796–803.

Bird, H.R., Gould, M.S., and Staghezza, B. (1992). Aggregating data from multiple informants in child psychiatric epidemiological research. *Journal of the American Academy of Child and Adolescent Psychiatry*, **31**, 78–85.

Caspi, A., Moffitt, T., Newman, D.L., and Silva, P.A. (1996). Behavioral observations at age 3 years predict adult psychiatric disorders: longitudinal evidence from a birth cohort. *Archives of General Psychiatry*, **53**, 1033–1039.

Cohen, J. (1988). *Statistical power analysis for the behavioral sciences*, 2nd edn. New York, Academic Press.

Feehan, M., McGee, R., and Williams, S.M. (1995). Models of adolescent psychopathology: childhood risk and the transition to adulthood. *Journal of the American Academy of Child and Adolescent Psychiatry*, **34**, 670–679.

Ferdinand, R.F. and Verhulst, F.C. (1995). Psychopathology from adolescence into young adulthood: an 8-year follow-up study. *American Journal of Psychiatry*, **152**, 1586–1594.

Ferdinand, R.F., Verhulst, F.C., and Wiznitzer, M. (1995a). Continuity and change of self-reported problem behaviors from adolescence into young adulthood. *Journal of the American Academy of Child and Adolescent Psychiatry*, **166**, 680–90.

Ferdinand, R.F., Reijden, M. van der, Verhulst, F.C., Nienhuis, F.J., and Giel, R. (1995b). Assessment of the prevalence of psychiatric disorder in young adults. *British Journal of Psychiatry*, **166**, 480–488.

Ferdinand, R.F., Stijnen, Th., Verhulst, F.C., and Reijden, M. van der (1998). Associations between behavioral and emotional problems in adolescence and maladjustment in young adulthood. *Journal of Adolescence*, in press.

Loeber, R., Green, S.M., and Lahey, B.B. (1990). Mental health professionals perception of the utility of children, mothers, and teachers as informants on childhood psychopathology. *Journal of Clinical Child Psychology*, **19**, 98–104.

MacDonald, V.M. and Achenbach, T.M. (1996). Attention problems versus conduct problems as six year predictors of problem scores in a national sample. *Journal of the American Academy of Child and Adolescent Psychiatry*, **35**, 1237–1246.

McConaughy, S.H., Stanger, C., and Achenbach, T.M. (1992). Three year course of behavioral and emotional problems in a national sample of 4 to 16 year olds. *Journal of the American Academy of Child and Adolescent Psychiatry*, **31**, 932–940.

Orvaschel, H., Lewinsohn, P.M., and Seeley, J.R. (1995). Continuity of psychopathology in a community sample of adolescents. *Journal of the American Academy of Child and Adolescent Psychiatry*, **34**, 1525–1535.

Reich, W. and Earls, F. (1987). Rules for making psychiatric diagnoses in children on the basis of multiple information: preliminary strategies. *Journal of Abnormal Child Psychology*, **15**, 601–616.

Robins, L.N., Helzer, J.E., Croughan, J., and Ratcliff, K.S. (1981). *NIMH Diagnostic Interview Schedule*: Version III (May 1981). National Institute of Mental Health, Rockville, MD.

Schaughency, E., McGee, R., Nada Raja, S., Feehan, M., and Silva, P.A. (1994). Self reported inattention, impulsivity, and hyperactivity at age 15 and 18 years in the general population. *Journal of the American Academy of Child and Adolescent Psychiatry*, **33**, 173–184.

Shaffer, D., Gould, M.S., Brasic, J., Ambrosini, P., Fisher, P., Bird, H.R., and Aluwahlia, S. (1983). A childrens global assessment scale. *Archives of General Psychiatry*, **44**, 1228–1231.

Shaffer, D., Schwab-Stone, M., and Fisher, P. (1993). The Diagnostic Interview Schedule for Children-revised version (DISC-R). I. Preparation, field testing, interrater reliability, and acceptability. *Journal of the American Academy of Child and Adolescent Psychiatry*, **32**, 643–650.

Verhulst, F.C. and Ende, J. van der (1992). Agreement between parents' reports and adolescents' self reports of problem behavior. *Journal of Child Psychology and Psychiatry*, **33**, 1011–1023.

Verhulst, F.C. and Koot, H.M. (1992). *Child psychiatric epidemiology: concepts, methods and findings*, pp 77–78. Sage Publications, London.

Verhulst, F.C., Ende J. van der, Ferdinand, R.F., and Kasius, M.C. (1997a) The prevalence of DSM-III-R diagnoses in a national sample of Dutch adolescents. *Archives of General Psychiatry*, **54**, 329–336.

Verhulst, F.C., Dekker, M.C., and Ende, J. van der (1997b) Parent, teacher, and self reports as predictors of signs of disturbance in adolescents: whose information caries the most weight? *Acta Psychiatrica Scandinavica*, **96**, 75–81.

WHO (1991). *SCAN. Schedules for Clinical Assessment in Neuropsychiatry*. World Health Organization, Division of Mental Health, Geneva.

2 Children of schizophrenic parents

Jennifer B. Watson, Sarnoff A. Mednick, Su-chin Serene Olin, Tyronne D. Cannon, Josef Parnas, and Fini Schulsinger

Paradigms and models

The high risk (HR) method was developed in the 1950s in response to the difficulties in examining the etiology of schizophrenia by comparing hospitalized schizophrenics with normal controls. The HR research design provides a method for investigating premorbid risk factors that relate to the development of schizophrenia and other psychotic illnesses. Among the many HR studies examining the premorbid characteristics of schizophrenia (Erlenmeyer-Kimling and Cornblatt 1987, Fish 1987, Marcus *et al.* 1987, Mednick *et al.* 1987, Tienari *et al.* 1987), most follow the Copenhagen HR project and define risk by selecting offspring of parents (usually mothers) who are schizophrenic. In an HR design, the offspring of the schizophrenic parents are then followed longitudinally with assessments of the at risk children continuing into adulthood. Since a number of these HR children will later develop schizophrenia, the data ascertained from these future schizophrenics provides researchers with a developmental perspective of schizophrenia. In addition the assessments yield information about the HR children who do not develop schizophrenia, which allows investigators to consider factors that may protect these children from negative outcomes.

One of the most valuable aspects of the HR design is that the early assessments of the behavior and biological reactions of the HR subjects are not biased by the consequences of their illness. Thus, the study of children of schizophrenic parents has resulted in the identification of premorbid indicators that may have some relevance for primary intervention. In this chapter we provide an overview of HR studies focusing on the Copenhagen HR project and discuss some of the premorbid predictors of adult mental breakdown which have been identified by these HR longitudinal studies.

Most of the HR studies began in the 1960s and 1970s. Only a few of these studies have followed their subjects for long enough to obtain diagnostic outcomes. Much data have been collected on the differences between the HR children and controls; however, not all children of schizophrenics go on to develop schizophrenia themselves. For a child whose mother has chronic schizophrenia, the risk of developing schizophrenia is 16%; thus, researchers face the challenge of distinguishing the HR children who will develop schizophrenia from those who will not.

The HR studies have elucidated several premorbid characteristics which have been identified as potential risk markers for future psychosis. These premorbid attributes of schizophrenia roughly fall into two categories:

- the first category consists of precursors involving early etiological factors such as family history of schizophrenia, neurobehavioral deficits, and delivery complications
- the second category relates to social and behavioral precursors of mental illness identified by teachers and parents as well as personality variables revealed by interviews and questionnaires.

Methods and design

There are numerous advantages to studying children of schizophrenic parents in the context of a genetic high-risk paradigm:

- A higher incidence of psychopathology has been noted among children of schizophrenics as compared to the general population. The general population risk for schizophrenia is 1%, but the risk for offspring of schizophrenic mothers is 10–16% and even higher if the father has schizophrenia or schizophrenia spectrum illness (Kallmann 1938, Parnas *et al.* 1993).

- When the HR subjects are examined, they are young, without mental illness, and their behavioral and biological reactions are not heavily colored by the consequences of illness.

- The experimenters, parents, teachers, and the subjects are unaware of who will develop schizophrenia; therefore, the premorbid data are not biased.

- Information gathered concerning behaviors and life events is current rather than retrospective.

- Ideal controls subjects may be found among the HR children who do not develop schizophrenia.

- The inclusion of a low risk (LR) control group in the research design makes it possible to examine whether a given environmental stressor affects the HR and LR groups differently. That is, the design encourages the investigation of gene–environment interactions in the etiology of the illness.

Findings

Table 2.1 provides a summary of the HR projects which have yielded much information about predictors of schizophrenia. The HR studies of children at risk for schizophrenia have produced a tremendous range of potential factors which may be markers of future schizophrenia including: obstetric complications and birthweight, family relations, motor functioning, and school behavior.

Obstetric complications and low birthweight

Mednick (1970) presented data indicating the increased risk for schizophrenia associated with birth complications. McNeill and Kaij (1978) later noted that adult schizophrenics have a

Table 2.1 High risk studies with offspring of schizophrenics

Study	Investigators/ reference	Date begun	HR (N)	LR (N)	Diagnostic outcome in HR group at most recent follow-up
Copenhagen HR Project	Mednick *et al.* (1987)	1962	207	104	31 schizophrenia 7 atypical psychosis 41 schizotypal and paranoid personality disorder
Finnish Adoptive Family Study	Tienari (1985)	1984	91	91	9 schizophrenia 4 spectrum psychosis
New York Infant Study	Fish (1987)	1952	10	12	1 schizophrenia 6 schizotypal or paranoid personality disorder
New York High Risk Project	Erlenmeyer-Kimling and Cornblatt (1987)	1971	63	143	6 schizophrenia 6 schizoaffective 3 unspecified functional psychosis 10 schizotypal and paranoid personality disorder
NIMH Israeli Kibbutz–City Study	Marcus and Auerbach (1981)	1967	50	50	5 schizophrenia 1 probable schizophrenia 3 schizoid personality disorder
Obstetric Copenhagen HR Project	Mednick and Schulsinger (1971)g	1972	72	193	16 schizophrenia 11 schizophrenia-spectrum disorder

Note: Additional HR studies include Grunebaum *et al.* 1974, Rieder *et al.* 1975, Wrede *et al.* 1984, Garmezy *et al.* 1984, Hanson *et al.* 1987, Worland *et al.* 1984, Weintraub *et al.* 1984.

history of serious obstetric complications more often than do controls. The HR studies have since produced evidence supporting the finding that obstetric complications and low birthweight may be a risk-increasing factor for schizophrenia. Findings from the Copenhagen HR study indicate that children of schizophrenic parents who later developed schizophrenia experienced significantly more perinatal complications than those HR subjects who later developed schizotypal personality disorder (SPD) or no mental illness (NMI) (Parnas *et al.* 1982). The NIMH Israeli Kibbutz–City Study has linked low birthweight to the later development of schizophrenia spectrum illnesses in children of schizophrenic parents (Marcus *et al.* 1981). It has been hypothesized that obstetric complications and low birthweight indicate a less than optimal pregnancy and birth process which may result in developmental disturbances and damage to critical neuroanatomical structures in HR children. Furthermore, these perinatal complications may interact with genetic risk factors to increase the risk for schizophrenia.

Family relations

Result of longitudinal HR studies have demonstrated that poor family functioning and/or instability of family rearing environment are associated with later development of schizophrenia. In the Finnish Adoptive Family Study, almost all of the adopted-away HR children who later became schizophrenic were reared by disturbed adoptive families (Tienari *et al.* 1985). Rearing in a secure stable adoptive home may serve as a protective factor for HR offspring. It is difficult to determine the direction of causality in relation to functionality, as it is feasible that the distressed child contributes to the observed disturbances in his adoptive family. In the NIMH Israeli Kibbutz–City Study, poor parenting behaviors (defined as inconsistency, overinvolvement with the child, and expressions of hostility toward the child) were predictors of later schizophrenia spectrum outcomes in offspring of schizophrenic parents (Marcus *et al.* 1987).

An unstable family rearing environment is also associated with the later development of schizophrenia in HR children. Results from the Copenhagen HR project reveal that the children of schizophrenics who later become schizophrenic were more likely than HR children who did not have negative outcomes to have been institutionalized in early childhood (Gutkind *et al.*, in press. Similarly, in the New York Infant Study the three HR children who experienced periods in institutions or a series of foster homes had the worst outcomes (Fish 1987).

Motor functioning

In the field of motor functioning, observational and neurological studies of children who later developed schizophrenia have demonstrated that preschizophrenic children evidence significant motor deficits when compared to control subjects who did not develop mental illness. An investigation of childhood home videos of future schizophrenics by Walker *et al.* (1994) revealed that preschizophrenic infants had significantly more movement abnormalities than controls including siblings with no mental illness. The motor dysfunctions included abnormal tonicity, dystonic posturing of hands, and choreoathoetoid movements (Walker *et al.* 1994).

We conducted a study (the Obstetric Copenhagen HR Project) of subjects who were at high risk for schizophrenia (had a schizophrenic parent) and found that data from a neurological examination at ages 11–13 could distinguish those who later (age 31) developed schizophrenia from those who did not develop mental illness (LaFosse 1994). In addition, LaFosse (1994) also reported that the preschizophrenic subjects had significantly more problems of motor coordination than subjects who later developed affective disorders.

The NIMH Israeli Kibbutz–City study examined neurobehavioral functioning (i.e. hyperkinesis, cognitive control, motor coordination, and cognitive coordination) of children who were genetically at high risk for developing schizophrenia. At a 13 year follow-up of these HR children, it was found that all children who later experienced a psychotic breakdown had exhibited poor neurobehavioral functioning in childhood (Marcus *et al.* 1987).

School behavior

One of the most powerful premorbid predictors of adult mental breakdown is teacher ratings of school behavior (Olin *et al.* 1995, 1997a,b). Teachers have been shown to be excellent judges of who will later have schizophrenia or a schizophrenia spectrum illness. Although it has been argued that there is a lack of clear prodromal signs of schizophrenic disorder (Betz 1973), the research looking at school records and teachers' comments argues otherwise. It may be that distinctive antecedents exist premorbidly in the social behavior of many schizophrenics; however, these signs are frequently overlooked by clinicians. Teachers, on the other hand, spend a large amount of concentrated time, often for a period of years, with their students and have the opportunity to observe their students functioning in many domains including academics and social interactions. They can also compare them with the other children in the class.

Of the four potential markers of future schizophrenia we have mentioned (obstetric complications and low birthweight, family relations, motor functioning, and school behavior), we will take one, school behavior, and discuss it in depth. We have selected school behavior because it has proved to be a powerful marker of later schizophrenia in offspring of schizophrenics. In addition, teacher ratings of HR children's behavior provide a useful guide for researchers and clinicians who are selecting participants for primary intervention.

Retrospective studies of early school behavior in schizophrenics

Beginning in 1972, Watt reviewed childhood school records for a group of hospitalized adult schizophrenics and a group of matched adult controls. He discovered that the teachers' annual comments on student performance differentiated the children destined to become schizophrenic adults. By systematically coding the childhood school records of adult schizophrenics, Watt (1972) found that in late childhood about one half of the boys exhibited more behavior that was irritable, aggressive, negativistic, and defiant of authority. In addition the school records of adult female schizophrenics revealed that the girls were more compliant, shy, and introverted (Watt 1972).

In 1978 Watt replicated his initial findings with a population of schizophrenics and matched control subjects. Teachers' comments in school reports showed once again that future schizophrenics were behaviorally distinguishable from their classmates. The preschizophrenic girls were identified by teachers' comments as being more passive, emotionally unstable, and introverted than controls, whereas the boys were described as more violent, emotionally unstable, and disagreeable than controls (Watt 1978). Thus, in both the 1972 and 1978 studies by Watt, the major prodromal sign for many adult female schizophrenics was introversion; the major prodromal signs for the adult male schizophrenics were irritability and disagreeable behavior.

Longitudinal studies of early school behavior in children at high risk for schizophrenia

The New York high risk project

In 1971, Erlenmeyer-Kimling and Cornblatt initiated a longitudinal study of 63 children of schizophrenics (HR), 100 children of normal parents (LR), and 43 psychiatric controls. The subjects for this study were drawn from the New York metropolitan region, and the children in both HR and LR groups were between the ages of 12 and 17 during the first assessment (see Erlenmeyer-Kimling and Cornblatt 1987 for details).

Data related to school behavior were collected when the children were between the ages of 12 and 15. Classroom teachers rated the behavior of 44 HR children and 70 LR children. Four teachers, who held a class with the students at least four times per week, completed the Pupil Rating Form (PRF) (Watt *et al.* 1982). The PRF was created from a coding system developed by Watt (1972) for the quantification of school records (The 1972 and 1978 studies by Watt discussed earlier used this system for quantifying school data.) The PRF has four clusters: scholastic motivation, extroversion, harmony, and emotional stability. The teachers were reported to have limited awareness of which children had a parent with schizophrenia.

The results of the New York HR study indicate that children at high risk for schizophrenia were perceived by their teachers as having less harmonious relations at school and as being less emotionally stable than control subjects. In addition, teachers noted that the HR children were less scholastically motivated; however, the researchers acknowledged that low motivation may be mediated by the lower intelligence that was observed in the HR group. These findings from the New York HR project provide noteworthy information about the children of schizophrenic parents, but these HR subjects are a heterogeneous group in regards to their future psychological outcomes.

The Copenhagen High Risk Project

The Copenhagen HR project was launched in 1962 by Mednick and Schulsinger to study children at high risk for schizophrenia (Mednick *et al.* 1987). The HR sample was obtained by screening psychiatric hospitals in the Copenhagen area for severe and chronic schizophrenic women with children. The children of the severely, chronic schizophrenic mothers who were between the ages of 9 and 20 years were included in the HR group ($N = 207$, 86 females). The low risk (LR) sample of 104 (44 females) consisted of individuals who were in the same age range but did not have a family history of psychiatric diagnosis for two generations (i.e. parents and grandparents). The LR sample was matched to the HR sample on a variety of variables including age, gender, parental social class, years of formal education, institutionalization versus family rearing, and urban versus rural residence (see Mednick and Schulsinger 1968 for details).

During the initial assessment in 1962, the subjects were between the ages of 9 and 20 with an average age of 15.1 years. At that time, none of the subjects had a psychiatric diagnosis. Since 1962, two subsequent diagnostic assessments have been performed, the first in 1972 and the second in 1986. The second diagnostic follow-up was conducted between 1986 and 1989 when the subjects averaged 39–42 years of age. A lifetime diagnosis was derived by reviewing the interview summaries both from diagnostic follow-ups and from hospital records. The lifetime diagnoses were derived from the (DSM-III-R; APA 1987). The overall attrition rate was low: 98% of the HR (excluding those who died and emigrated) and 98.1% of the LR subjects were successfully diagnosed.

The diagnostic follow-up with the Copenhagen 1962 HR cohort resulted in 12% of the subjects whose mothers, but not fathers, had schizophrenia developing schizophrenia themselves (see Table 2.2.) For subjects who had both mother and father in the schizophrenia spectrum, 25% developed schizophrenia. If broad spectrum diagnoses (schizophrenia, schizotypal personality disorder (SPD), or atypical psychosis) are included for the offspring of schizophrenic mothers, 30% of those whose mothers had schizophrenia. This broad spectrum outcome rate increases to 55% in those who have two parents with schizophrenia or schizophrenia spectrum (Parnas *et al.* 1993). To date, the Copenhagen 1962 HR study has the largest number of schizophrenia and schizophrenia spectrum outcomes. This is due to the early and start of the project and the investigators' ability to follow subjects almost 35 years and to determine lifetime diagnostic outcomes.

Table 2.2 Copenhagen 1962 HR project. Hierarchical frequencies of lifetime DSM-III-R diagnoses in high risk (HR) and low risk (LR) subjects (adapted from Table 3 in Parnas *et al.* 1993.)

DSM-III-R[a] diagnosis	HR (N = 207)	LR (N = 104)
Axis I functional psychosis		
Schizophrenia	31	2
Schizoaffective disorder	1	0
Schizophreniform psychosis	1	0
Atypical psychosis	7	1
Total	40	3
Cluster A personality disorders		
Schizotypal personality	36	5
Paranoid personality	5	5
Schizoid personality	1	0
Total	42	5
Other Axis I and II disorders		
Major depression	9	8
Organic brain syndrome	5	5
Substance abuse	12	5
Other Axis I disorder	6	7
Other Axis II disorder	10	8
Total	42	33

[a] DSM-III-R is the *Diagnostic and Statistical Manual of Mental Disorder*, 3rd edn, revised (American Psychiatric Association 1987).

Teacher-rated behaviors

All subjects in the Copenhagen HR study were extensively assessed on many measures, including a teacher report of school behavior. The teachers who knew the students best filled out the 26-item questionnaire. For each subject, the teacher who completed the questionnaire, had known the student for at least 3 years. Figure 2.1 shows the 26-item questionnaire filled out by teachers. (Item 1 is informational and not used for research purposes.) Items 5–24 required teachers to provide true–false responses regarding the student's behavior in the classroom. True scores are rated as deviant for these items. Item 4 involved a rating by the teacher of the student's intelligence as high, average, or low. A low score was considered deviant. Questions 2, 3, and 26 required a yes–no response to questions involving the student's academic experience. Item 25 asked teachers to predict the child's future psychological health. For all items, a 'don't know' response was allowed.

It should be noted that some of the items on the teacher questionnaire are subjective and require the teacher to respond to questions that may be difficult to define precisely. However, the Danish teachers are highly trained professionals who knew the student for at least 3 years before completing the questionnaires.

1. Descriptional
2. Repeated a grade
3. Tested by psychologist
4. Intelligence: low, average, high
5. Performance poorer than abilities
6. Quiet and unengaged
7. Rarely takes initiative
8. Rarely participates in spontaneous activity
9. Seldom laughs or smiles with others
10. Lonely and rejected by peers
11. Contented with isolation
12. Shy, reserved and silent
13. Anxious and restrained wth classmates
14. Anxious and restrained with teachers
15. Uneasy about criticism
16. Does not react when praised or encouraged
17. Easily excited or irritated
18. Emotional reaction persists, high strung
19. Disturbs class with inappropriate behavior
20. Extremely violent and aggressive
21. Disciplinary problem
22. Strong activity
    Normal activity
    Passivity
23. Reacts sensitively
    Reacts normally
    Reacts insensitively
24. Nervous
25. Future psychotic or emotional problem
26. Remedial instruction

Fig. 2.1 School report questionnaire.

Predictive value of teacher reports for schizophrenia

In the Copenhagen HR study, the teacher reports of student behavior were examined to determine how teachers, in 1962, had described those who were identified in the 1989 diagnostic follow-up as having schizophrenia or schizotypal personality disorder. Olin *et al.* (1995) attempted three types of discrimination within those offspring whose mothers had schizophrenia:

• schizophrenics versus subjects with no mental illness
• schizophrenics versus subjects with nonpsychotic disorders
• schizophrenics versus those with schizotypal personality disorder or paranoid personality disorder.

The school behavior was analyzed separately for males and females, since previous studies have reported gender differences in the premorbid behavior of schizophrenics (Watt 1972, Watt and Lubensky 1976, Watt 1978, Schwartzman *et al.* 1985). A likelihood ratio approach was employed to identify school behaviors that distinguished the schizophrenics from other diagnostic groups. The behaviors that distinguish schizophrenics from other outcomes are presented in Table 2.3.

Table 2.3 School behaviors that distinguish future schizophrenics from other outcomes (in decreasing order of discriminative power)

Schizophrenics vs. no mental illness

Distinguishing characteristics of schizophrenic females
>> Teacher predicts future emotional or psychotic problems
>> Nervous

Distinguishing characteristics of schizophrenic males
>> Disciplinary problem
>> Teacher predicts future emotional or psychotic problems
>> Repeated a grade
>> Disturbs class with inappropriate behavior
>> Emotional reaction persists; high strung
>> Lonely and rejected by peers
>> Treated by psychologist for problem
>> Easily excited or irritated

Schizophrenics versus schizotypal or paranoid personality disorders

Distinguishing characteristics of schizophrenic females
>> Normal emotional reaction (is not overly sensitive or insensitive)
>> Not uneasy about criticism

Distinguishing characteristics of schizophrenic males
>> Disciplinary problem
>> Disturbs class with inappropriate behavior
>> Lonely and rejected by peers
>> Less nervous

Schizophrenics versus non-psychotic disorders

Distinguishing characteristics of schizophrenic females
>> Lonely and rejected by peers
>> Nervous
>> Uneasy about criticism
>> Rarely takes part in spontaneous activity
>> Teacher predicts future emotional or psychotic problems
>> Average intelligence
>> Passivity

Distinguishing characteristics of schizophrenic males
>> Lonely and rejected by peers
>> Repeated a grade
>> Passivity
>> Teacher predicts future emotional or psychotic problems
>> Emotional reaction persists; high strung

Schizophrenia versus no mental illness

Females

For the female schizophrenics versus those with no mental illness, it was found that teachers predicted future psychotic problems for the young adolescents who later became schizophrenic women. In addition the teachers also noted that the future schizophrenic females were nervous.

Males

Compared to those who had normal outcomes, the adolescent males were more likely: to disturb the class, be emotionally reactive, to have been treated by a school psychologist, and to be a disciplinary problem. In addition, teachers also reported that these subjects were more lonely and rejected by peers.

Schizophrenics versus non-psychotic disorders

Females

The preschizophrenic females were distinctly different from those women with non-psychotic psychiatric outcomes in school behavior. The preschizophrenic women were more likely to be viewed by their teachers as lonely, rejected by peers, nervous, uneasy about criticism, and passive. The teachers also deemed the preschizophrenic females to be more susceptible to psychotic or emotional problems and to have either high or low intelligence rather than average intelligence.

Males

The preschizophrenic males were more often perceived as lonely and rejected by peers, more passive, more emotionally high strung and more likely to have repeated a grade than males who later developed other diagnoses. Also, teachers predicted (correctly) that the preschizophrenic males were more likely to experience future psychotic or emotional problems and to be emotionally high strung compared to their non-psychotic contemporaries.

Schizophrenia versus Schizotypal or Paranoid Personality Disorder

Females

Relative to the female adolescents who later developed schizophrenia, the future SPD or schizophrenia spectrum girls were more uneasy regarding criticism and either highly sensitive or insensitive.

Males

The preschizophrenic males were more frequently seen by teachers as disruptive in class and were deemed a disciplinary problem. These future schizophrenic males were more likely to be lonely and rejected by their peers. The future SPD or schizophrenia spectrum males were frequently perceived as nervous when compared to the preschizophrenic males.

Diagnostic efficacy of the entire teacher report

In a paper by Olin *et al.* (1995) on the Copenhagen HR project, a standard receiver operating characteristic (ROC) analysis was applied to the teacher report in an attempt to determine the efficacy of the school report in differentiating the HR who later developed schizophrenia from those HR children with more benign outcomes. Specific school behaviors were merged to create aggregated markers for discriminating the future schizophrenics from those who develop no mental illness, those with other non-psychotic disorder and schizotypals. Such an analysis provides an assessment of the efficacy level of the teacher reports for correctly identifying subjects who will develop schizophrenia, given the level of false positives, i.e. those individuals who are incorrectly predicted to later suffer from schizophrenia.

The study by Olin *et al.* (1995) demonstrated that the aggregated school behaviors have a greater predictive power than the individual items on the school report. Overall the results of the ROC analysis revealed that the male adolescents who later developed schizophrenia were distinguishable from those who later had no mental illness and from HR males who later developed schizotypy. In comparison the preschizophrenic females were more distinguishable from those who later developed an other non-psychotic illness; however, the preschizophrenic females were not as easily distinguished from subjects who had no adult mental illness. Thus, the ROC analyses demonstrated that discrimination between future schizophrenics, those with no mental illness, or SPD subjects was more powerful for males than females. This finding may be due to the fact that the preschizophrenic males were exhibiting more easily observed antisocial behaviors, which is congruent with findings from a number of reports that document poorer premorbid social competence in males (Klorman *et al.* 1977, Kokes *et al.* 1977, Ziegler *et al.* 1977, Goldstein 1988).

Summary and implications of teacher report findings

The findings related to teacher's ratings of student behavior have several implications. First, the substantive findings we reported differentiating schizophrenics from those with no mental illness are quite similar to other findings reported (e.g. Offord and Cross 1969, Watt 1972, Watt and Lubensky 1976, Watt 1978, Watt *et al.* 1982). These investigators have located school or child guidance records of individuals with schizophrenia and controls from a general population and reported the differences we have noted. The similarities of our findings to the results of these studies (which did not involve HR subjects) suggest that the teacher report findings are most likely generalizable to an unselected population. Secondly, the accuracy of the teachers' predictions intimates that such ratings may be useful in other settings in helping identify children vulnerable to future psychosis.

Conclusions

The findings from these studies of teachers' reports contribute to a growing body of literature supporting the hypothesis that schizophrenia is not an illness which appears suddenly in adulthood. The results of a number of studies indicate that future schizophrenics may be presenting deviant behaviors before early adulthood (Watt 1972, Watt 1978, Olin *et al.* 1995). Furthermore, results of additional analyses with the Copenhagen HR project revealed that the type of premorbid behavioral deviance is highly congruent with the schizophrenia symptomatology that is evidenced later. Among those who develop schizophrenia, the children who were characterized by teachers as aggressive and disruptive in school later developed predominantly positive symptoms; those who were passive and withdrawn in school develop predominately negative symptoms (Cannon *et al.* 1990).

The identification of premorbid behaviors that distinguishes preschizophrenics from their peers adds support to the theory that schizophrenia is a developmental disorder. In addition, it seems that the readily available data from teacher reports of school behavior, an assessment of perinatal complications, and evaluations of motor functioning and family functioning may be used to detect those at especially high risk for schizophrenia. A combination of risk indicators (such as family history of schizophrenia, perinatal complications, behavior deviance, low birthweight, and motor abnormalities) could be used to target individuals for early intervention programs.

References

Betz, B.J. (1973). Childhood status and adult schizophrenia. *American Journal of Psychotherapy* **27**, 27–33.

Cannon, T.D., Mednick, S.A., and Parnas, J. (1990). Antecedents of predominantly negative and predominantly positive schizophrenia in a high risk population. *Archives of General Psychiatry*, 47, 622–632.

Erlenmeyer-Kimling, L. and Cornblatt, B.A. (1987). The New York High-Risk Project: A follow-up report. *Schizophrenia Bulletin*, **13**(3), 451–461.

Fish, B. (1987). Infant predictors of the longitudinal course of schizophrenic development. *Schizophrenia Bulletin*, **13**(3), 395–409.

Goldstein, J. M. (1988). Gender differences in the cause of schizophrenia. *American Journal of Psychiatry*, **145**, 684–689.

Gutkind, D., Mednick, B., Cannon, T.D., Parnas, J., Schulsinger, F., and Mednick, S.A. (in press). Parental absence and schizophrenia—a 27-year follow-up of the Copenhagen high-risk cohort. *Archives of General Psychiatry.*

Kallman, F.J. (1938). *The Genetics of Schizophrenia.* Augustin Publisher, New York.

Klorman, R., Strauss, J.S., and Kokes, R.F. (1977). Premorbid adjustment in schizophrenia: Concepts, measures, and implications: III. The relationship of demographic and diagnostic factors to measures of premorbid adjustment in schizophrenia. *Schizophrenia Bulletin*, **3**(2), 214–225.

Kokes, R.F., Strauss, J.S., and Klorman, R. (1977). Premorbid adjustment in schizophrenia: Concepts, measures, and implications: II. Measuring premorbid adjustment: The instruments and their development. *Schizophrenia Bulletin*, **3**(2), 186–213.

LaFosse, J.M. (1994). Motor coordination in adolescence and its relationship to adult schizophrenia. Unpublished Dissertation, University of Southern California, Los Angeles;

Marcus, J., Auerbach, J., Wilkinson, L., and Burack, C.M. (1981). Infants at risk for schizophrenia. *Archives of General Psychiatry*, **38**, 703

Marcus, J., Hans, S.L., Nagler, S.A., J.G., Mirsky, A., and Subrey, A. (1987). Review of the NIMH Israeli Kibbutz–City Study and the Jerusalem Infant Development Study. *Schizophrenia Bulletin*, **13**(3), 425–438.

McNeill, T.F. and Kaij, L. (1978). Obstetric factors in the development of schizophrenia: Complications in the birth of preschizophrenics and in reproduction by schizophrenic parents. In *Schizophrenia: New Approaches to Research and Treatment*, ed. L.C. Wynne, R.L.

Cromwell, and S. Matthysse, pp. 401–429. Wiley, New York.

Mednick, S.A. (1970). Breakdown in individuals at high risk for schizophrenia: predispositional factors. *Mental Hygiene*, **54**, 50–63.

Mednick, S.A., and Schulsinger, F. (1968). Some premorbid characteristics related to breakdown in children with schizophrenic mothers. *Journal of Psychiatric Research*, **6**, 267–291.

Mednick, S.A. Parnas, J., and Schulsinger, F. (1987). The Copenhagen High-Risk Project, 1962–86. *Schizophrenia Bulletin*, **13**(3), 485–495.

Offord, D.R. and Cross, L.A. (1969). Behavioral antecedents of adult schizophrenia. *Archives of General Psychiatry*, **21**, 267–283.

Olin, S.S., John, R., and Mednick, S.A. (1995). Assessing the predictive value of teacher reports in a high risk sample for schizophrenia: a ROC analysis. *Schizophrenia Research*, **16**, 53–66.

Olin, S.S., Mednick, S.A., Cannon, T., Jacobsen, B., Parnas, J., Schulsinger, F., and Schulsinger, H. (1997a). School teachers ratings predictive of psychiatric outcome 25 years later. *British Journal of Psychiatry*, **172**, suppl. 33, 7–13.

Olin, S.S., Raine, A., Cannon, T., Parnas, J., Schulsinger, F., and Mednick, S.A. (1997b). Childhood behavior precursors of schizotypal disorder. *Schizophrenia Bulletin*, **23**(1), 93–103.

Parnas, J., Schulsinger, F., Teasdale, T.W., Schulsinger, H., Feldman, P.H., and Mednick, S.A. (1982). Perinatal complications and clinical outcome within the schizophrenia spectrum. *British Journal of Psychiatry*, **140**, 416.

Parnas, J., Cannon, T., Jacobsen, B., Schulsinger, H., Schulsinger, F., and Mednick, S.A. (1993). Lifetime diagnostic outcomes in offspring of schizophrenia mothers: Results from the Copenhagen High-Risk Study. *Archives of General Psychiatry*, **50**, 707–714.

Schwartzman, A.E., Ledingham, J.E., and Serbin, L.A. (1985). Identification of children at risk for adult schizophrenia: A longitudinal study. *International Review of Applied Psychology*, **34**, 363–380.

Tienari, P., Sorri, A., Lahti, I., Naarala, M., Wahlberg, K.-E., Moring, J., Pohjola, J., and Wynne, L.C. (1987). Genetic and psychosocial factors in schizophrenia: The Finnish Adoptive Family Study. *Schizophrenia Bulletin*, **13**(3), 477–484.

Tienari, P., Sorri, A., Lahti, I., Naarala, M., Wahlberg, K.E., Ronkko, T., Pohjola, J., and Moring, J. (1985). The Finnish adoptive family study of schizophrenia. *Yale Journal of Biological Medicine*, **58**, 227.

Walker, E., Savoie, T., and Davis, D. (1994). Neuromotor precursors of schizophrenia. *Schizophrenia Bulletin*, **20**, 453–480.

Watt, N.F. (1972). Longitudinal changes in the social behavior of children hospitalized for schizophrenia as adults. *Journal of Nervous and Mental Disease*, **155**, 42–54.

Watt, N.F. (1978). Patterns of childhood social development in adult schizophrenics. *Archives of General Psychiatry*, **35**, 160–165.

Watt, N.F. and Lubensky, A.W. (1976). Childhood roots of schizophrenia. *Journal of Consulting and Clinical Psychology*, **44**, 363–375.

Watt, N.F., Grubb, T.W., and Erlenmeyer-Kimling, L. (1982). Social, emotional, and intellectual behavior at school among children at high risk for schizophrenia. *Journal of Consulting and Clinical Psychology*, **50**, 171–181.

Ziegler, E., Levine, J., and Ziegler, B. (1977). Premorbid social competence and paranoid-nonparanoid status in female schizophrenic patients. *Journal of Nervous and Mental Disease*, **164**, 333–339.

3 Children of affectively ill parents

Constance Hammen

Depression runs in families. Indeed, children of depressed parents have a high likelihood of developing both behavioral and emotional disorders including depression, and also experience a variety of other adverse outcomes. Studies of offspring of bipolar parents are less common, but also consistently indicate elevated risk for dysfunction and disorders. Despite the consistency of findings, the meaning of such patterns is far less clear. The goal of the present chapter is to report briefly on the results of high risk research in terms of children's diagnoses and adjustment, and much of the chapter is devoted to recent research on processes and mechanisms of the effects. A final section highlights some of the unresolved empirical and conceptual issues that may guide future research in this area.

Paradigms and models

The initial studies in this field at least implicitly examined genetic models of intergenerational transmission of affective disorders. Cross-sectional case–control designs essentially compared children of ill parents with children of normal parents. However, since family aggregation of disorders cannot illuminate the relative contributions of genetic and environmental factors, such studies began to explore the *environmental* contributions of children's risk, particularly those related to the qualities of the relationship between the ill parent and the child. At the same time, investigators observed that in families of women with unipolar depression, for example, there were also high rates of marital discord and other adversities affecting the child's psychosocial adjustment. Consequently, most recent paradigms have shifted to a multiple risk factor approach, attempting to examine and evaluate various factors influencing the child, including environmental factors such as parent–child and spousal relationships and stressors, as well as psychological ones, such as children's acquisition of positive self-concept or other cognitive styles. It should be noted that many contemporary models primarily assess mechanisms of effects of parental depression in non-clinical samples, often using laboratory paradigms to test specific hypotheses about the influence of maternal depressed mood on children's behavior—especially that of infants.

Thus, to a great extent the questions moving this field have shifted from *what* effects do parental mood disorders have, to *how* these effects come about. This chapter provides a brief review of the findings of both types of studies, with a focus on unanswered questions that call for multiple research efforts on many fronts.

Methods and designs

Over the past 25 years, studies of children of depressed parents have generally been conducted in several overlapping phases defined by different goals and methods. One of the first attempts was primarily focused on high risk for schizophrenia, with mood disorders serving as comparison groups, such as the Stony Brook High-Risk Study (Weintraub and Neale 1984) and the Rochester Longitudinal Study (Sameroff *et al.* 1984). The studies were designed to compare various diagnostic groups and normal controls, and typically included measures of children's cognitive and social competence that were intended to identify early signs of schizophrenia.

Next came the first generation of case–control studies primarily focused on children of parents with affective disorders. Most were implicitly if not explicitly based on models of genetic high risk, and rarely included evaluations of potential mechanisms of children's risk (e.g. Weissman *et al.* 1972) Eventually, unipolar offspring studies began to use direct interview assessment of the children as a means of establishing diagnostic status (e.g. Hammen *et al.* 1987, Beardslee *et al.* 1988, Radke-Yarrow et al. 1992). Some of these studies were designed to help clarify the contribution of environmental risk factors.

A relatively recent development in mood disorder high risk has been focus on infants and toddlers of clinically depressed (unipolar) parents (e.g. Radke-Yarrow *et al.* 1985, Teti *et al.* 1995) Several studies of clinically ill mothers and their infants and toddlers have evaluated *attachment security* as a potentially crucial marker of maladaptation.

The most recent and active wave of studies of the effects of depression on youngsters has focused largely on non-clinical samples of women with elevated scores on depression questionnaires. Some of these investigations actually commenced in the early 1980s or so, and represent the efforts of developmental psychopathologists to explore the effects of negative affect and non-optimal parenting styles on children's development. These studies have focused largely on infants and young children.

Finally, a relatively small number of studies have been conducted on children of bipolar parents. Recently, most have included direct-interview methods, and some have included comparisons with other psychiatric groups including unipolar disorder (e.g. Klein *et al.* 1985, Hammen *et al.* 1987, Radke-Yarrow *et al.* (1992). The majority of these studies have been designed on the basis of assumptions of genetic mechanisms of risk, and have tested relatively few questions abut processes and mechanisms of children's adjustment.

Review of findings of high risk studies

Diagnoses and adjustment among children of unipolar parents

The schizophrenia high risk studies with depression as a comparison group have been reviewed by Hammen (1991) and Downey and Coyne (1990), among others, who report outcomes in detail. The early studies appeared to indicate that children of parents with mood disorders were impaired by comparison with offspring of normal parents, and typically as impaired as children of schizophrenic parents (e.g. Sameroff *et al.* 1984, Weintraub and Neale 1984). Unfortunately, however, the early studies did not have diagnostic instruments available for evaluating children's disorders. Moreover, samples were typically defined by DSM-II or DSM-III criteria, which often blurred the boundaries between unipolar and bipolar disorder, or between schizophrenia and bipolar disorder. Nonetheless, these high risk studies established the potential impact of parental depressive disorders on children, and foretold the development of separate lines of research to explore such issues.

The early case–control studies that focused specifically on mood disorders (e.g. Weissman *et al.* 1972) were reviewed by Beardslee *et al.* (1983) and Downey and Coyne (1990). Most such investigations found signs of impairment in the offspring of affectively ill parents, as rated by observers and parents, but did not use direct interview methods of assessing the children.

Findings from the direct interview studies of children of unipolar parents clarified diagnostic outcomes and other maladjustment. Studies of school age children based on direct interview methods have been consistent in displaying relatively high rates of disorder in general, and *depressive disorders* in particular. For instance, current or lifetime *major depression* rates ranged between 45% in the 8–16 year old offspring in Hammen *et al.* (1991), to 38% among 6–23 year olds in Weissman *et al.* (1987) to 24% in Keller *et al.* (1986) and Beardslee *et al.* (1988), and 20% in Goodman *et al.* (1994). In contrast, children of normal comparison families reported depression rates of 4–24% depending on the age of the sample. Rates of other disorders were also significantly higher than in comparison groups, with children of depressed parents displaying elevated rates of anxiety disorders, disruptive disorders, and substance use disorders, as well as high proportions of comorbid disorders. For instance, rates of *any diagnosis* ranged from 65% (Beardslee/Keller) to 73% (Weissman), 80% (Goodman), or 82% (Hammen).

Additionally, apart from children's diagnostic status, ample evidence attests to dysfunction among offspring of unipolar parents in multiple domains. School age children have been found to have marked academic and social difficulties (Anderson and Hammen 1993), intellectual impairment (Kaplan *et al.* 1987), negative cognitions about the self, including self-concept and attribution style (Jaenicke *et al.* 1987), and deficiencies in social and emotional competence including peer difficulties (Goodman *et al.* 1993).

Studies of infant offspring of parents with unipolar disorder also yield evidence of dysfunction. Several studies indicate higher rates of insecure attachment in offspring of depressed women compared to controls (e.g. Radke-Yarrow *et al.* 1985). Several studies have observed that insecure attachment is especially pronounced with chronic or severe maternal disorder (e.g. Frankel *et al.* 1991, Campbell *et al.* 1993). Adverse conditions along with maternal depression were especially associated with 'disorganized' attachment (e.g. Lyons-Ruth *et al.* 1990 with a non-clinically depressed sample; DeMulder and Radke-Yarrow 1991). The largest study of attachment to date, with 61 depressed women (in treatment) and 43 non-depressed controls, found high rates of insecure attachment in infants (80%) and preschoolers (87%) among the children of the depressed women (Teti *et al.* 1995).

Infants and toddlers of clinically depressed women have also been shown to display problems regulating emotional reactions including aggression, as well as peer interaction difficulties (e.g. Zahn-Waxler *et al.* 1984). Toddlers of unipolar depressed mothers also had emotional and behavioral disturbances and delayed expressive language or lower cognitive developments (Cox *et al.* 1987, Whiffen and Gotlib 1989).

Relatively few of the offspring diagnosis studies included a longitudinal follow-up of children's risk for the development or continuation of disorders. Nevertheless, those that have followed children over a period of time have provided evidence of persisting problems (e.g. Hammen *et al.* 1990, Warner *et al.* 1992).

Studies of non-clinical, dysphoric mothers interacting with their infants have fairly consistently observed that the babies display distress. In general, face-to-face interactions have shown that infants respond with withdrawal, anger, and reduced activity to maternal displays of flat affect, withdrawn behavior or intrusiveness (e.g. Cohn and Tronick 1989, Field *et al.* 1990). These difficulties may persist over time (Field *et al.* 1996).

Diagnosis and adjustment in children of bipolar parents

The research on children at risk for bipolar disorders is much less extensive than that for unipolar offspring, and includes mostly case–control studies with and without direct interviews of the children. A complete review of this research is reported in Hammen (1991). Several of six direct interview studies, for example, have generally reported elevated rates of disorders (e.g. 52% in Decina *et al.* 1983; 72% in Gershon *et al.* 1985; 43% in Klein *et al.* 1985). Offspring display not only mood disorders but behavior and anxiety disorders as well. Relatively few studies have reported bipolar outcomes, potentially limited by difficulties in assessing such problems in children.

One observation of particular note regarding bipolar offspring is that their outcomes are often more positive than those of similarly aged children of unipolar depressed parents. Hammen *et al.* (1987) found that the bipolar offspring had moderate amounts of diagnosable disorders, but significantly lower levels of major depression than did the unipolar offspring (Hammen *et al.* 1990). Their social and academic functioning was significantly superior to that of unipolar offspring (Anderson and Hammen 1993). Radke-Yarrow and colleagues (1992) also observed that overall, bipolar children fared better than unipolar offspring in terms of clinically significant problems, except in later childhood when the unipolar and bipolar youngsters had similar high rates of any disorder (68% and 61% respectively).

There have been very few recent studies of bipolar offspring. The most recently published study by Todd *et al.* (1996) examined the genetic risk for bipolar disorder by studying offspring in extended bipolar pedigrees. Twelve of 50 school-aged offspring received diagnoses, and the children of a parent with a mood disorder had a 5.1-fold risk compared with children of healthy parents. The youngsters had elevated risks particularly for bipolar or anxiety disorders. Considerably more research is needed to answer important questions concerning children at risk for bipolar disorders.

Results of studies of mechanisms and modifiers of risk in unipolar offspring

In recent years there has been increased emphasis on mechanisms of risk, and on development of theoretical models. Most of the recent research has explored topics which are reviewed below.

Parent–child interactions and children's risk

A considerable amount of research has documented evidence of dysfunctional interactions and deficient parenting skills (reviewed in Downey and Coyne 1990, Gelfand and Teti 1990,

Hammen 1991, Cummings and Davies 1994). Echoing early clinical observation of mother–child friction and decreased involvement, themes of hostility, detachment, and unresponsiveness are the most typical characteristics reported in the large volume of direct observation studies.

Observations of depressed women with their infants and toddlers, for example, have shown that the women display flat affect, provide less touching, contingent responding, and less positive affection compared with non-depressed women interacting with infants (e.g. Field *et al.* 1990). Maternal depression has also been associated with increased anger and hostility and intrusiveness during mother–infant interactions (e.g. Cohn *et al.* 1986). Similar problems also characterize depressed mothers with preschool age children (e.g. Goodman and Brumley 1990, Kochanska *et al.* 1987).

Studies of older children and adolescents have been somewhat more scarce. In the UCLA Family Study the unipolar women showed significantly higher rates of criticism and negativity toward their children, less positive comments, and more off-task (uninvolved) comments compared to the other groups (except that they were not less positive than the bipolar women) (Gordon *et al.* 1989; see also Hops *et al.* 1987, Webster-Stratton and Hammond 1988, Tarullo *et al.* 1994).

Mechanisms of dysfunctional parent–child interactions

Observations studies reveal that depressed women are typically unresponsive or negative (or both) with their youngsters. Investigators have suggested several possible mechanisms by which dysfunctional interaction patterns may have negative consequences for the children. One is attachment quality (e.g. Cummings and Cicchetti 1990, Gelfand and Teti 1990). A woman who is preoccupied, or disinterested in or even hostile toward her baby, and fails to respond sensitively and contingently, may have a child who grows to conceive itself as unworthy and the world and other people as untrustworthy, uncaring, or unpredictable. Insecure attachment, in turn, may perhaps interfere with youngsters' development of capacities to regulate affect, behavior, and arousal (Cummings and Davies 1994). Children exposed to inconsistent and emotionally fluctuating mothers may themselves have difficulty in managing their emotions and acquiring and displaying appropriate behaviors under stressful conditions.

Another process by which maladaptive parenting associated with depression might have a negative impact on children is through dysfunctional parenting skills (e.g. Gelfand and Teti 1990, Cummings and Davies 1994). Parental depression may reduce the parent's attentiveness and energy, and increase irritability and hostility that arouse and provoke the child—as well as reinforcing maladaptive behaviors. Depressed parents have indeed been found to be not only more negative and less positive in verbal interactions with their children, as noted earlier, but also more inconsistent and ineffectual in child discipline (e.g. Forehand *et al.* 1986, Zahn-Waxler *et al.* 1990). They use more forceful control strategies (Fendrich *et al.* 1990) or avoidant, less effortful discipline and conflict resolution strategies (e.g. Kochanska *et al.* 1987, Gordon *et al.* 1989).

A third mechanism that may account for children's maladjustment as a consequence of negative interactions is the child's acquisition of maladaptive skills and cognitions. Depression theorists, in particular, have extended cognitive vulnerability models of adult depression to children, suggesting that acquired negative cognitions about the self and the world create a diathesis for depression. For instance, Jaenicke *et al.* (1987) found that children of unipolar depressed women had the most negative cognitions about themselves of all groups in the UCLA Family Stress Project, and that their negative self-cognitions were associated with the degree to which their mothers expressed actual criticism and negative comments during an interaction task. Nolen-Hoeksema *et al.* (1995) demonstrated that depressed mothers behaved toward their children during a puzzle-solving task in a way that promoted 'learned helplessness'. They observed that women who expressed relatively more negativity and hostility had children who responded to a frustrating task with low persistence and less enthusiasm, and displayed fewer problem-solving responses and lower competence in related situations. A study by Goodman *et al.* (1994) found that maternal negative attitudes expressed toward the child affected global self-worth; children of depressed mothers who also expressed more negative attitudes toward them had the lowest self-worth scores.

A fourth potential mechanism accounting for the link between poor quality of interacting and children's disorders in offspring of depressed parents is a 'stress-buffering' effect. The low availability or supportiveness of an unresponsive or critical parent to help the child deal with stressors (including the stress of dysfunctional parenting) might result in children's difficulties in managing stress. Hammen *et al.* (1991) found partial support for this hypothesis, reporting that among youngsters who experienced high levels of personally stressful events, only those who also had a mother who was depressed during the stressor period became depressed following the negative events.

Clearly, the experience of negatively toned, less sensitive, or non-contingent responding by depressed mothers is a powerful ingredient in children's maladaptive outcomes. Further studies will help to clarify the mechanisms of the effects, and the related issues of timing and chronicity of exposure, as well as the specificity of the patterns to depressed parents and their families.

Biological approaches

Many of the studies of children at risk due to parental depression were conceived with the assumption of genetic mechanisms of risk. Obviously, familial patterns do not themselves indicate genetic pathways, since family environmental factors may also contribute to outcomes. To date there have been no studies that directly address the issue of genetic transmission in offspring studies, although increasing evidence points to heritable factors in at least some forms of depressive disorders (Kendler *et al.* 1993, McGuffin *et al.* 1996).

Another major approach to understanding potential biological pathways to children's risk has focused on electroencephalogram (EEG) patterns of depressed women and their infants. Research on depressed adults has revealed a pattern of asymmetrical EEG recordings in the frontal lobe areas (e.g. Henriques and Davidson 1990). In particular, depression appears to be associated with less activation of the left frontal region, suggesting decrements in expression of 'approach' or positive-related emotions. Recently, studies have found similar patterns in inhibited or withdrawn children (reviewed in Field *et al.* 1995). Several investigators explored the patterns of depressed mothers and their infants. Field *et al.* (1995) found the predicted asymmetry in both depressed mothers and their 3–6 month old infants, but were unable to determine whether the effect was an indicator of current negative affect associated with being in an interaction with their depressed mothers, or whether it might reflect a marker of chronic negative affect potentially portending subsequent behavioral disorders. Dawson *et al.* (1994) also demonstrated that more infants of depressed mothers showed relative right frontal asymmetry (lower left frontal activation).

Fox *et al.* (1994) speculated that hemispheric asymmetry may reflect temperamental patterns associated with emotion regulation and behavioral styles, such that maladaptive patterns may eventually give rise to internalizing or externalizing disorders. Such patterns may reflect the complex transactions between genetically determined predispositions and experiences with the environment (e.g. a depressed mother). Dawson *et al.* (1994) also emphasize the role of parental behavior as an influence on the shaping of cortical reactions and emotional responses. Dawson's group is presently engaged in a longitudinal study to determine whether children's physiological patterns are stable or relative to mothers' current mood states.

A related emphasis on biological elements of risk for depression among children of depressed parents focuses on abnormal stress responses. Several developmental psychopathologists (e.g. Tronick and Gianino 1986, Dawson *et al.* 1994) speculated that depressed parents fail to respond adaptively to their children's emotional signals, resulting in poor self-regulation strategies and increased negative affect. According to Dawson *et al.* (1994), this may lead to an overly inward or self-focused style of emotion regulation instead of seeking support from others. This self-focused style may be accompanied by elevations in physiological arousal (even if outwardly passive). Consistent with this model, Field *et al.* (1988) showed that during interactions with their depressed mothers, 3–6 month old infants displayed higher heart rates than infants interacting with non-depressed mothers. Dawson *et al.* (1994) also found that infants of clinically depressed mothers showed significantly elevated heart rates when engaged in face-to-face interactions with their mothers (but not during a baseline period).

These studies offer promising leads for integrating biological and psychological processes in accounting for children's risk for psychopathology as offspring of depressed parents. Additional work is needed, of course, to clarify these processes, their specificity to depression, and their potential contribution to children's disorders.

Multiple risk factor models

In the search to clarify the determinants of maladaptive outcomes among children of depressed parents, a number of investigators have noted the co-occurrence of multiple risk factors in many such families. Downey and Coyne (1990), for example, have particularly emphasized the role of marital distress as an ingredient affecting children's outcomes, and one that is often confounded with parental depression. They have proposed different versions of a model in which the link between parental depression and child distress is mediated or moderated by the level of marital conflict. Fendrich *et al.* (1990) examined the presence and contribution of marital discord, parent–child discord, low family cohesion, and divorce in samples of depressed and non-depressed families and their children. They observed that all of the risk factors were more prevalent among children of depressed parents than among children of non-depressed parents. The presence of such factors was associated with major depression, conduct disorder, and any diagnosis. With the exception of conduct disorder, parental depression did not add significantly to the prediction of negative child outcomes beyond that contributed by the family risk factors.

Goodman *et al.* (1993) examined parent marital status and presence of fathers' psychiatric disorder in addition to maternal depression as factors affecting children's social and emotional competence. They found that in some analyses maternal depression added little to predicting children's outcomes once paternal diagnosis and divorce status had been taken into account. On the other hand, the combination of maternal depression and fathers' psychiatric disorder was associated with children's lower competence levels.

Hammen and colleagues have emphasized multiple risk factors in families with a depressed parent. One common ingredient is high levels of chronic and episodic stress; psychiatric disability often contributes to—as well as results from—poor marital, occupational, family, and financial functioning and accompanying stress. Hammen *et al.* (1987) demonstrated that chronic stress and depressed mood, factors that cut across the boundaries of diagnosis, contributed more to children's adverse outcomes than did maternal psychiatric history as such. Children of unipolar depressed women were especially challenged by exposure to high rates of both maternal chronic stress and their own stressful life events (Adrian and Hammen 1993). In addition to stress and high levels of divorce or marital discord, Hammen (1991) also noted that the majority of the biological fathers of children of depressed mothers had diagnosable disorders, and also that the majority of the depressed mothers themselves had parents with psychopathology. These patterns were speculated to expose children to a mother who herself might have received dysfunctional parenting, and whose social and interpersonal deficiencies might have contributed to mate selection of a dysfunctional man whose pathology virtually ensures marital disruption. Hammen (1991) offered a multifactorial model of intergenerational transmission of disorder in offspring as a complex outcome of mothers' own family history, dysfunctional mate selection, and consequent chronic stress in marital and other domains contributing in part to negative or uninvolved interactions with the child. Such factors contribute both directly and indirectly to children's maladaptive outcomes (which are also influenced by the child's own dysfunctional skills and resources in coping with stressful circumstances).

Cummings and Davies (1994) have also proposed a multifactorial model of children's risk. The generic model includes parental characteristics, marital functioning, and parent–child relationships as factors influencing child characteristics, and interacting in bidirectional fashion with maternal depression.

Factors that modify or clarify children's risk

There are numerous unresolved issues regarding the characteristics of the depression or the family that potentially modify children's risk. Owing to limitations of space, only two key issues are discussed briefly, characteristics of maternal depression and the role of fathers.

Characteristics of parental depression

As noted, offspring studies have varied widely in criteria for selection, ranging from individuals in treatment of unipolar depressive disorders to individuals with mildly elevated depression scores on mood measures. However, depression differs not only in severity, but it also in frequency or chronicity, in timing of occurrence in relation to children's age and development, in terms of co-occurrence with other psychiatric disorders, and in symptom characteristics (e.g. lethargy and withdrawal versus irritability and hypersensitivity). The surface has barely been scratched in addressing these questions that are essential to understanding the role of exposure to parental depressive experiences.

A few studies of offspring determined that it is chronicity and severity of parental disorder that predicted adverse outcomes in children (e.g. Sameroff *et al.* 1984, Keller *et al.* 1986). Hammen (1991) reported that children whose mothers had more depressive episodes were themselves more likely to have more severe diagnoses. Warner *et al.* (1995) in their most recent offspring study demonstrated that only recurrent, early-onset major depression in the parent was significantly associated with major depression in the offspring. In a recent study focused on depressed mothers and their infants, Campbell *et al.* (1995) demonstrated that relatively less positive interactions between mothers and their babies were observed only among women whose depressions had lasted through six months postpartum. Those who were depressed at 2 months postpartum but whose depressions remitted over time did not differ from non-depressed comparison women. Frankel and Harmon (1996) found that many depressed women who had more severe or chronic depressions were seen as significantly less emotionally available and had higher rates of insecurely attached children than women with episodic depression only. Also, Teti *et al.* (1995) found that the most chronically and severely depressed women had infants and preschoolers with insecure attachments marked by less coherent and organized strategies.

These studies suggest that mild and transient depressive symptoms have insignificant effects on children, compared to more severe and chronic conditions. Nevertheless, it remains to be seen whether it is the depression of more severely ill parents—or coexisting factors such as psychosocial adversity, impaired functioning, comorbidity, and the like—that account for children's risk. Also, the *timing* of maternal depression may be critical. It is certainly speculated that maternal depression during the development of attachment relationships may be particularly disruptive for long-term functioning, but further research is needed to explore this topic.

The father's role

The great majority of studies of effects of parental depression on children have examined the influence of maternal depression. This has been both a theoretically based and a practical choice in most cases, reflecting the relative importance assigned to the mother–child relationship as well as the often noted difficulty of obtaining fathers' cooperation in research studies. It is also more difficult to locate men with significant depression, compared to the numbers of women, and who also have either intact families or, if divorced, have substantial contact with children. Several earlier studies with relatively small numbers of depressed fathers tended to find little effect of paternal depression, or no difference between the impact of paternal or maternal depression (Keller *et al.* 1986, Orvaschel *et al.* 1988).

Another issue about the father's role is the strikingly high rate of disorder in men whose partners are depressed. Several studies found that the majority of fathers had diagnoses (e.g. Merikangas *et al.* 1988, Hammen 1991, Radke-Yarrow *et al.* 1992, Goodman *et al.* 1993,

Warner *et al.* 1995). Commonly, father's diagnoses include substance abuse, antisocial personality disorder, or mood disorders. Moreover, most of these studies found that paternal diagnoses were risk factors for children's negative outcomes—especially depending on marital status or discord. Presence of paternal illness along with maternal depression might compound children's risk, for example, whereas having a well father at home might reduce the ill effects of maternal depression. Similarly, in non-clinical samples of depressed women, children with non-depressed fathers appeared to interact more positively with their fathers than their mothers (e.g. Hossain *et al.* 1994), or to have fewer problems (Tannenbaum and Forehand 1994).

This small body of research on fathers provides at least three questions that need urgent pursuit:

- What is the impact of fathers' depressive disorders on youngsters?
- What role does a healthy father play in families of depressed mothers (or the role of a healthy coparent when one has a depressive disorder)?
- What is the process—and consequence—of mate selection that results in two parents with diagnosable conditions?

Conclusions

This brief and selective review of children of parents with mood disorders has observed remarkable consistency in findings about children's outcomes. However, further advances in this field are needed to address several methodological and conceptual limitations.

Methodological gaps in high risk research

Although use of standardized diagnostic criteria is no longer a significant problem, there remains the issue of sample selection. If treatment samples are used, are such parents representative of depression as it most commonly exists in the community? Some argue that those who seek treatment may be especially likely to have multiple problems including comorbid diagnoses and the most severe clinical conditions—factors that may yield unrealistic pictures of the typical risk to children of having a depressed parent. The use of depression questionnaires and non-diagnostic criteria for sample selection often arises in current studies: are mildly depressed parents a reasonable target group for gaining clearer understanding of the effects of depression on children? To a large extent, this is an empirical question requiring actual data rather than the assumption of continuity between clinical and subclinical conditions.

Another design problem is the selection of comparison groups to address the issue of specificity. A limited number of research designs have attempted to determine whether depression has unique effects due to the disorder itself, or whether parental psychopathology in general, or stressful life conditions in various forms, account for children's adverse outcomes. Several studies have provided some evidence that children of unipolar parents fare worse than those with medically ill parents (e.g. Hammen *et al.* 1987, Klein *et al.* 1988, Lee and Gotlib 1989). Limited information also suggests that offspring of unipolar parents may fare worse on some outcomes than children of parents with other psychiatric disorders such as bipolar or psychotic disorders.

Few studies except as noted have used longitudinal designs to explore children's outcomes over time. Such designs are needed to address questions such as the stability of children's dysfunction, as well as the influence of parent current mood versus ongoing characteristics. Longitudinal studies may also help to address critical questions of the role of timing of parental depression in relation to children's age and development.

An additional limitation concerns outcome assessments. There has been emphasis on children's diagnoses and a relative neglect of areas of functioning such as academic, cognitive, and interpersonal competencies and vulnerabilities. Many further issues concerning empirical and conceptual gaps are raised in sections of this chapter.

Conceptual and empirical issues for future research

A central conceptual issue requiring further exploration is the extent to which it is depression as such that contributes to children's risk for maladaptive outcomes. This issue has several inter-related aspects.

Depression versus relational pathology?

Lyons-Ruth (1995) noted that many of the adverse outcomes of children of depressed mothers are shared by other groups, and may be related to a variety of both contextual and emotional factors. She has raised the intriguing possibility that dysphoria clusters with relational problems—marital, parent–child, attachment—that may themselves reflect a more basic underlying process. She proposes that rather than mood, a better conceptual explanation might be defects in the relational mechanisms that interfere with healthy child development. Although there is insufficient evidence to verify this hypothesis, it raises a critical question about the central mechanisms responsible for children's difficulties and serves to remind us that depressed mood might itself be a marker rather than the central ingredient of maladaptive processes.

Depression versus other affects or impairments?

Relatedly, further research is needed to clarify precisely what it is about depression that might influence children in maladaptive ways: as noted previously, depression symptoms include withdrawal—or irritability—or a host of other manifestations. Additionally, many of the studies of depressed mothers have not evaluated specificity of the effects of depression, rather than other affects or pathologies. For instance, depressed mood symptoms often covary with anxiety or other distress symptoms. Depression often co-occurs with others disorders, including pervasive Axis II pathology. Specificity of effects due to depression has rarely been addressed in a satisfactory way.

If depression, how much? how often? when?

If depressive states are responsible for children's adverse outcomes, we still have little understanding of how much depression, or how much exposure over time, relate to the impact on children. Moreover, the matter of potential critical periods of exposure, or different effects at different developmental levels of effects, require study. Recent research suggests that transitory depression is uninformative, but basic issues remain of whether even mild but persistent depression has the same impact as severe but intermittent disorder. Also, little is known about the functioning of parents between periods or episodes of depression.

Even if depression is critical, what about the correlated risk factors?

As emphasized throughout, depression rarely occurs in a vacuum; it is typically accompanied by adverse environmental conditions, stress, marital difficulties or disruption, and history of intergenerational pathology. These issues have been addressed to a limited extent, but rarely studied more than one variable at a time. Large-scale studies are clearly needed to include multiple and interacting risk factors, and to evaluate the relative contributions of such variables along with parental depression.

Additional unresolved issues

Even beyond core conceptual issues as noted, there remain many specific questions to study:

- what is the effect of depression in fathers?
- What are the specific outcomes for children of exposure to depressed parents (in contrast to other forms of exposure to parental dysfunction)?
- How stable are children's difficulties, and what factors account for variability in outcomes (e.g., resilience factors)?

Overall, the legacy of research on children of depressed parents has been exceedingly rich in information about normal and maladaptive outcomes. In recent years in particular the topic has proven to be a virtual laboratory for studying mother–child interaction processes, and the contexts that shape them. The complexity of the questions posed by this line of research suggests that grand conceptual models at this moment are premature. Nevertheless, we look forward to the future development of integrated biological–psychosocial models of the impact of parental affective disorder on children.

References

Adrian, C. and Hammen, C. (1993). Stress exposure and stress generation in children of depressed mothers. *Journal of Consulting and Clinical Psychology*, **61**, 354–359.

Anderson, C.A. and Hammen, C.L. (1993). Psychosocial outcomes of children of unipolar depressed, bipolar, medically ill, and normal women: A longitudinal study. *Journal of Consulting and Clinical Psychology*, **61**, 448–454.

Beardslee, W.R., Bemporad, J., Keller, M.B., and Klerman, G.L. (1983). Children of parents with major affective disorder: A review. *American Journal of Psychiatry*, **140**, 825–832.

Beardslee, W., Keller, M., Lavori, P., Klerman, G., Dorer, D., and Samuelson, H. (1988). Psychiatric disorder in adolescent offspring of parents with affective disorder in a non-referred sample. *Journal of Affective Disorders*, **15**, 313–322.

Campbell, S.B., Cohn, J.F., Meyers, T.A. Ross, S., and Flanagan, C. (1993). Chronicity of maternal depression and mother-infant interaction. Paper presented at the meetings of the Society for Research in Child Development, New Orleans, LA.

Campbell, S.B., Cohn, J.F., and Meyers, T.A. (1995). Depression in first-time mothers: Mother-infant interaction and depression chronicity. *Developmental Psychology*, **31**, 349–357.

Cohn, J.F. and Tronick, E. (1989). Specificity of infants' response to mothers' affective behavior. *Journal of the American Academy of Child and Adolescent Psychiatry*, **28**, 242–248.

Cohn, J.F., Matias, R., Tronick, E., Connell, D., and Lyons-Ruth, K. (1986). Face-to-face interactions of depressed mothers and their infants. In *Maternal depression and infant disturbance*, ed. E. Tronick and T. Field (New Directions for Child Development No. 34), pp. 31–46. Jossey-Bass, San Francisco.

Cox, A., Puckering, C., Pound, A., and Mills, M. (1987). The impact of maternal depression in young children. *Journal of Child Psychology and Psychiatry*, **28**, 917–928.

Cummings, E.M. and Cicchetti, D. (1990) Toward a transactional model of relations between attachment and depression. In *Attachment in the preschool years: Theory, research and intervention*, ed. M. Greenberg, D. Cicchetti and E.M. Cummings, pp. 339–372. University of Chicago Press, Chicago.

Cummings, E.M. and Davies, P.T. (1994). Maternal depression and child development. *Journal of Child Psychology and Psychiatry*, **35**, 73–112.

Dawson, G., Hessl, D., and Frey, K. (1994). Social influences on early developing biological and behavioral systems related to risk for affective disorder. *Development and Psychopathology*, **6**, 759–779.

Decina, P., Kestenbaum, C.J., Farber, S. Kron, L., Gargan, M., Sackheim, H.A. and Fieve, R.R. (1983). Clinical and psychological assessment of children of bipolar probands. *American Journal of Psychiatry*, **140**, 548–553.

DeMulder, E.K. and Radke-Yarrow, M. (1991). Attachment with affectively ill and well mothers: Concurrent behavioral correlates. *Development and Psychopathology*, **3**, 227–242.

Downey, G. and Coyne, J.C. (1990). Children of depressed parents: An integrative review. *Psychological Bulletin*, **108**, 50–76.

Fendrich, M., Warner, V., and Weissman, M.M. (1990). Family risk factors, parental depression, and psychopathology in offspring. *Developmental Psychology*, **26**, 40–50.

Field, T., Healy, B., Goldstein, S., Perry, S., Bendall, D., Schanberg, S., Zimmermann, E., and Kuhn, C. (1988). Infants of depressed mothers show depressed behavior even with non-depressed adults. *Child Development*, **59**, 1569–1579.

Field, T., Healy, B., Goldstein, S., and Guthertz, M. (1990). Behavior-state matching and synchrony in mother-infant interactions of nondepressed versus depressed dyads. *Developmental Psychology*, **26**, 7–14.

Field, T., Fox, N.A., Pickens, J., and Nawrocki, T. (1995). Relative right frontal EEG activation in 3- to 6-month-old infants of "depressed" mothers. *Developmental Psychology*, **31**, 358–363.

Field, T., Lang, C., Martinez, A., Yando, R., Pickens, J., and Bendell, D. (1996). Preschool follow-up of infants of dysphoric mothers. *Journal of Clinical Child Psychology*, **25**, 272–279.

Forehand, R., Lautenschlager, G.J., Faust, J., and Graziano, W.G. (1986). Parent perceptions and parent–child interactions in clinic-referred children: A Preliminary investigation of the effects of maternal depressive moods. *Behaviour Research and Therapy*, **24**, 73–75.

Fox, N.A., Calkins, S.D., and Bell, M.A. (1994). Neural plasticity and development in the first two years of life: Evidence from cognitive and socioemotional domains of research. *Development and Psychopathology*, **6**, 677–696.

Frankel, K.A. and Harmon, R.J. (1996). Depressed mothers: They don't always look as bad as they feel. *Journal of the American Academy of Child and Adolescent Psychiatry*, **35**, 289–298.

Gelfand, D.M. and Teti, D.M. (1990). The effects of maternal depression on children. *Clinical Psychology Review*, **10**, 320–354.

Gershon, E.S., McKnew, D., Cytryn, L., Hamovit, J., Schreiber, J., Hibbs, E., and Pelligrini, D. (1985). Diagnoses in school-age children of bipolar affective disorder patients and normal controls. *Journal of Affective Disorders*, **8**, 283–291.

Goodman, S.H. and Brumley, H.E. (1990). Schizophrenic and depressed mothers: Relational deficits in parenting. *Developmental Psychology*, **26**, 31–39.

Goodman, S.H., Brogan, D., Lynch, M.E., and Fielding B. (1993). Social and emotional competence in children of depressed mothers. *Child Development*, **64**, 516–531.

Goodman, S.H., Adamson, L.B., Riniti, J., and Cole, S. (1994). Mothers' expressed attitudes: Associations with maternal depression and children's self-esteem and psychopathology. *Journal of the American Academy of Child and Adolescent Psychiatry*, **33**, 1265–1274.

Gordon, D., Burge, D., Hammen, C., Adrian, C., Jaenicke, C., and Hiroto, D. (1989). Observations of interactions of depressed women with their children. *American Journal of Psychiatry*, **146**, 50–55.

Hammen, C. (1991). *Depression runs in families: The social context of risk and resilience in children of depressed mothers*. Springer-Verlag, New York.

Hammen, C., Adrian, C., Gordon, D., Burge, D., Jaenicke, C., and Hiroto, D. (1987). Children of depressed mothers: Maternal strain and symptom predictors of dysfunction. *Journal of Abnormal Psychology*, **96**, 190–198.

Hammen, C., Burge, D., Burney, E., and Adrian, C. (1990). Longitudinal study of diagnoses in children of women with unipolar and bipolar affective disorder. *Archives of General Psychiatry*, **47**, 1112–1117.

Hammen, C., Burge, D., and Adrian, C. (1991). Timing of mother and child depression in a longitudinal study of children at risk. *Journal of Consulting and Clinical Psychology*, **59**, 341–345.

Henriques, J.B. and Davidson, R.J. (1990). Regional brain electrical asymmetries discriminate between previously depressed and healthy control subjects. *Journal of Abnormal Psychology*, **99**, 22–31.

Hops, H., Biglan, A., Sherman, L., Arthur, J., Friedman, L., and Osteen, V. (1987). Home observations of family interactions of depressed women. *Journal of Consulting and Clinical Psychology*, **55**, 341–346.

Hossain, Z., Field, T., Gonzalez, J., Malphurs, J., and Del Valle, C. (1994). Infants of "depressed" mothers interact better with their nondepressed fathers. *Infant Mental Health Journal*, **15**, 248–257.

Jaenicke, C., Hammen, C., Zupan, B., Hiroto, D., Gordon, D., Adrian, C., and Burge, D. (1987). Cognitive vulnerability in children at risk for depression. *Journal of Abnormal Child Psychology*, **15**, 559–572.

Kaplan, B., Beardslee, W., and Keller, M. (1987). Intellectual competence in children of depressed parents. *Journal of Clinical Child Psychology*, **16**, 158–163.

Keller, M.B., Beardslee, W.R., Dorer, D.J., Lavori, P.W., Samuelson, H., and Klerman, G.R. (1986). Impact of severity and chronicity of parental affective illness on adaptive functioning and psychopathology in children. *Archives of General Psychiatry*, **43**, 930–937.

Kendler, K.S., Kessler, R.C., Neale, M.C., Heath, A.C., and Eaves, L.J. (1993). The prediction of major depression in women: Toward an integrated etiologic model. *American Journal of Psychiatry*, **150**, 1139–1148.

Klein, D.N., Depue, R.A., and Slater, J.F. (1985). Cyclothymia in the adolescent offspring of parents with bipolar affective disorder. *Journal of Abnormal Psychology* **94**, 115–127.

Klein, D., Clark, D., Dansky, L., and Margolis, E. (1988). Dysthymia in offspring of parents with primary unipolar affective disorder. *Journal of Abnormal Psychology*, **97**, 265–274.

Kochanska, G., Kuczynski, L., Radke-Yarrow, M., and Welsh, J.D. (1987). Resolutions of control episodes between well and affectively ill mothers and their young children. *Journal of Abnormal Child Psychology*, **15**, 441–456.

Lee, C. and Gotlib, I. (1991). Adjustment of children of depressed mothers: A 10-month follow-up. *Journal of Abnormal Psychology*, **100**, 473–477.

Lyons-Ruth, K. (1995). Broadening our conceptual framework: Can we reintroduce relational strategies and implicit representational systems to the study of psychopathology? *Developmental Psychology*, **31**, 432–436.

Lyons-Ruth, K., Connell, D.B., Grunebaum, H., and Botein, S. (1990). Infants at social risk: Maternal depression and family support services as mediators of infant development and security of attachment. *Child Development*, **61**, 85–98.

McGuffin, P., Katz, R., Watkins, S., and Rutherford, J. (1996). A hospital-based twin register of the heritability of DSM-IV unipolar depression. *Archives of General Psychiatry*, **53**, 129–136.

Merikangas, K., Weissman, M., Prusoff, B., and John, K. (1988). Assortative mating and affective disorders: Psychopathology in offspring. *Psychiatry*, **51**, 48–57.

Nolen-Hoeksema, S., Wolfson, A., Mumme, D., and Guskin, K. (1995). Helplessness in children of depressed and nondepressed mothers. *Developmental Psychology*, **31**, 377–387.

Orvaschel, H., Walsh-Allis, G., and Ye, W. (1988). Psychopathology in children of parents with recurrent depression. *Journal of Abnormal Child Psychology*, **16**, 17–28.

Radke-Yarrow, M., Cummings, E.M., Kuczynski, L., and Chapman, M. (1985). Patterns of attachment in two-and-three-year olds in normal families and families with parental depression. *Child Development*, **56**, 884–893.

Radke-Yarrow, M., Nottelmann, E., Martinez, P., Fox, M.B., and Belmont, B. (1992). Young children of affectively ill parents: A longitudinal study of psychosocial development. *Journal of the American Academy of Child and Adolescent Psychiatry*, **31**, 68–77.

Sameroff, A.J., Barocas, R., and Seifer, R. (1984). The early development of children born to mentally ill women. In *Children at risk for schizophrenia*, ed. N. Watt, E.J. Anthony, L. Wynne, and J. Rolf, pp. 482–514. Cambridge University Press, New York.

Tannenbaum, L. and Forehand, R. (1994). Maternal depressive mood: The role of the father in preventing adolescent problem behaviors. *Behavior Research and Therapy*, **32**, 321–325.

Tarullo, L.B., DeMulder, E.K., Martinez, P.E., and Radke-Yarrow, M. (1994). Dialogues with preadolescents and adolescents: Mother–child interaction patterns in affectively ill and well dyads. *Journal of Abnormal Child Psychology*, **22**, 33–51.

Teti, D.M., Gelfand, D.M., Messinger, D.S., and Isabella, R. (1995). Maternal depression and the quality of early attachment: An examination of infants preschoolers, and their mothers. *Developmental Psychology*, **31**, 364–376.

Todd, R.D., Reich, W., Petti, T.A., Joshi, P., DePaulo, J.R., Nurnberger, J., and Reich, T. (1996). Psychiatric diagnoses in the child and adolescent members of extended families indentified through adult bipolar affective disorder probands. *Journal of the American Academy of Child and Adolescent Psychiatry*, **35**, 664–671.

Tronick, E.Z. and Gianino, A.F. (1986). The transmission of maternal disturbances to the infant. In *Maternal depression and infant disturbance*, ed. E.Z. Tronick and T. Field, pp. 5–11. Jossey-Bass, San Francisco.

Warner, V., Weissman, M., Fendrich, M., Wickramaratne, P., and Moreau, D. (1992). The course of major depression in the offspring of depressed parents. *Archives of General Psychiatry*, **49**, 795–801.

Warner, V., Mufson, L., and Weissman, M.M. (1995). Offspring at high and low risk for depression and anxiety: Mechanisms of psychiatric disorder. *Journal of the American Academy of Child and Adolescent Psychiatry*, **34**, 786–797.

Webster-Stratton, C. and Hammond, M. (1988). Maternal depression and its relationship to life stress, perceptions of child behavior problems, parenting behaviors, and child conduct problems. *Journal of Abnormal Child Psychology*, **16**, 299–315.

Weissman, M.M., Paykel, E.S., and Klerman, G.L. (1972). The depressed woman as a mother. *Social Psychiatry*, **7**, 98–108.

Weissman, M., Gammon, G., John, K., Merikangas, K., Warner, V., Prusoff, B., and Sholomskas, D. (1987). Children of depressed parents: Increased psychopathology and early onset of major depression. *Archives of General Psychiatry*, **44**, 847–853.

Weissman, M.M., Wickramarantne, P., Adams, P.B., Lish, J.D., Horwath, E., Charney, D., Woods, S.W., Leeman, E., and Frosch, E. (1993). The relationship between panic disorder and major depression. *Archives of General Psychiatry*, **50**, 767–780.

Whiffen, V. and Gotlib, I. (1989). Infants of postpartum depressed mothers: Temperament and cognitive status. *Journal of Abnormal Psychology*, **98**, 274–279.

Zahn-Waxler, C., Cummings, E.M., Iannotti, R., and Radke-Yarrow, M. (1984). Young offspring of depressed parents: A population at risk for affective problems. *New Directions for Child Development*, **26**, 81–105.

Zahn-Waxler, C., Iannotti, R.J., Cummings, E.M., and Denham, S. (1990). Antecedents of problem behaviors in children of depressed mothers. *Development and Psychopathology*, **2**, 271–291.

4　Children of alcoholic parents

Hans-Christoph Steinhausen

Although transcultural data on the prevalence of alcoholism based on representative samples is lacking, it is quite clear that alcoholism is one of the most common and deleterious psychiatric disorders throughout the world. It has devastating effects on the patients themselves, the more personal social environment of the immediate family, relatives and friends, and society and the community at large. Children of alcoholics represent a large proportion of the population throughout the western world and are the unfortunate victims of the disorder of their parents. In contrast to most other psychiatric disorders, alcoholism may affect both the mother and the father. In fact, for a substantial proportion of children, their immediate family environment is characterized by not one but two addicted parents. The distress for the developing child is thereby increased because of the lack of any buffering effects from a healthy parent.

Paradigms and models

There are three main risk factors that influence development in the offspring of alcoholic parents. These three risk factors are also the guiding principles for the paradigms and models that have been used in research.

- First, largely but not entirely due to genetic risk factors, children of alcoholic parents themselves develop alcoholism later during adolescence or adulthood.
- A second source of risk factors for the developing child of alcoholic parents originates in the teratogenicity of alcohol. Owing to intrauterine exposure to alcohol, children born to alcoholic mothers are at further specific developmental risk.
- Finally, children of alcoholic parents are exposed to an increased risk of developing other or comorbid psychiatric disorders during their lifetime that manifest themselves as a consequence of genetic or environmental risk factors or an interaction of the two.

Methods and design

According to the three models described above, the various studies differ considerably in methods and design. Most commonly, the studies are based on cohorts or random samples stemming from various sources. The latter may include treatment facilities for the parents or even the (grown up) children themselves, self-help groups, clinical settings, or institutions for delinquents. As a consequence, there is a danger of overgeneralization of findings coming from these different types of samples. For example, psychopathology in the parents will be higher in samples in which the parents are in treatment as compared to samples recruited from self-help groups. Unfortunately, there is a scarcity of community studies that could buffer against this bias of sample selection.

The cross-sectional design is the major model for the vast majority of studies; the potential of the more expensive and complicated longitudinal design still has to be implemented to a greater extent into future research. The latter approach would be much better suited to studying developmental processes as a function of risk status in the children of alcoholic parents.

Further variation in the studies derives from differences in the ascertainment of alcoholism in the parents. Studies relying on the family history method are jeopardized by poor reporting due to the identification of false positives and even more of false negatives, whereas studies with direct assessment of the alcoholic parent are not affected by this bias.

Another methodological problem in many studies is caused by the heterogeneity of alcoholism. Certainly, there are various types of alcoholism. However, the relatively recent of research interest in subtyping alcoholism according to age at onset, course, clinical characteristics, and comorbidity has not yet affected projects on the offspring of alcoholics to a great extent. This could also include the density of alcoholism in other first- and second-degree relatives. Furthermore, so far, most research has focused on children of alcoholic fathers; the impact of maternal alcoholism has been studied mainly in the context of fetal alcohol effects.

Other basic design issues discussed in the monograph by Sher (1991) include the insufficiently controlled effects of spousal psychopathology, the common lack of control groups, the problems of inclusion and exclusion criteria, the quality of matching procedures, the variation in age of the samples, and the sample sizes that might lead to both type 1 and type 2 errors of statistical analysis.

In conclusion, the following review of findings is plagued by a substantial list of potential methodological shortcomings of past and recent research, and in many instances the findings must therefore be regarded as tentative. The following sections on the findings begin with a brief summary of genetic influences and continue with a review of findings on the effects of prenatal exposure to alcohol. This is followed by a description of the family environment and the psychopathology found in children of alcoholic parents. A shorter section attempts to summarize the findings on the cognitive and neuropsychological functioning in children of alcoholics before the chapter closes with some general comments.

Genetic influences

It is quite clear from a large series of studies that alcohol use and abuse are genetically determined (for reviews see Searles 1988, Merikangas 1990, Sher 1991). The evidence of the familial transmission of alcoholism has been scientifically supported by family studies, twin studies, and adoption studies.

- *Family studies* indicate that there is an average seven-fold increase in the risk of children of alcoholism among the first degree relatives of children of alcoholics as compared to children of non-alcoholic parents. The relative risk of alcoholism is greater in male than in female relatives. This sex difference obviously cannot be attributed to transmissible genetic factors.

- Furthermore, *twin studies* based both on registries of normal twins or on pairs in which one member was identified through an alcoholism treatment program revealed that the concordance rates for monozygotic pairs are significantly higher than for dizygotic pairs.

- Finally, a series of *adoption studies* performed in Scandinavia (Goodwin *et al.* 1974, 1977, Bohman *et al.* 1981, Cloninger *et al.* 1981,1987) documented that there is a two-and-a-half times greater chance of an adoptee developing alcoholism—irrespective of exposure to the alcoholic parent—if a biological parent is alcoholic. In these studies two subtypes of alcoholism were delineated:

  - *Type I* is comprised of an equal number of males and females with onset after the age of 25 and is associated with anxiety and depression syndromes.

  - In contrast, *Type II* predominantly affects of men and is basically a heritable form with early onset heavy drinking and comorbid antisocial personality and criminality.

One may conclude from these family, twin, and adoption studies that a considerable proportion of the familial aggregation of alcoholism can be attributed to genetic factors. However, the specific inherited components of alcoholism are still unknown, and a critical analysis of the findings in the literature suggests that environmental influences in their interaction with the genetic transmission have been under emphasized in their potential as further significant factors (Searles 1988).

The effects of prenatal alcohol exposure

Studies on the effects of intrauterine exposure to alcohol were largely stimulated after Jones and Smith (1973) described a distinct pattern of abnormal morphogenesis and CNS dysfunction called *fetal alcohol syndrome* (FAS). The syndrome is characterized by craniofacial malformations, stunted growth, delayed psychomotor maturation, and impaired intellectual development. The incidence of FAS is estimated at 1–2 per 1000 live births (Abel and Sokol 1987). The less serious diagnosis of *fetal alcohol effects* (FAE) (Clarren and Smith 1978, Rosett 1980) is applied to patients exposed to alcohol *in utero* with some partial FAS phenotype and or CNS dysfunction. FAE is estimated to occur several times more often than FAS.

Since it was first described, FAS has been documented in a large series of clinical reports on individual children (for a review see Clarren and Smith 1978). In the recent past, most notably European groups in Germany (Steinhausen *et al.* 1982b, 1984, Spohr and Steinhausen 1987, Majewski and Majewski 1988, Spohr *et al.* 1993, Steinhausen *et al.* 1993, 1994) and Sweden (Aronson *et al.* 1985), and also the Seattle group in the US (Streissguth 1992), reported on larger series of patients.

All these studies show that FAS is associated with an extremely high rate of mental retardation and borderline intelligence. This was known even before children suffering from FAS were systematically studied. For instance, Hagberg *et al.* (1981) found alcohol fetopathy in 8% of an unselected series of 91 Swedish schoolchildren with mild mental retardation. Majewski and Majewski (1988) described 83% of a series of 175 children with FAS of varying ages, including about 50 school aged children, as being mentally retarded. In our Berlin follow-up study of 158 children, including 70 school aged children, we found that 34% of the patients had borderline intelligence and 31% were mentally retarded. In the Swedish series from

Gothenburg, one half of the children had borderline or retarded mental development and, in general, they had significantly lower mental abilities than their mothers (Aronson *et al.* 1985). Finally, in the first major report on adolescents and adults with FAS the Seattle group (Streissguth *et al.* 1991) found that a little more than half of the patients were mentally retarded.

With regard to the behavioral features of FAS, early reports always stressed the delayed development and a high frequency of hyperkinetic disorders in the afflicted children (Steinhausen and Spohr 1986). Our own studies in Berlin were the first to systematically assess developmental history and psychopathology in these children. In addition to maternal and even paternal alcoholism, there was an increased rate of neonatal risk factors and indices of retarded development throughout infancy and the toddler period (Steinhausen *et al.* 1982a,b). Structured psychiatric assessment including FAS children and matched controls revealed that eating and sleeping problems, stereotypies, retarded speech and language development, hyperkinetic disorders, relationship problems, and emotional disorders were significantly more frequent in FAS children (Steinhausen *et al.* 1982a,b). It became evident that, in terms of dysmorphic features, the most severely damaged children were also the ones with the most marked psychiatric symptoms.

So far, the Berlin study also comprises the largest cohort with the most extended follow-up periods to have been analyzed. These studies revealed that in a 10-year follow-up the characteristic craniofacial malformations diminished with time, but microcephaly and, to a lesser degree, short stature and underweight (in boys) persisted. The outcome was less favorable in terms of psychopathology and intelligence (Spohr *et al.* 1993, Steinhausen *et al.* 1993, 1994). After extended follow-up periods, extending into late adolescence in some cases, hyperkinetic disorders, emotional disorders, sleep disorders, and abnormal habits and stereotypies persisted over time. Even in the longitudinal perspective, the severe morphological damage was correlated with a high number of psychiatric symptoms and greater impairment of intelligence. There was no indication in the Berlin study that either postnatal milieu or remedial therapy contributed to the outcome.

FAS certainly represents the most deleterious effects of intrauterine exposure to alcohol. It results from chronic maternal alcoholism and persistent and relatively high doses of alcohol during pregnancy. However, there are also long-term consequences of prenatal exposure to lower levels of alcohol. They have been analyzed in various studies, most notably in the Seattle Longitudinal Prospective Study on Alcohol and Pregnancy (for reviews see Forrest *et al.* 1992, Streissguth 1992) and the Detroit Studies (Jacobson *et al.* 1993).

The Seattle study on so-called 'social drinkers' is based on a cohort of approximately 500 children who were examined at various ages and whose mothers were interviewed during pregnancy regarding alcohol and other drug use. Adverse effects of alcohol consumption during pregnancy were shown on various levels. In neonates it was manifested by poor newborn learning and behaviors, decreased sucking pressure, poor habituation, and low arousal. During infancy the signs were poor mental and motor development. At preschool age the indictors were poor attention, slower reaction time, and a decrement of 5 IQ points in children of mothers drinking more than 250 g alcohol per week. At the age of 7 years the adverse effects were still apparent in terms of poor attention, distractibility, slower reaction time, poor performance in further neurobehavioral tests, and a decrement of 7 IQ points when the mother drank more than 165 g alcohol per week. A recent further follow-up assessment of this cohort indicates that, even at the age of 14 years, prenatal alcohol exposure was significantly related to deficits in attention and memory in a dose-dependent fashion (Steissguth *et al.* 1994).

Both the Seattle and the Detroit studies addressed the issue of thresholds for specific areas of function, which are likely to vary in their sensitivity to different toxic agents. In the Detroit study the threshold for gross motor development at 13 months was established as 28 standard drinks per week, whereas it was only 7 standard drinks only for cognition, fine motor coordination, and language skills (Jacobson *et al.* 1993). The Seattle study revealed threshold effects on IQ at 4 years at 21 standard drinks per week, whereas it was only 14 drinks at 7 years; the discrepancy is presumably due to the superior reliability of the test at the older age (Streissguth *et al.* 1989, 1990). Obviously, neurobehavioral threshold values depend on both the sensitivity and the reliability of the testing instruments.

Although neonatal problems as a consequence of prenatal alcohol exposure were universally observed in other studies, the evidence for adverse effects beyond the neonatal stage is less convincing, as indicated by a recent analysis of the literature by Forrest *et al.* (1992). Based on this critique, and with the aim of studying the dose–response curve at high consumption levels, a collaborative European study with 9 participating centers, including more than 8400 subjects, recently studied the relation between maternal alcohol consumption and pregnancy outcome. This study showed an association between infant's body size and maternal alcohol consumption at levels of about 140 g per week (i.e. 14 standard drinks) or more, either before or in early pregnancy. From this study it was recommended that women should abstain from drinking alcoholic beverages during pregnancy. If this is not possible because of social pressures, pregnant women should not drink more than one standard drink a day (Euromac Project Group 1992). The study, however, was limited to body size parameters only.

In addition to the study of the effects of prenatal exposure to alcohol, the question as to the confounding effects of cigarettes or other drugs has been raised, because many alcoholics also abuse these substances. However, the issue of disentangling these various effects is very complicated. Various studies have concluded that exposure to nicotine during pregnancy is associated with deficits in physical growth, neurological functioning, cognitive development, school achievement, and even behavioral adjustment (Naeye 1992, Tong and McMichael 1992, Olds *et al.* 1994). However, exposure to nicotine is not associated with any dysmorphic syndrome, and the cognitive and behavioral abnormalities are only slight.

Interestingly, the effects of illegal street drugs are also remarkably different from alcohol insofar as there are no clear teratogenic effects leading to a distinct dysmorphic syndrome. Perinatal problems such as prematurity or small size for gestational age are quite common in the offspring, and certain drugs lead to withdrawal symptoms in the newborn. However, the effects on cognitive and behavioral functioning are again only slight. There is no knowledge of the long-term development of these children (see Chapter 5, Neuspiel and Hamel 1991, Zuckerman and Bresnahan 1992, Brooks-Gunn *et al.* 1994).

From an impressive amount of research it has to be concluded that maternal alcoholism during pregnancy has devastating effects on child development. The affected children continue to manifest developmental disabilities, psychiatric disorders, and cognitive impairment as they mature. The more severely they are affected morphologically, the more they suffer from impaired development. Their attentional and cognitive deficits render them vulnerable for learning difficulties and poor school careers. Their psychiatric problems and deficits in adaptive behavior impose specific burdens on their care-givers and high costs on the community at large.

In contrast to these consequences of maternal alcoholism, the issue of the effects of maternal social drinking during pregnancy is less clear. Nevertheless there is no doubt that there are adverse effects on the neonate, so drinking alcohol during pregnancy should be avoided.

The family environment with an alcoholic parent

Etiological studies of genetic and environmental factors in the development of alcoholism and other psychiatric morbidity clearly indicate that psychosocial determinants are operative. However, the specific environmental variables that may contribute to alcoholism and other psychopathology still have to be identified by further research. It must also be borne in mind that certain characteristics of the home environment of the alcoholic parent do not necessarily imply causality in the development of disorders in the children. With this caveat in mind, the following description of the family environment of alcoholic parents addresses the most salient features that create further risk factors for the developing child.

The assumption of a strong relation between family violence and parental alcoholism is derived from clinical experience. However, the empirical evidence is less convincing because studies suffer from a number of methodological shortcomings pertaining to the ascertainment of violence and alcohol abuse, the sampling procedures, and the lack of adequate controls. From these studies it appears that the relation between alcoholism and spouse abuse is stronger than the relation to child abuse, including sexual abuse, and that this relation is stronger for the lower social class (Sher 1991, 1992).

Family interactions in alcoholic families were assessed in a large series of studies using self-reports or behavioral observations. Reviews of these approaches (Jacob and Seilhamer 1987, Sher 1991, 1992) indicate that alcoholic families are characterized by higher levels of conflict and lower levels of cohesion, impaired problem-solving, and more negative and hostile communications relative to non-alcoholic families. However, one should also not overlook that there is a great deal of heterogeneity in the interaction patterns among alcoholic families and that disturbed family interaction is not specific to these families. Furthermore, it is difficult to generalize from these laboratory studies using volunteers to the community where the comorbidity is higher and the rate of intact nuclear families is expected to be lower.

Unfortunately, most of the research on family interaction in alcoholic families has, so far, not analyzed the relation between family characteristics and offspring adjustment. From the limited knowledge, it seems that relapse of alcoholism (particularly in fathers), the ongoing stress due to a drinking parent, and the severity of the alcoholism are crucial variables that are related to problems of adjustment in children.

Finally, it has to be assumed that modeling of parents' drinking could, in principle, represent an important factor of causality for at least some alcoholics. Parental alcohol use has been proved to be an important correlate of alcohol use in adolescence (Sher 1991).

In conclusion, there is some evidence that certain families with an alcoholic parent are marked by a negative milieu with adverse effects on the family members. However, one has to conclude that most of these effects are characteristic for the periods of active alcoholism. Recovering alcoholics do not have the same effects on family life. Active alcoholism leads to disturbed family interaction patterns that are also found in other kinds of parental psychopathology.

Psychopathology in the offspring of alcoholic parents

Various reviews have recently summarized the current knowledge on the association of parental alcoholism with a wide range of behavioral problems and psychopathology in the offspring. (Earls 1987, West and Prinz 1987, von Knorring 1991, Sher 1991, 1992). The offspring are at risk for the development of a variety of disorders, although only a minority of all children of alcoholic parents are affected and such outcomes are not specific to this group of children. These disorders do not necessarily have to progress to adult manifestations of psychiatric disorders. Furthermore, little is known about protective factors that might explain why the majority of children of alcoholic parents do not develop psychiatric disorders. According to findings from the Kauai study, the offspring of alcoholics who did not develop any serious coping problems in childhood and adolescence were characterized by temperamental features that elicited positive attention from primary care-givers, higher intelligence and communication skills, achievement orientation, a responsible and caring attitude, a positive self-concept, a more internal locus of control, and a belief in self-help (Werner 1986).

A study by Curran and Chassin (1996) examined whether maternal parenting behavior might serve to buffer a child from the potentially negative effects associated with paternal alcoholism. The study was based on a community sample and matched control group and tested the hypothesis in both cross-sectional and longitudinal analyses. Whereas the cross-sectional approach produced only limited support for the buffering hypothesis, there was no support from the longitudinal analysis.

Certain disorders are most likely to be associated with parental alcoholism. These types of psychopathology will be considered in the following sections: they include conduct disorders and delinquency, hyperkinetic disorders, substance abuse, anxiety and depression, and somatic problems.

Conduct disorders and delinquency

A considerable number of studies have found a strong relation between parental alcoholism and conduct disorders, especially in sons (Rydelius 1981, Steinhausen *et al.* 1984, Earls *et al.* 1988, Reich *et al.* 1993). However, the parental disharmony and the environmental disruption caused by parental alcoholism may be more influential than any direct influence of alcoholism. Similarly, adolescent delinquency in the children of alcoholics is more closely related to family discord (West and Prinz 1987). In addition, there is a better chance that delinquent acts in these subjects are detected because of greater awareness of various social agencies supervising families with an alcoholic parent (Rydelius 1981).

Hyperkinetic disorder

Early family studies of hyperkinetic children showed a higher prevalence of alcoholic and sociopathic fathers in the respective pedigrees, and a genetic relation was postulated (for review see Cantwell 1976). However, findings from more recent studies have been mixed. When studies began with alcoholic parents and then assessed the children, some association with hyperactivity was found. In contrast, this association did not emerge in studies in which the index sample consisted of hyperkinetic children (West and Prinz 1987). None of the studies obtaining a positive association has controlled for prenatal exposure to alcohol and its strong association with hyperactivity. Furthermore, the lack of differentiation between hyperkinetic disorders prevents clear conclusions. Several studies indicate that the association of conduct disorder with parental alcoholism is stronger than that of hyperkinetic disorders (Steinhausen *et al.* 1984, Knop *et al.* 1985, Merikangas *et al.* 1985).

Substance abuse

The relation between parental alcoholism and alcohol abuse in adolescents has been documented in various studies (e.g. Rydelius 1983, Merikangas *et al.* 1985) but has not been confirmed in others (Knop *et al.* 1985, Johnson *et al.* 1989). In contrast, one study revealed that children of alcoholic parents were more likely to report abuse of various other substances, i.e. cannabis, speed, and cocaine (Johnson *et al.* 1989). In a recent study, Reich *et al.* (1993) also reported a higher use of alcohol and other substances but no abuse or dependence.

Emotional disorders

There is also sufficient evidence from various studies to indicate that children of alcoholic parents suffer from an increased rate of emotional disorders and symptoms (for reviews see West and Prinz 1987, von Knorring 1991). Only a few studies have gone beyond the level of reporting a variety of emotional problems and have assessed the prevalence of emotional disorders as defined by the major international classification schemes. Accordingly, the most recent study reported an increased rate of over anxious disorders, as defined by DSM-III criteria, in the offspring of alcoholics, whereas the rate of depression did not differ from that of controls (Reich *et al.* 1993). In another study Steinhausen *et al.* (1984) found that 67% of the children with alcoholic mothers had an emotional disorder according to ICD-9. The rate was 59% in children with two alcoholic parents and only 31% in the children with alcoholic fathers.

However, as in previously described psychopathology, one should caution against attributing emotional disorders in the offspring directly or entirely to parental alcoholism. Psychiatric comorbidity in the parents, disharmony in the family, and other environmental stress factors certainly have a confounding effect on the development of anxiety, depression, and further emotional problems in the offspring.

Somatic and other problems

The physical health status in children of alcoholic parents has received only limited interest in research. Although Moos and Billings (1982) found only a trend for children of relapsed alcoholics to have a higher number of physical problems, there are several studies reporting a significant relation between impaired child physical health and parental alcoholism. In the study by Roberts and Brent (1982), female subjects had significantly higher physician utilization rates and diagnoses than matched controls. Steinhausen *et al.* (1982a) found higher rates of outpatient therapy, eating problems, headaches, and sleeping problems in children of alcoholics when compared to children of epileptic or of healthy mothers, respectively.

In the study by Biek (1981), which used a predominantly female sample, adolescent medical clinic outpatients with a problem-drinking parent were found to have nearly twice as many somatic complaints and health concerns as those without a problem-drinking parent. Significantly higher prevalence rates of eating-disordered symptoms were found in another study on female adolescents of parents who misused alcohol (Chandy *et al.* 1995). Again, none of these studies report on further family stressors that may play a role in the development of physical symptoms.

Cognitive and neuropsychological functioning in the offspring

Lower IQ scores for children of alcoholics than for controls were reported in various studies (reviewed by West and Prinz 1987). However, the majority of these studies were undertaken to analyze the effects of prenatal exposure to alcohol, whereas others did not control for these effects. Unfortunately, this lack of control for prenatal exposure to alcohol also applies to a recent longitudinal, controlled population-based study in which children of alcoholic parents had poorer mental development up to the end of their fourth year of life (Nordberg *et al.* 1993). In other samples, there is less evidence of impaired intelligence. When Johnson and Rolf (1988) studied children of recovering alcoholics from a non-disadvantaged background, they did not find statistically significant differences in intelligence. Similarly, Tarter *et al.* (1984) did not reveal differences in intelligence when they studied the adolescent sons of alcoholic fathers and matched controls. One may hypothesize that the neurotoxic effect of alcohol in prenatal life is the critical variable for any impairment of intelligence.

The study of further cognitive and neuropsychological functioning has also been the aim of various studies. As reviewed by Sher (1992), there is evidence that children of alcoholics have poorer verbal ability than controls, although the performance is within normal limits and the deficit is only relative. Studies for a similar deficit in visuospatial abilities are less consistent, whereas learning and memory are not affected. Besides verbal ability, abstraction and conceptual reasoning are other areas in which deficits in children of alcoholics were detected. These deficits may contribute to school failure and, consequently, to an impairment in self-esteem and problems in behavior and adaptation as well. In fact, several studies have shown that academic performance and school careers are more frequently negatively affected in children of alcoholic parents than in controls (for reviews see West and Prinz 1987, Sher 1992). However, the complex net of interactions between neuropsychological deficits, school failure, and behavioral problems in these children at risk has not been sufficiently disentangled.

Concluding comments

There are clearly a number of inconsistencies resulting from the heterogeneity of the studies, and the various methodological shortcomings outlined earlier in the chapter. However, there is abundant evidence that children of alcoholic parents are children at risk. A large series of studies originating from the new field of behavioral teratology has convincingly shown that prenatal exposure to alcohol has devastating effects on development. Fortunately, this is also an area of research in which the consequences in terms of prevention and intervention in the fields of medical policy and practice are easy to delineate. This is far more difficult for our current understanding of the findings coming from genetic research. Although there is no doubt that a significant proportion of the familial aggregation of alcoholism can be attributed to genetic factors, the specific components of alcoholism that may be inherited and the mechanisms for the transmission of alcoholism have yet to be identified. Thus, consequences for prevention are more difficult to delineate.

With regard to the environmental risks for the development of the offspring of alcoholic parents, it is far more complicated to derive similar action-oriented conclusions from a complex field of research. Here we are confronted with a large body of both knowledge and ignorance. As previous reviews of the field have stated, there is considerable evidence that parental alcoholism is disruptive to family life and that a large proportion of children of alcoholic parents suffer from externalizing or internalizing types of psychiatric disorder. However, as concluded by West and Prinz (1987) in their excellent review, we need to find out more about the individual differences and the impact of the developmental level and gender of the offspring of alcoholic parents. As in other fields of research in child psychopathology, comorbidity of disorders and specificity of disorders are largely neglected topics in the study of children of alcoholics. Similarly, a widely ignored area of research concerns the resiliency found in a large number of children who manage to cope positively, despite apparent distress from the environment.

Unfortunately, most of the research literature has so far ignored the fact that in a considerable number of families both parents are alcoholics. This may have potentiating adverse effects in terms of an extremely disorganized milieu with an increase of risk factors to the child. Besides the obvious environmental deficits in terms of negligent and abusive or violent rearing, in these families an interaction with further biological risk factors operates. The latter include the consequences of maternal ingestion of alcohol during pregnancy and may also be hypothetically extended to damage to paternal germ cells or gonads from alcohol with still unknown consequences to the child.

Currently, the most complicated issue for research in this area of studies on the children of alcoholics is the inference of causal pathways. Both mediating and moderating (buffering) factors have to be assumed and deserve carefully designed investigations. Mediating factors pertaining to the family (e.g. disrupted family interactions or marital discord) or characterizing the sick parents (e.g. severity of the alcoholism or sex-specific drinking patterns) still have to be isolated when studying the development and outcome of children of alcoholic parents. Similarly, the potential moderating effects of social class, family life, social support, personality features, and other individual characteristics deserve further investigation. Scientific progress in the understanding of these complex issues will certainly contribute to interventions aimed at reducing the various risks that children of alcoholic parents are exposed to.

Acknowledgment

This chapter is in part a revised version of an earlier review by the author on the same topic (Steinhausen 1995).

References

Abel, E.L. and Sokol, R.J. (1987). Incidence of the fetal alcohol syndrome and economic impact of FAS-related anomalies. *Drug and Alcohol Dependancy*, **19**, 51–70.

Aronson, M., Kyllerman, M., Sabel, K.G., Sandin, B., and Olegard, R. (1985). Children of alcoholic mothers. Developmental, perceptual and behavioural characteristics in children of alcoholic mothers compared to matched controls. *Acta Paediatrica Scandinavica*, **74**, 27–33.

Biek, J. (1981). Screening test for identifying adolescents adversely affected by a parental drinking problem. *Journal of Adolescent Health Care*, **2**, 107–113.

Bohman, M., Sigvardsson, S., and Cloninger, C.R. (1981). Maternal inheritance of alcohol abuse. Cross-fostering analysis of adopted women. *Archives of General Psychiatry*, **38**, 965–969.

Bohman, M., Cloninger, R., Sigvardsson, S., and von Knorring, A-L. (1987). The genetics of alcoholism and related disorders. *Journal of Psychiatric Research*, **21**, 447–452.

Brooks-Gunn, J., McCarton, C., and Hawley, T. (1994). Effects of in utero drug exposure on children's development—Review and recommendations. *Archives of Pediatrics and Adolescent Medicine*, **148**, 33–60.

Cantwell, D.P. (1976). Genetic factors in the hyperkinetic syndrome. *Journal of the American Academy of Child Psychiatry*, **15**, 214–223.

Chandy, J.M., Harris, L., Blum, R.W., and Resnick, M.D. (1995). Female adolescents of alcohol misusers: Disordered eating features. *International Journal of Eating Disorders*, **17**, 2833–2839.

Clarren, S.K. and Smith, D.W. (1978). The fetal alcohol syndrome. *New England Journal of Medicine*, **298**, 1036–1037.

Cloninger, C.R., Bohman, M., and Sigvardsson, S. (1981). Inheritance of alcohol abuse—cross-fostering analysis of adopted men. *Archives of General Psychiatry*, **38**, 861–868.

Curran, P.J. and Chassin, L. (1996). A longitudinal study of parenting as a protective factor for children of alcoholics. *Journal of Studies on Alcohol*, **57**, 305–313.

Earls, F. (1987). On the familial transmission of child psychiatric disorder. *Journal of Child Psychology and Psychiatry and Allied Disciplines*, **28**, 791–802.

Earls, F., Reich, W., Yound, K.G., and Cloninger, C.R. (1988). Psychopathology in children of alcoholic and antisocial parents. *Alcoholism: Clinical and Experimental Research*, **12**, 481–487.

Euromac Project Group (1992). The Euromac Project Group. Euromec: Maternal alcohol consumption and its relation to the outcome of pregnancy and development at 18 months. *International Journal of Epidemiology* **21** (Suppl. 1), ed. C.d.V. Florey, F. Bolumar, M. Kaminski, and J. Olsen).

Forrest, F., Florey, C.d.V., and Taylor, D. (1992). Maternal alcohol consumption and child development. *International Journal of Epidemiology* **21** (Suppl. 1), ed. C.d.V. Florey, F. Bolumar, M. Kaminski, and J. Olsen), pp. 17–23.

Goodwin, D.W., Schulsinger, F., Møller, N., Hermansen, L., Winokur, G., and Guze, S.B. (1974). Psychopathology in adopted and nonadopted sons of alcoholics. *Archives of General Psychiatry*, **31**, 164–169.

Goodwin, D.W., Schulsinger, F., Knop, J., Mednick, S., and Guze, S.B. (1977). Psychopathology in adopted and nonadopted daughters of alcoholics. *Archives of General Psychiatry*, **34**, 1005–1009.

Hagberg, B., Hagberg, G., Lewerth, A., and Lindberg, U. (1981). Mild mental retardation in Swedish school children. *Acta Psychiatrica Scandinavica*, **70**, 445–452.

Jacob, T. and Seilhamer, R.A. (1987). Alcoholism and family interaction. In *Family interaction and psychopathology: Theories, methods and findings*, ed. T. Jacob, pp. 535–580. Plenum, New York.

Jacobson, J.L., Jacobson, S.W., Sokol, R.J., Martier, S.S., Ager, J.W., and Kaplan-Estrin, M.G. (1993). Teratogenic effects of alcohol on infant development. *Alcoholism: Clinical and Experimental Research*, **17**, 174–183.

Johnson, J.L. and Rolf, J.E. (1988). Cognitive functioning in children from alcoholic and non-alcoholic families. *British Journal of Addiction*, **83**, 849.

Johnson, S., Leonard, K.E., and Jacob, T. (1989). Drinking, drinking styles, and drug use in children of alcoholics, depressives, and controls. *Journal of Studies on Alcohol*, **50**, 427–431.

Jones, K.L. and Smith, D.W. (1973). Recognition of the fetal alcohol syndrome in early infancy. *Lancet*, **2**, 999–1001.

Knop, J., Teasdale, T.W., Schulsinger, F., and Goodwin, D.W. (1985). A prospective study of young men at high risk for alcoholism: School behavior and achievement. *Journal of Studies on Alcohol*, **46**, 273–278.

Majewski, F., and Majewski, B. (1988). Alcohol embryopathy: Symptoms, auxiological data, frequency among the offspring and pathogenesis. *Excerpta Medica, International Conference Series* **805**, 837–844.

Merikangas, K.R. (1990). The genetic epidemiology of alcoholism. *Psychological Medicine*, **20**, 11–22.

Merikangas, K.R., Weissman, M.M., Prusoff, B.A., Pauls, D.L., and Leckman, J.F. (1985). Depressives with secondary alcoholism—psychiatric disorders in offspring. *Journal of Studies of Alcohol*, **46**, 199–204.

Moos, R.H. and Billings, A.G. (1982). Children of alcoholics during the recovery process: Alcoholic and matched control families. *Addictive Behaviors*, **7**, 155–163.

Naeye, R.L. (1992). Commentary. Cognitive and behavioral abnormalities in children whose mothers smoked cigarettes during pregnancy. *Developmental and Behavioral Pediatrics*, **13**, 425–428.

Neuspiel, D.R. and Hamel, S.C. (1991). Cocaine and infant behavior. *Journal of Developmental and Behavioral Pediatrics*, **12**, 55–64.

Nordberg, L., Rydelius, P.A., and Zetterstöm, R. (1993). Children of alcoholic parents: Health, growth, mental development and psychopathology until school age. *Acta Pediatrica*, **82** (Suppl. 387), 1–25.

Olds, D.L., Henderson, C.R., and Tatelbaum, R. (1994). Intellectual impairment in children of women who smoke cigarettes during pregnancy. *Pediatrics*, **93**, 221–227.

Reich, W., Earls, F., Frankel, O., and Shayka, J.J. (1993). Psychopathology in children of alcoholics. *Journal of the American Academy of Adolescent Psychiatry*, **32**, 995–1002.

Roberts, K., and Brent, E. (1982). Physician utilization and illness patterns in families of alcoholics. *Journal of Studies of Alcohol*, **43**, 119–128.

Rosett, H.L. (1980). A clinical perspective of the fetal alcohol syndrome. *Alcoholism: Clinical and Experimental Research*, **4**, 119–122.

Rydelius, P-A. (1981). Children of alcoholic fathers. Their social adjustment and their mental status over 20 years. *Acta Paediatrica Scandinavica*, Suppl. 286, 1–89.

Rydelius, P-A. (1983). Alcohol-abusing teenage boys—testing a hypothesis on the relationship between alcohol abuse and social background factors, criminality and personality in teenage boys. *Acta Psychiatrica Scandinavica*, **68**, 368–380.

Searles, J.S. (1988). The role of genetics in the pathogenesis of alcoholism. *Journal of Abnormal Psychology*, **97**, 153–167.

Sher, K. (1991). *Children of alcoholics*. University of Chicago Press, Chicago.

Sher, K.J. (1992). Psychological characteristics of children of alcoholics—Overview of research methods and findings. In *Recent developments in alcoholism* Vol. 9, ed. M. Gallanter, pp. 301–326. Plenum, New York.

Spohr, H-L. and Steinhausen, H-C. (1987). Follow-up studies of children with fetal alcohol syndrome. *Neuropediatrics*, **18**, 13–17.

Spohr, H-L., Willms, J., and Steinhausen, H-C. (1993). Prenatal alcohol exposure and long-term developmental consequences. *Lancet*, **341**, 907–910.

Steinhausen, H-C. (1995). Children of alcoholic parents. *European Child and Adolescent Psychiatry*, **4**, 143–52.

Steinhausen, H-C. and Spohr, H-L. (1986). Fetal alcohol syndrome. In *Advances in clinical child psychology* Vol. 9, eds. B.B. Lahey and A.E. Kazdin. Plenum, New York.

Steinhausen, H-C., Göbel, D., Nestler, V., and Huth, H. (1982a). Psychopathology and mental functions in the offspring of alcoholic and epileptic mothers. *Journal of the American Academy of Child Psychiatry*, **21**, 268–273.

Steinhausen, H-C., Nestler, V., and Spohr, H-L. (1982b). Development and psychopathology of children with fetal alchohol syndrome. *Journal of Developmental Behavioral Pediatrics*, **3**, 49–54.

Steinhausen, H-C., Göbel, D., and Nestler, V. (1984). Psychopathology in the offspring of alcoholic parents. *Journal of the American Academy of Child Psychiatry*, **23**, 465–471.

Steinhausen, H-C., Willms, J., and Spohr, H-L. (1993). Long-term psychopathological and cognitive outcome of children with fetal alcohol syndrome. *Journal of the American Academy of Child and Adolescent Psychiatry*, **32**, 990–994.

Steinhausen, H-C., Willms, J., and Spohr, H-L. (1994). Correlates of psychopathology and cognitive outcome of children with fetal alcohol syndrome. *Journal Child Psychology and Psychiatry*, **35**, 323–331.

Steissguth, P.P., Sampson, P.D., Olson, H.C., Bookstein, F.L., Barr, H.M., Scott, M., Feldman, J., and Mirsky, A.F. (1994). Maternal drinking during pregnancy: Attention and short-term memory in 14-year-old offspring: A longitudinal prospective study. *Alcoholism: Clinical and Experimental Research*, **18**, 202–218.

Streissguth, A.P. (1992). Fetal alcohol syndrome and fetal alcohol effects. In *Maternal substance abuse and the developing nervous system*, ed. I.S. Zagon and T.A. Slotkin, pp. 5–24, Academic Press, San Diego, C.A.

Streissguth, A.P., Barr, H.M., Sampson, P.D., Darby, B.L., and Martin, D.C. (1989). IQ at age 4 in relation to maternal alcohol use and smoking during pregnancy. *Developmental Psychology*, **25**, 3–11.

Streissguth, A.P., Barr, H.M., and Sampson, P.D. (1990). Moderate prenatal alcohol exposure: Effects on child IQ and learning problems at age 7½ years. *Alcoholism: Clinical and Experimental Research*, **14**, 662–69.

Streissguth, A.P., Aase, J.M., Clarren, S.K., Randels, S.P., La Due, R.A., and Smith, D.F. (1991). Fetal alcohol syndrome in adolescents and adults. *Journal of the American Medical Association*, **265**, 1961–1967.

Tarter, R.E., Hegedus, A.M., Goldstein, G., and Shelly, C. (1984). Adolescent sons of alcoholics: neuropsychological and personality characteristics. *Alcoholism: Clinical and Experimental Research*, **8**, 216–222.

Tong, S. and McMichael, A.J. (1992). Maternal smoking and neuropsycological development in childhood: A review of the evidence. *Developmental Medicine and Child Neurology*, **34**, 191–197.

von Knorring, A-L. (1991). Annotation: Children of alcoholics. *Journal of Child Psychology and Psychiatry*, **32**, 411–421.

Werner, E.E. (1986). Resilient offspring of alcoholics—A longitudinal study from birth to age 18. *Journal of Studies on Alcohol*, **47**, 34–40.

West, M.O. and Prinz, R.J. (1987). Parental alcoholism and childhood psychopathology. *Psychological Bulletin*, **102**, 204–218.

Zuckerman, B., and Bresnahan, K. (1992). Developmental and behavioural consequences of prenatal drug and alcohol exposure. *Pediatric Clinics of North America*, **38**, 1387–1406.

5 Children of drug-addicted parents

Anneloes L. van Baar

Children of drug-addicted parents (CDAP) are at risk for developmental problems, including psychopathology. Most drug-addicted parents use cocaine, heroin, or methadone, and other drugs such as tranquillizers or amphetamines. Some parents also smoke marijuana and almost all are heavy cigarette smokers. Some also take alcohol regularly, although apparently this is not a popular combination (van Baar 1991). For the children of these drug-addicted parents, biological as well as social risk factors are important.

Risk factors

Biological risk factors

The biological risk factors for CDAP consist of direct drug-related factors, such as prenatal drug exposure and its concomitant withdrawal period, as well as perinatal problems and genetic dispositions.

The development of the fetus may be affected by prenatal drug exposure. The effect depends upon variations in maternal drug abuse, in amounts and frequency of use, and also in combinations and way of use. Also important are individual differences in metabolic processes, affected by the mothers' habits and history of drug abuse, amount of cigarettes smoked, regularity of eating and sleeping, and maternal health in general. The effect of prenatal drug exposure could also vary with the developmental phase of the fetus, as reflected in the three trimesters of pregnancy.

The neonatal abstinence syndrome (NAS) in infants prenatally exposed to heroin and methadone clearly shows that the fetus has been affected by the drugs the mother has used. Of these infants, 60–95% show abstinence symptoms such as tremors, sleeping problems, high-pitched crying, hyperactivity, feeding and respiratory problems, yawning, sneezing, and sweating (Finnegan 1980). Newborn babies of mothers who used mainly cocaine and no opioids during pregnancy do not consistently show signs of withdrawal and do not need pharmaceutical treatment (Singer *et al.* 1993). However, Tronick *et al.* (1996) have reported on dose–response relationships reflecting higher neurobehavioural risk in heavier exposed infants, who show poorer motor capacities and state regulation, lesser autonomic stability, and greater excitability on the Neonatal Behavioral Assessment Scale (NBAS; Brazelton 1984).

Studies on pregnancy outcomes of CDAP report higher rates of prematurity, intra-uterine growth retardation, low birthweight, small head circumference, and perinatal complications besides NAS (Householder *et al.* 1982, Deren 1986, Miller 1996). One study described some specific facial characteristics in cocaine-exposed infants (Fries *et al.* 1993).

Genetic factors may also increase the risk of CDAP, such that these children are even at risk for later substance abuse problems themselves. Genetic factors are, for instance, important for expression of attention deficit hyperactivity disorder (ADHD) symptoms, especially in socioeconomically disadvantaged environments (Biederman *et al.* 1995). Children with ADHD have been found to be five times more likely to have an ongoing drug abuse disorder at adult follow-up (Manuzza *et al.* 1993).

Social risk factors

It is possible that CDAP are not seriously affected by biological risk factors at birth and do not develop NAS, or fully recover from it. For some CDAP the biological risk factors are less important, as their parents became drug-addicted after their birth. Probably all of these children still have to cope with the social risk factors involved in these families. The social risk factors for CDAP result from the socioeconomic situation and social problems of the addicted parents and their specific lifestyle or from a transition to foster parents or other care-givers.

Financial difficulties, and problems regarding housing and contact with partners, family, and friends, are common among drug users. They have also been found to hold less conventional values than non-users, which can be expected to influence all areas of their lives, including child rearing (Kandel 1990). Drug-addicted women often have to work as prostitutes or resort to illegal and criminal activities to get the drugs they need in order to prevent their own withdrawal and illness. The physical and psychological wellbeing of a pregnant addicted woman is stressed by many non-optimal circumstances besides her drug dependency. After the delivery these drug-dependent mothers have to cope with their usual problems as well as guilt concerning, for example, their infant's illness due to withdrawal problems (Rosenbaum 1979). The lifestyle of the parents may contribute to an intergenerational cycle of drug abuse, as discussed by Deren (1986) who emphasizes parental modelling. When the parents do not succeed in adequate care-giving, the infants are placed in children's homes, or with foster parents or members of the extended family of the parents, often after having stayed some time with their own parents.

The social risk factors in combination with the biological risk factors may have aggravated effects on the development of the children.

Paradigms and models

In studies on development of CDAP, paradigms and models have often remained implicit. Studies differ in the risk factors taken into consideration. Three different approaches can be distinguished concerning identification of chemical drug effects, family and social problems, or description of any developmental problem realizing the myriad of interrelated risk factors.

Emphasis on biological risk

First, studies have attempted to evaluate specific and direct effects on the fetus or infants of the substances used by the mothers. These studies tried to describe the prenatal exposure accurately, and were especially interested in the functioning of the infants. The social risk factors involved were considered to be confounding factors that needed to be controlled (Neuspiel 1994). More specific theories concerning prenatal exposure to cocaine have stated that it has vasoconstrictive effects on placental and fetal blood vessels, which may result in fetal hypoxemia and decreased nutrient transfer and consequently decreased fetal (brain) growth, which may have specific effects too, e.g. hyperexcitable or depressed behaviour (Lester *et al.* 1991). Cocaine may also affect the monoaminergic neurotransmitter system, which is involved in the regulation of arousal and attentional states (Mayes 1994).

Emphasis on social risk

Another approach has focused on the social risk factors and studied, for instance, the occurrence of maltreatment of children born to cocaine-dependent mothers (Wasserman and Leventhal 1993). The evaluation of (drug) treatment effects combined with a socioeducational program for the addicted parents also focused more on the postnatal mother–infant interaction and environment (Black *et al.* 1994). The comparison of subgroups of CDAP being reared by (one of) their own parents or reared by foster parents also fits into this category (Groeneweg and Lechner 1988).

Emphasis on interrelationship of biological and social risk

Finally, some studies have been based upon awareness of all different kinds of risk factors and the interrelationships between them. Our own Amsterdam study in the Netherlands was designed from a perspective on human development as based on multilevel, reciprocal functioning of systems evolving over time (van Baar 1991). In such a study assessments of different facets of development have to be carried out concurrently and repeatedly, in order to get an adequate impression of development. Potential causes of developmental problems are *a priori* considered to be multifactorially determined. As a matched control group can only be provided for a few of the many specific risk factors involved, it is considered inappropriate for determining the importance and weight of the different causal factors involved. The combination and interaction of drug addiction and social and biological risk factors may have different consequences for the development of the infants than such factors would have by themselves, or in combinations without drug abuse. Consequently 'comparison' groups or normative 'reference' groups are used in this area of research instead of 'control' groups. Studies using this approach have focused on identifying what kind of developmental problems are found in CDAP. In the Amsterdam study we used a reference group consisting of infants without specific risk factors, expected to show normal variation in development. Comparisons between CDAP and such a reference group can provide indications of specific developmental problems and processes in need of extra support, when significant group differences are found (van Baar 1991). Sometimes standardized measurements are used in comparing outcome of CDAP to population norms (e.g. Soepatmi 1994). Other authors have used a contrast comparison group that was characterized by other perinatal risk factors or other substances used during pregnancy (Rodning *et al.* 1989, Chassnof *et al.* 1992).

Subgroups

In order to study the consequences of a naturally occurring phenomenon such as drug abuse, it is essential that research follows what happens in 'real life'. Studies on infants of drug-addicted parents published in the 1970s and early 1980s originated mainly from the US and concerned prenatal exposure to heroin or methadone (Householder *et al.* 1982). During the 1980s, however, the main drug of abuse in the US became (crack) cocaine and there was a large increase in drug users. Prevalence rates of cocaine use during pregnancy vary from 8% to 45%, with the high rates applying to impoverished inner-city populations (Ostrea *et al.* 1992, Martin *et al.* 1996). In the US, children prenatally exposed to heroin and methadone have become a subgroup within the total population of CDAP. As a consequence, the focus of US studies on the development of infants of drug-addicted mothers changed to prenatal exposure to cocaine; many of the mothers did not use heroin or methadone (Barton *et al.* 1995). In Europe drug addicts are still mainly polydrug users, using cocaine as well as opioids. In our hospital in Amsterdam, with 1500 births per year, just 21 drug-addicted women abusing only cocaine were found from 1987 to 1994 (Smit *et al.* 1994). However, the number of heroin- and methadone-dependent women who also used cocaine during pregnancy showed an increase in the Netherlands too during the 1980s (van Baar *et al.* 1993).

The difference in patterns of drug addiction, and the resulting prenatal exposure, justifies a distinction between studies on development of CDAP mainly exposed to cocaine, and CDAP exposed to heroin, methadone, and cocaine. A third subgroup of CDAP that may need to be distinguished consists of children who were not prenatally exposed, as their mothers became addicted after their birth. However, not much research has yet been done on the development of this subgroup.

For the sake of clarity, results of follow-up studies on prenatal exposure to marijuana or amphetamines are excluded from this chapter, as are studies on drug-exposed infants who are also infected by the human immunodeficiency virus (HIV). With regard to marijuana use during pregnancy, in a low risk sample of 12 and 24 month old infants Fried and Watkinson (1988) found a lesser effect of maternal marijuana use during pregnancy relative to cigarette and (low level) alcohol use. In Sweden, where amphetamine addiction is prevalent, prenatal ampheta-mine exposure has been found to be related to increased aggressive behaviour and poor school performance up to 10 years of age (Eriksson and Zetterström 1994). Infants of intravenous drug users are especially at risk for HIV infection. Mellins *et al.* (1994) concluded that infants who are HIV infected and prenatally exposed to drugs performed considerably worse in terms of mental and motor functioning than infants who have only one of these risk factors.

Findings

As a result of all the risk factors involved, problems of CDAP may appear in every developmental domain, i.e. somatic development, neuromotor, cognitive, and socioemotional development, including psychopathology. Psychopathology may result from a genetic predisposition, disturbances of brain functioning, or an extreme learning history; probability for all these factors is increased for CDAP. So far very little research has been done on psychopathology in CDAP. This is partly dependent on the age of CDAP studied; the older they are, the less known of their development. Development of psychopathology, however, may already be seen in studies using interaction observations or behavioural ratings, providing indications of attachment behaviour and regulation of emotion (Zeanah *et al.* 1997). The findings in the domain of socioemotional development therefore form the core of this section, but other problems may also be important for a child's emotional well-being.

Somatic and neuromotor development

Several studies have been done on growth of CDAP, and health is mentioned in a few. The results are summarized briefly here.

Studies on growth of CDAP resulted in inconsistent findings. Some showed group differences in growth parameters (Wilson 1989, Hurt *et al.* 1995) in favour of the comparison groups, but not so much that it might affect self-perception of CDAP. In addition, CDAP (prenatally exposed to heroin or methadone) generally appeared to be healthy (Rosen and Johnson 1985, Soepatmi 1994). Therefore, in general, development of CDAP is not expected to be influenced by serious somatic problems.

Although some inconsistent findings have been reported, most studies did not show difficulties in gross motor development of CDAP (Rosen and Johnson 1985, van Baar 1991, Bender *et al.* 1995). Consequently, development of CDAP is not expected to be influenced by serious neuromotor problems.

Cognitive development

·As serious problems of CDAP have indeed been found in cognitive development, these results are reported more extensively for different subgroups.

Prenatal cocaine exposure

The Bayley mental scale (Bayley 1969) showed no group differences during the first 2½ years (Chasnoff *et al.* 1992, Hurt *et al.* 1995). Struthers and Hansen (1992) found that infants prenatally exposed to cocaine and/or amphetamine had lower scores in visual recognition memory at 8 months of age than their reference infants. Griffith *et al.* (1994) found that cocaine-exposed children had lower scores in verbal reasoning at 3 years than non-exposed children, but no differences in overall results on the intelligence test (mean = 94, SD = 9). However, Beckwith *et al.* (1995) report that children of mothers using phencyclidine (PCP) and cocaine showed more immature play behaviour at 24 months of age than their reference children. For 16 drug-exposed children at 3½–4½ years, they reported a low mean score (mean = 70, SD = 18) on the McCarthy general cognitive index (McCarthy 1972).

Language development turns out to be a vulnerable domain for these CDAP (Johnson *et al.* 1997). Specifically receptive language difficulties were found in children prenatally exposed to cocaine (Malakoff *et al.* 1994, Bender *et al.* 1995, Mentis and Lundgren 1995).

Prenatal heroin, methadone, and cocaine exposure

Rosen *et al.* (1985) and Chasnoff *et al.* (1986) found differences in mental development between CDAP and comparison infants, with means in the low normal range. Significant group differences are not found in all studies, reflecting the fact that the comparison group is from a deprived socioeconomic background (Strauss *et al.* 1979, Kaltenbach and Finnegan 1984, Lifschitz *et al.* 1985, Rosen and Johnson 1985). In the Amsterdam study following a group of CDAP and a reference group longitudinally with nine assessments of cognitive functioning during the first 5½ years, specifically difficulties in early language development were found (van Baar and de Graaff 1994). At 4½ and 5½ years, around 50% of the CDAP have low scores (> 1 SD below the norm) on an intelligence test. Language problems of CDAP are also mentioned by other researchers (Kaltenbach and Finnegan 1984, Rosen and Johnson 1985).

Rodning *et al.* (1989) and Metosky and Vondra (1995) studied play of CDAP at 18 months and reported that they showed fewer representational events during play (such as combing hair of a doll). The CDAP had lower scores in simple and elaborate pretend play, and in a total score of symbolic play, and they also had shorter periods of such play activities.

At school age de Cubas and Field (1993) found no difficulties in cognitive development in children of methadone-maintained mothers, but Wilson (1989) reports worrying results for heroin-exposed school age children (6–11 years), showing that 30% has repeated a grade.

No prenatal drug exposure, but addicted parent

For a sample of children between 6 and 14 years of age, Herjanic *et al.* (1979) reported that they did less well on a cognitive task than their opiate-addicted fathers. Davis and Templer (1988) reported that children who were not prenatally exposed, but whose mother lived with a narcotic-addicted partner, had a higher total and performance IQ and less difficulties in perceptual, motor, and attention realms, than children prenatally exposed to narcotics.

In summary, many prenatally exposed CDAP have difficulties in cognitive development, especially in symbolic and language development. Such problems may be related to difficulties in socioemotional development.

Socioemotional development and psychopathology

Studies on socioemotional development differ in their emphasis on the dynamic processes of interpersonal relationships or on outcome concerning socioemotional characteristics of the children. The presentation of these results is therefore grossly divided into data on early mother–infant interaction and attachment observations, and results of assessments of temperament, behaviour problems, and personality characteristics.

Prenatal cocaine exposure

Concerning parent–child interaction observations, Woods *et al.* (1996) reported that 32 mothers who used cocaine during pregnancy were less confident and had a lower quality of physical contact, when compared to 57 comparison dyads during a videotaped feeding in the first 4 days. No differences were seen between the infants, and their most striking finding was how few differences there were between the groups. Neuspiel *et al.* (1991) found no differences in maternal or infant interaction at 2–3 months postpartum between 51 cocaine users and 60 comparison dyads. Olson *et al.* (1996) reported on 100–126 chemically dependent women

(48% cocaine, 12% opioids) that one quarter showed at-risk teaching interactions with their infants at 4 months. A recent report on 47 non-users, 73 substance users (mainly cocaine) in drug treatment, and 20 mothers rejecting drug treatment, studied at 4, 9, 12, 18, and 24 months, showed slightly higher HOME scores (Home Observation and Measurement of the Environment; Caldwell and Bradley 1978) for the non-users and no differences on a mother–infant interaction scale. The HOME scores of all three groups compared favorably to the norm (Myers *et al.* 1996).

More serious socioemotional problems have also been seen. In a study of 38 mothers abusing PCP and cocaine, Beckwith *et al.* (1995) report on attachment assessments of the mothers and their children at 15 months of age. Only 7 (18%) showed secure attachment, and a high number (39%) showed avoidant attachment behaviour; 68% were found to show disorganized attachment. At 3 months the addicted mothers were found to be less responsive and at 9 months the exposed children were found to experience more rejection, neglect, interference, and insensitivity to communications, less response to distress, and had less physical contact. At 2 years deviant and immature behaviour during symbolic play was observed in these children, indicating vulnerability concerning social cognition. The study-group also made fewer positive social bids. At 3½–4½ years of age 13 drug-exposed and 4 comparison children were seen again, and this sample was supplemented with 3 additional drug-exposed subjects and 14 non-exposed comparison children. The drug-exposed children were more non-compliant and needed more assistance to complete the tasks, and they were more insensitive and inexperienced in playing with peers.

Wasserman and Leventhal (1993) studied the occurrence of maltreatment and placement in foster care or with a substitute care-giver over the first 2 years in 47 CDAP and 47 matched comparison children in an impoverished mainly African-American inner-city population. They found an incidence of 23% versus 4% of maltreatment and 20% versus 2% of changes in placement to the disadvantage of the CDAP. Barton *et al.* (1995) report frequent referrals to child protective agencies and high incidences of foster placements of CDAP.

With regard to temperament, behaviour problems and personality characteristics, the following results were found.

- Mayes *et al.* (1996) found impaired regulation of arousal, evidenced by more crying and showing more negative affect responding to novel stimulus presentation in 36 exposed compared to 27 non-exposed 3 month old infants.

- Less interest and arousal and reduced emotional responsivity was seen during contingency learning as well as lower activity levels and less emotional reactivity on the Infant Behavior Questionnaire (IBQ; Rothbart 1981) in 36 cocaine-exposed 4–8 month old infants, when compared to 36 non-exposed infants (Alessandri *et al.* 1995).

- Using a temperament questionnaire with 29 cocaine-exposed and 30 comparison infants at 6 months, Edmondson and Smith (1994) reported that the CDAP were less cooperative, more difficult to manage, and more arrhythmic, according to their mothers.

- Lewkowicz *et al.* (1996) found equal preference for infant-directed speech as opposed to adult-directed speech up to 6–7 months, but diminished preference at 10 months in 54–26 cocaine-exposed infants, differing in this from both 49–30 normal comparison children and 203–172 children with brain damage.

- Azuma and Chasnoff (1993) found no group differences with the Child Behavior Checklist (CBCL; Achenbach 1988) and in perseverance at a task at the age of 3 years between 92 children exposed to cocaine, 25 children exposed to multiple drugs but not cocaine, and 45 drug-free comparison children. Poor perseverance was related to lower IQ scores, small head circumference and to higher estimates of externalizing behaviour. Later they did report a difference on the CBCL, with the drug-exposed groups showing more externalizing problems than 25 drug-free comparisons (Griffith *et al.* 1994).

- Beckwith *et al.* (1995) found no group differences in parental temperament and behaviour problem ratings at preschool age. During play with peers the exposed children were more often to be assessed as intrusive.

- Anecdotal reports of teachers of school-age children suggested that cocaine-exposed children exhibit many of the behaviours of attention deficit hyperactivity disorder (ADHD), and that they tend to be mean and have little empathy and remorse or awareness of repercussions of their aggressive behaviour (Field 1995). She therefore compared 18 CDAP and 16 ADHD children, all in special education classes, on the CBCL for teachers (TRF; Achenbach 1991b) and found more behaviour problems for the exposed children in this selected group.

Prenatal heroin, methadone, and cocaine exposure

Already in the neonatal period more neurobehavioural difficulties or non-optimal functioning were found in CDAP, especially in those prenatally exposed to heroin and methadone (Hans *et al.* 1984). CDAP specifically showed less visual orientation abilities, which may affect care-giver–infant attachment (van Baar 1991). During unstructured play interaction at 2 weeks of age, Schuler *et al.* (1995) found no differences between 20 CDAP and 20 drug-free infants in irritability of the infants, perceived irritability by the mothers, perception of social support by the mothers, and positive involvement of both mothers and infants. Jeremy and Bernstein (1984) used standardized interaction observations and found that 17 methadone-aintained mothers were less able to help their 4 month old infants to organize their communicative efforts. Bauman and Levine (1986) found that both partners in the study group of 70 methadone-aintained mothers and their children from 3–6 years old showed more aversive behaviour patterns, with the mothers having an authoritarian parenting style and the children having higher scores on behaviour codes such as teasing, yelling, hitting, and hyperactivity than the 70 comparison children. In an intervention study Black *et al.* (1994) found a marginally favourable difference on the HOME at 30 months, indicating that the 31 drug-addicted mothers in the experimental group who had been visited every 2 weeks from pregnancy until their children were 18 months old were more involved with their children than the 29 comparison mothers. In a study on 33 CDAP and a socioeconomically matched comparison group of 30 children, no group differences were found on the preschool version of the HOME interview or in interactive behaviours of mothers and infants during a period in a waiting room situation (Strauss *et al.* 1979).

In the Netherlands, Groeneweg and Lechner-Van de Noort (1988) found that 26 drug-dependent mothers reacted less sensitively towards verbalizations of their infants between 0 and 7 years, and less positively and also later to negative utterances than 27 foster mothers of CDAP. No differences were seen in social behaviour during interactions, nor in exploration or behaviours showing attachment of the infants towards their care-givers. A number of group differences were also found in the Amsterdam study following 30–16 CDAP and 35–30 drug-free reference children and their mothers and (once) fathers at 1, 6, 9, 12, and 18 months with the HOME, interaction, and attachment observations. The results suggest less smooth and positive interaction and communication processes and somewhat more avoidant, indifferent behaviour of the children within the CDAP group. Specific risk factors of CDAP such as neonatal withdrawal problems and short attention span of the mothers appear to affect the interaction processes (van Baar 1999).

Concerning temperament and behaviour problems, 16 methadone-exposed infants were more tense, active, and poorly coordinated than 23 comparisons (Marcus *et al.* 1984). No differences were found on the IBQ between 19 exposed and 32 reference children at 9 months in the Amsterdam study (van Baar 1991). Sowder and Burt (1980) reported more emotional problems in 34 3–7 year old CDAP. They also studied 126 CDAP and 126 comparison children between 8 and 17 years of age and found more behavioral and school problems in the CDAP. CDAP did have positive self-images (Sowder and Burt 1980). Not all children in this study rom were prenatally exposed, and Sowder and Burt (1980) did find prenatal exposure to be of importance within their index group.

Observing waiting room behaviour, Strauss *et al.* (1979) found 33 CDAP at 5 years to be more active than 30 comparison children. Wilson (1989) observed disturbances of activity level and attention span in infants of heroin-addicted mothers over the first 2½ years. In a later study she observed more adjustment problems at the age of 3–6 years in 22 CDAP exposed to heroin. At school age (6–11 years) 65% of 40 heroin-exposed children showed behaviour problems, indicating especially inattention and poor self-discipline (Wilson 1989). Olofsson *et al.* (1983) found 56% of 72 CDAP between 1 and 10 years of age to be hyperactive and aggressive. De Cubas and Field (1993) found more behaviour problems according to the CBCL (Achenbach 1991a), reflecting internalizing as well as externalizing problems in 20 CDAP of methadone-maintained mothers when compared to 20 non-exposed children between 6 and 13 years. In the Netherlands, Soepatmi (1992) examined 98 CDAP between 4 and 12 years of age using the Dutch version of the CBCL (Verhulst 1985) and found that 28 (32%) had total problem scores above the 90th percentile; in this study the boys of 4–5 years of age especially had many behaviour problems. In another Dutch study, Groeneweg and Lechner (1988) found for 16 fostered CDAP and 18 CDAP in the care of one of their own parents between 4 and 7 years of age that according to the CBCL respectively 7 (44%) and 6 (33%) had high 'clinical' total problem scores, based on internalizing as well as externalizing behaviour problems. At preschool age the Amsterdam study longitudinally followed 25–22 CDAP and 32–31 reference children between 4 and 5½ years using the CBCL twice along with a temperament questionnaire and the California Child Q-sort (CCQ; Block and Block 1980). The results showed higher activity levels, more attention and externalizing behaviour problems, and a less controlled behavioural style in the CDAP, which particularly reflects their relative lack of conscientiousness. The pattern of behaviour problems suggests more antisocial personality characteristics for the CDAP (van Baar and Briët 1999).

Concerning foster placement, Soepatmi (1992) reported a rate of 36% in 91 children between 3 and 12 years and in the Amsterdam study 50% was found in the CDAP group by 5½ years (van Baar and de Graaff 1994).

No prenatal drug exposure, but addicted parent

On psychiatric interviews with 32 children 6–17 years of age in 14 families of opiate addicts (7 teenagers) and 37 children (15 teenagers) in the same age range, referred to a pediatric clinic, Herjanic *et al.* (1979) found that the 7 target teenagers showed earlier and stronger antisocial trends. These authors concluded, to their surprise, that they found no other psychopathology. Davis and Templer (1988) studied 28 narcotic-exposed children aged 6–15 years (mean 8.5) and compared them to 28 children who were not prenatally exposed, but whose mother lived with a narcotic-addicted partner. All the group differences found showed that the narcotic-exposed children were less capable or more pathological than the non-exposed comparison group. According to behavior rating scales answered by the teachers, the exposed children were impulsive, undersocialized, inattentive, and prone to school adjustment problems and disturbed interpersonal relationships. Wilens *et al.* (1995) studied 44 children of opioid-dependent parents (18 mothers and 9 fathers) treated in a methadone clinic (including 15 girls) between 4 and 18 years of age (mean age 10.4), without specifying if they were already prenatally exposed. They were compared to a group of medically referred boys without ADHD and a group of boys with ADHD and comorbid psychiatric disorders. No differences were found between the latter 'psychiatric' group and the CDAP, and the CDAP had more internalizing, as well as externalizing problems, especially delinquency and attention problems, than the medical comparison group. High problem scores ($T \geqslant 59$) for any of the dimensions were found in 55% of the CDAP.

In summary, serious problems in socioemotional development of CDAP have emerged, in particular in the prenatally exposed groups. Difficulties in modulation of arousal were seen, as were less emotional responsivity during play, avoidant attachment behaviour, communication difficulties, attentional problems, and externalizing, aggressive, antisocial behaviour. The results do not indicate group differences and problems of the CDAP of a more internalizing and neurotic, depressed nature. Concerning behaviour of the mothers during interaction with their children, study results varied greatly, from no group differences at all to more insensitive care-giving. Only a few studies reported a high incidence of maltreatment and neglect, but referrals to child protective agencies or foster placements of CDAP are frequently necessary.

Conclusions

In all developmental domains, differences between CDAP and comparison groups have been found. Inconsistent data evolve from different studies, partly explained of course by differences in sample size, age, social background, and methods used. The group of CDAP prenatally exposed to cocaine as well as heroin and methadone seems to show the most problems, which become clearer when the children studied are older. In somatic growth and neuromotor development generally subtle differences were seen. More serious delays were seen in cognitive development of CDAP after infancy, especially in language capacities.

CDAP have serious difficulties in socioemotional development from infancy onwards. The kind of problems seen in socioemotional development of CDAP vary from subtle differences in interactive behaviour during play, avoidant attachment behaviour, and communication difficulties, to less emotional responsivity and attentional problems and externalizing, aggressive, antisocial behaviour. With regard to psychopathology, reflecting the problematic end of the spectrum of emotional development, no definite conclusions can yet be drawn, owing to the paucity of research in this area. More CDAP than comparison children do indeed have many serious behaviour problems. However, many CDAP have only slightly more problems than comparison children. The adverse outcomes for which the CDAP are most probably at risk are language impairments, conduct disorders, and hyperkinetic and attentional disorders; at older ages, they may also themselves be at risk of substance abuse disorders. Generally the CDAP studied were still too young to enable strong conclusions to be drawn with regard to the incidence of clear psychiatric disorders.

Research on development of CDAP has to deal with specific methodological problems, partly of course also dependent on the specific questions and hypotheses studied. The subgroups distinguished in this chapter also reflect such problems. The subdivision can easily be elaborated into subgroups of CDAP in foster care or CDAP with perinatal problems. Our own research, however generally showed the same outcome for such subgroups as for the total group of CDAP studied (van Baar 1991). In particular, studies attempting to investigate the significance of a causal factor, such as the substance used during gestation, are fraught with difficulties concerning all confounding factors. Usually prenatal exposure involves not only cocaine or any one substance; usually at least tobacco (known to potentially affect the development of the fetus) was also used, and was positively related to the amount of cocaine used (Tronick *et al.* 1996). Even if comparison groups did for instance use alcohol and tobacco, but not cocaine, these women took less alcohol and tobacco than the cocaine-abusing mothers (e.g. Mayes *et al.* 1995). The same holds for the socioeconomic circumstances of the comparison groups (Schutter and Brinker 1992). So, despite careful matching procedures and sophisticated statistical analyses, it remains questionable to ascribe causal effects only to chemical effects of one substance used during pregnancy.

Another characteristic methodological problem that bothers all longitudinal studies is the high attrition rate in groups of CDAP. Reports stating that less than 50% of the original sample could be followed are not unusual (Azuma and Chasnoff 1993, Landry and Whitney 1996). Erratic attendence for appointments is a common problem (van Baar and de Graaff 1994). Researchers should of course try to keep as many subjects in longitudinal studies as possible, but they should also indicate if their original sample differs from their final sample, in order to allow comparisons between studies in this respect too.

Studies and publications on development of CDAP not always are based solely on scientific criteria. Political, societal, emotional, and ethical questions have also been posed, for example:

- Is it desirable to prescribe methadone during pregnancy, or the other way around, to withhold methadone treatment during pregnancy?
- Should drug-dependent parents be allowed to take care of their own children?
- Are the developmental problems of CDAP any different from the difficulties encountered by children growing up in impoverished environments?

The issue of confounding factors in trying to determine the chemical effects of drugs is a methodological problem, but if poor outcomes are considered drug effects, it can have serious societal and individual consequences with termination of pregnancies and labeling of irreparably damaged children (Neuspiel 1994).

In my opinion, the emphasis in studies on development of CDAP needs to be on the fact that all specific risk factors are interrelated. In particular, the relatively small group of CDAP prenatally exposed to opioids, with the concomitant neonatal abstinence syndrome, deserves attention and further efforts to prevent the occurrence of developmental problems and psychopathology. Obviously more studies have to be done in order to evaluate the indications that many CDAP have behaviour problems and antisocial personality characteristics. The imminent risk of an intergenerational cycle of addiction and psychopathology needs to be evaluated and taken into account. Attempts to design effective intervention programmes to improve communication skills and socioemotional development of CDAP from early ages onwards are already worthwhile. Finally, for clinical practice it is important to realize that the results presented in this chapter mainly reflect group differences. As so many specific risk factors are involved in development of CDAP, individual circumstances, history, and experiences have to be considered in detail for each child and its family against the background of available research results, in order to make a careful diagnosis and provide optimal, individually adjusted, care.

References

Achenbach, T.M. (1988). *Child Behavior Checklist for age 2–3*. University of Vermont, Burlington, VT.

Achenbach, T.M. (1991a). *Manual for the Child Behavior Checklist/4–18 and 1991 profiles*. University of Vermont, Burlington, VT.

Achenbach, T.M. (1991b). *Manual for the Teachers Report Form*. University of Vermont, Burlington, VT.

Alessandri, S.M., Sullivan, M.W., Bendersky, M., and Lewis, M. (1995). Temperament in cocaine exposed infants. In *Mothers, babies and cocaine: The role of toxins in development*, ed. M. Lewis and M. Bendersky, pp. 273–286. Erlbaum, Hillsdale, N.J.

Azuma, S. and Chasnoff, I.J. (1993). Outcome of children prenatally exposed to cocaine and other drugs: a path analysis of three-year data. *Pediatrics*, **92**, 396–402.

Barton, S.J., Harrigan, R., and Tse, A.M. (1995). Prenatal cocaine exposure: implications for practic, policy, development and needs for future research. *Journal of Perinatology*, **15**, 10–22.

Bauman, P.S. and Levine, S.A. (1986). The development of children of drug addicts. *International Journal of Addictions*, **21**, 849–863.

Bayley, N. (1969). *Bayley Scales of Infant Development*. Psychological Corporation, New York.

Beckwith, L., Crawford, S., Moore, J.A., and Howard, J. (1995). Attentional and social functioning of preschool-age children exposed to PCP and cocaine in utero. In *Mothers, babies and cocaine: the role of toxins in development*, ed. M. Lewis and M. Bendersky, pp. 287–303. Erlbaum, Hillsdale, N.J.

Bender, S.L., Word, C.O., DiClemente, R.J., Crittenden, M.R., Persaud, N.A., and Ponton, L.E. (1995). The developmental implications of prenatal and/or postnatal crack cocaine exposure in preschool children: a preliminary report. *Journal of Developmental and*

Behavioral Pediatrics, **16**, 418–424.

Biederman, J., Milberger, S., Faraone, S.V., Kiely, K., Guite, J., Mick, E., Ablon, S., Warburton, R., and Reed, E. (1995). Family-environment risk factors for attention-deficit hyperactivity disorder. *Archives of General Psychiatry*, **52**, 464–470.

Black, M.M., Nair, P., Kight, C., Wachtel, R., Roby, P., and Schuler, M. (1994). Parenting and early development among children of drug-abusing women: Effects of home intervention. *Pediatrics*, **94**, 440–448.

Block, J.H. and Block, J. (1980). The role of ego-control and ego-resiliency in the organization of behavior. In *Development of cognition, affect and social relations*, ed. W.A. Collins. Erlbaum. Hillsdale, N.J.

Brazelton, T.B. (1984). *Neonatal Behavioural Assessment Scale*, 2nd edn. Clinics in Developmental Medicine No. 50. Heinemann, London.

Caldwell, B.M. and Bradley, R.H. (1978). *The Home Observation and Measurement of the Environment*. University Press Little Rock, A.K.

Chasnoff, I.J., Burns, K.A., Burns, W.J., Schnoll, S.H. (1986). Prenatal drug exposure: effects on neonatal and infant growth and development. *Neurobehavioral Toxicology and Teratology*, **8**, 357–362.

Chasnoff, I.J., Griffith, D.R. Freier, C., and Murray, J. (1992). Cocaine/polydrug use in pregnancy: two-year follow up. *Pediatrics*, **89**, 284–289.

Cubas, de, M. and Field, T.F. (1993). Children of methadone-dependent women: developmental outcomes. *American Journal of Orthopsychiatry*, **63**, 266–276.

Deren, S. (1986). Children of substance abusers: a review of the literature. *Journal of Substance Abuse Treatment*, **3**, 77–94.

Edmondson, R. and Smith, T.M. (1994). Temperament and behavior of infants prenatally exposed to drugs: clinical implications for the mother-infant dyad. *Infant Mental Health Journal*, **15**, 368–379.

Eriksson, M. and Zetterström, R. (1994). Amphetamine addiction during pregnancy: 10-year follow up. *Supplement for Acta Paediatrica*, **404**, 27–31.

Field, T.M. (1995). Cocaine exposure and intervention in early development. In *Mothers, babies and cocaine: the role of toxins in development*, ed. M. Lewis and M. Bendersky, pp. 355–368. Erlbaum, Hillsdale, NJ.

Finnegan, L.P. (ed.) (1980). *Drug dependence in pregnancy: clinical management of mother and child*. Castle House Publications, Tunbridge Wells.

Fried, P.A. and Watkinson, B. (1988). 12- and 24 months neurobehavioral follow up of children prenatally exposed to marihuana, cigarettes and alcohol. *Neurotoxicology and Teratology*, **10**, 305–313.

Fries, M.H., Kuller, J.A., Norton, M.E., Yankowitz, J., Kobori, J., Good, W.V., Ferriero, D., Cox, V., Seto Donlin. S., and Golabi, M. (1993). Facial features of infants prenatally exposed to cocaine. *Teratology*, **48**, 413–420.

Griffith, D.R., Azuma, S.D., and Chasnoff, I.J. (1994). Three year outcome of children exposed prenatally to drugs. *Journal of the American Academy of Child and Adolescent Psychiatry*, **33**, 20–27.

Groeneweg, B.F. and Lechner-van de Noort, M.G. (1988). *Kinderen van drugverslaafde ouders: opvoeding en ontwikkeling*. Eburon, Delft.

Hans, S.L., Marcus, J., Jeremy, R.J., and Auerbach, J.G. (1984). Neurobehavioral development of children exposed in utero to opioid drugs. In *Neurobehavioral Teratology*, ed. J. Yanai. Elsevier.Amsterdam,

Householder, J., Hatcher, R., Burns, W., and Chasnoff, I. (1982). Infants born to narcotic addicted mothers. *Psychological Bulletin*, **92**, 453–468.

Hurt, H., Brodsky, N.L., Betancourt, L., Braitman, L.E., Malmud, E., and Gianetti, J. (1995). Cocaine-exposed children: follow up through 30 months. *Journal of Developmental and Behavioral Pediatrics*, **16**, 29–35.

Jeremy, R.J. and Bernstein, V.J. (1984). Dyads at risk: Methadone-maintained women and their four-month-old infants. *Child Development*, **55**, 1141–1154.

Johnson, J.M., Seikel, J.A., Madison, C.L., Foose, S.M., and Rinard, K.D. (1997). Standardized test performance of children with a history of prenatal exposure to multiple drugs/cocaine. *Journal of Communicative Disorders*, **30**, 45–73.

Kandel, D.B. (1990). Parenting styles, drug use, and childrens adjustment in families of young adults. *Journal of Marriage and the Family*, **52** 183–196.

Kaltenbach, K. and Finnegan, L.P. (1984). Developmental outcome of children born to methadone maintained women: a review of longitudinal studies. *Neurobehavioral Toxicology and Teratology*, **6**, 271–275.

Landry, S.H. and Whitney, J. (1996). The impact of prenatal cocaine exposure: studies of the developing child. *Seminars in Perinatology*, **20**, 99–106.

Lester, B.M., Corwin, M.J., Sepkoski, C., Seifer, R., Peucker, M., McLaughlin, S., and Golub, H.L. (1991). Neurobehavioral syndromes in cocaine-exposed newborn infants. *Child Development*, **62**, 694–705.

Lifschitz, M.H., Wilson, G.S., OBrian Smith, E., and Desmond, M.M. (1985). Factors affecting head growth and intellectual function in children of drug addicts. *Pediatrics*, **75**, 269–274.

Malakoff, M.E., Mayes, L.C., and Schottenfield, R.S. (1994). Language abilities of preschool-ag children living with cocaine using mothers. *American Journal of Geriatric Psychiatry*, **2**, 346–354.

Manuzza, S., Klein, R.G., Bessler, A., Malloy, P., and Lapadula, M. (1993). Adult outcome of hyperactive boys. *Archives of General Psychiatry*, **50**, 565–576.

Marcus, J., Hans, S., and Jeremy, R.J. (1984). Children born to methadone maintained women. III: Effects of multiple risk factors on development at four, eight and twelve months. *American Journal of Drug and Alcohol Abuse*, **10**, 195–207.

Martin, J.C., Barr, H., Martin, D.C., and Streissguth, A. (1996). Neonatal neurobehavioral outcome following preatal exposure to cocaine. *Neurotoxicology and Teratology*, **18**, 617–625.

Mayes, L.C. (1994). Neurobiology of prenatal cocaine exposure: effect on developing monoamine systems. *Infant Mental Health Journal*, **15**, 121–133.

Mayes, L.C., Bornstein, M.H., Chawarska, K., Haynes, M., and Granger, R.H. (1996). Impaired regulation of arousal in 3-month-old infants exposed prenatally to cocaine and other drugs. *Development and Psychopathology*, **8**, 29–42.

McCarthy, D. (1972). *McCarthy Scales of Childrenss Abilities*. Psychological Corporation/ Harcourt Brace Jovanovich, New York

Mellins, C.A., Levenson, R., L., Zawadzki, R., Kairam, R., and Weston, M. (1994). Effects of pediatric HIV infaction and prenatal drug exposure on mental and psychomotor development. *Journal of Pediatric Psychology* **19**, 617–628.

Mentis, M. and Lundgren, K. (1995). Effects of prenatal exposure to cocaine and associated risk factors on language development. *Journal of Speech and Hearing Research*, **38**, 1303–1318.

Metosky, P. and Vondra, J. (1995). Prenatal drug exposure and play and coping in toddlers: a comparison study. *Infant Behavior and Develoment*, **18**, 15–25.

Miller, H. (1996). Prenatal cocaine exposure and mother-infant interaction: implicataions for occupational therapy intervention. *American Journal of Occupational Therapy*, **51**, 119–131.

Myers, B.J., Kavanaugh, V.M., Dawson, K.S., Lodder, D.E., Britt, G.C., Hagan, J.C., and Schnoll, S. (1996). Substance-exposed and nonexposed infants and toddlers: their home environments and teaching interactions. *Infant Behavior and Development*, **19**, 643.

Neuspiel, D.R. (1994). Behavior in cocaine-exposed infants and children: association versus causality. *Drug and Alcohol Dependence*, **36**, 101–107.

Neuspiel, D.R., Hamel, S.C., Hochberg, E., Green, J., and Campbell, D. (1991). Maternal cocaine use and infant behavior. *Neurotoxicology and Teratology*, **13**, 229–233.

Olofsson, M., Buckley, W., Andersen, G.E., and Friis-Hansen, B. (1983). Investigation of 89 children born by drug dependent mothers. II Follow up 1–10 years after birth. *Acta Pediatrica Scandinavica*, **72**, 407–410.

Olson, H.C., Toth-Sadjadi, S., and Hanna, E. (1996). Substance abusing women and their young infants: early child outcome and sources of vulnerability. *Infant Behavior and Development*, **19**, 373.

Ostrea, E., Brady, M., Gause, S., Raymundo, A.L., and Stevens, M. (1992). Drug screening of newborns by meconium analysis: a large scale, prospective, epidemiologic study. *Pediatrics*, **89**, 107–113.

Rodning, C., Beckwith, L., and Howard, J. (1989). Prenatal exposure to drugs: Behavioral distortions reflecting CNS impairment? *Neurotoxicology*, **10**, 629–634.

Rosen, T.S. and Johnson, H.L. (1985). Long term effects of prenatal methadone maintainance. In *Current research on the consequences of maternal drug abuse*, ed. T. Pinkert. NIDA Research Monograph 59, DHHS Pub. No. (ADM) 85–1400.

Rosenbaum, M. (1979). Difficulties in taking care of business; women addicts as mothers. *American Journal of Drug and Alcohol Abuse*, **6**, 431–446.

Rothbart, M.K. (1981). Measurement of temperament in infancy. *Child Development*, **52**, 569–578.

Singer, L., Arendt, R., and Minnes, S. (1993). Neurodevelopmental effects of cocaine. *Clinics in Perinatology*, **20**, 245–262.

Schuler, M.E., Black, M., and Starr, R.H. (1995). Determinants of mother–infant interaction: effects of prenatal drug exposure, social support and infant temperament. *Journal of Clinical Child Psychology*, **24**, 307–405.

Schutter, L.S. and Brinker, R.P. (1992). Conjuring a new category of disability from the prenatal cocaine exposure: are the infants unique biological or caretaking casuaties? *Topics in Early Childhood Special Education*, **11**, 84–111.

Smit, B.J., Boer, K., van Huis, A.M., Lie-a-Ling, I.S.E., and Schmidt, S.C. (1994). Cocaine use in pregnancy in Amsterdam. *Supplement to Acta Paediatrica*, **404**, 32–36.

Soepatmi, S. (1992). De ontwikkeling van kinderen van drugafhankelijke moeders. Thesis, University of Amsterdam.

Soepatmi, S. (1994). Developmental outcomes of children of mothers dependent on heroin or heroin/methadone during pregnancy. *Supplement for Acta Paediatrica*, **404**, 36–40.

Sowder, B.J. and Burt, M.R. (1980). *Children of heroin addicts*. Preager, New York

Strauss, M.E., Lessen-Firestone, J.K., Chavez, C.J., and Stryker, J.C. (1979). Children of methadone treated women at five years of age. *Pharmacology, Biochemistry and Behavior*, **11**, 3–6.

Struthers, J.M. and Hansen, R.L. (1992). Visual recognition memory in drug-exposed infants. *Developmental and Behavioral Pediatrics*, **13**, 108–111.

Tronick, E.Z., Frank, D.A., Cabral, H., Mirochnik, M., and Zuckerman, B. (1996). Late dose-response effects of prenatal cocaine exposure on newborn neurobehavioral performance. *Pediatrics*, **98**, 76–83.

van Baar, A.L. (1991). *Development of infants of drug dependent mothers*. Thesis, University of Amsterdam. Swets and Zeitlinger, Lisse.

van Baar, A.L. (1999). Socio-emotional development of children of drug dependent mothers I: Infancy and toddler age. Submitted.

van Baar, A.L., and Briët, J.M. (1999). Socio-emotional development of children of drug dependent mothers II: Preschool age. Submitted.

van Baar, A.L. Boer, K., Soepatmi, S. (1993). De gevolgen van drugsverslaving van de moeder voor haar kind: de huidige stand van zaken met betrekking tot kennis en zorgbeleid in Nederland. *Nederlands Tijdschrift voor Geneeskunde*, **36**, 1811–1815.

van Baar, A.L., and de Graaff, B.M.T. (1994). Cognitive development at preschool age of infants of drug dependent mothers. *Developmental Medicine and Child Neurology*, **36**, 1063–1075.

Verhulst, F.C. (1985). *Mental health in Dutch children; an epidemiological study*. Rotterdam, Thesis.

Wasserman, D.R., and Leventhal, J.M. (1993). Maltreatment of children born to cocaine-dependent mothers. *American Journal of Diseases in Children*, **147**, 1324–1328.

Wilens, T.E., Biederman, J., Kiely, K. Bredin, E., and Spencer, T.J. (1995). Pilot study of behavioral and emotional disturbances in the high-risk children of parents with opioid dependence. *Journal of the American Academy of Child and Adolescent Psychiatry*, **34**, 779–785.

Wilson, G.S. (1989). Clinical studies of infants and children exposed prenatally to heroin. *Annuals of the New York Academy of Science*, **562**, 183–194.

Woods, N.S., Eyler, F.D., Behnke, M., Conlon, M., Wobie, K., Peterson, K.M., Hatman, E., and Page, C. (1996). Cocaine-exposed infants and their mothers: patterns of interaction. *Infant Behavior and Development*, **19**

Zeanah, C.H., Boris, N.W., and Scheeringa, M.S. (1997). Psychopathology in infancy. *Journal of Child Psychology and Psychiatry*, **38**

6 Adopted children at risk

Frank C. Verhulst and Herma J.M. Versluis-den Bieman

Adoption by non-relatives is an accepted solution for the rearing of children whose biological parents are not able or willing to provide for them. Adoption is also a solution for the adoptive parents who wish for a family life that they cannot have because of infertility or other reasons. In contemporary society, adoption is incorporated into many mental health professionals' thinking as a good alternative for the rearing of unwanted children who might otherwise be raised in institutions.

Because adoption involves the loss of the biological parents and family ties, and because factors related to adoption may place the child at various risks for developing problems, the question arises of what the impact of the adoption situation is on the developing child. Although adoption seems to be in the best interest of children who would otherwise go on living in adverse circumstances, we need to know how adopted children fare in the long run, and how we can reduce the possible risks of developing psychological problems.

Apart from aspects concerning the rearing arrangement and the development of adopted children, adoption also gives the opportunity to study the extent to which familial resemblances are due to genetic or environmental similarity.

Paradigms and models

Genetic studies

Adoption studies provide a strong test of the contribution of genetic and environmental influences on behavior. By comparing different family types, it is possible to test the origin of familial resemblance. These family types are:

- biological parents and their adopted-away offspring
- adoptive parents and their adopted children
- non-adoptive parents and their biological children.

Resemblance between biological parents and their adopted-away offspring can be due only to shared genetic influences, whereas resemblance between adoptive parents and their adopted children can be due only to shared environmental influences.

The adoption design has been used to test the genetic and environmental contribution to psychopathology, such as schizophrenia, by comparing the frequency of the disorder in adopted-away relatives of affected individuals with the frequency of the disorder in relatives of unaffected individuals (Plomin *et al.* 1990). Recently, a quantitative genetic approach has been used to test the genetic influence, and shared and non-shared environmental influences, on problem behaviors of biologically related and unrelated adopted siblings as reported by their adoptive parents (Van den Oord *et al.* 1995). It was found that genetic influences were substantial for externalizing behaviors but unimportant for internalizing behaviors. Non-shared environmental influences were the strongest contributors to parent-reported problems.

Adoption outcome studies

Although the majority of adopted children seem to be well adjusted, clinical studies suggest that adopted children are overrepresented among children using mental health facilities (Jerome 1986). Non-clinical studies show that adopted children are at higher risk for developing problem behaviors than non-adopted children, but also that they are referred more readily than non-adopted subjects with similar levels of problems (Warren 1992, Lipman *et al.* 1993). Other non-clinical studies found little evidence for increased problem behaviors among adopted children (Bohman 1970).

A factor complicating the comparison of results from different studies, as well as the application of the results from earlier studies to the present situation, is that the practice of adoption is highly variable across time and across countries. Adoption typically used to involve the placement of an infant with parents of the same race. However, the increased availability of contraception and abortion resulted in a steep decline of infants available for adoption. Parents then increasingly chose to adopt children of a different race, or older or handicapped children.

Outcome studies pertaining to preadolescent children

Outcome studies pertaining to preadolescent children generally reported somewhat elevated levels of problem behaviors in adopted subjects. A Swedish study of 579 adopted children showed that teachers reported more maladjustment for adopted children than for non-adopted children in a comparison group at age 11 years (Bohman and Sigvardsson 1980). Seglow *et al.* (1972) found a higher prevalence of teacher-reported problem behavior in 108 7 year old adopted boys selected from a British national sample compared with non-adopted boys, but not for girls. This sex difference was not replicated by Brodzinsky *et al.* (1984), who found that parents reported more problems in adopted versus non-adopted children of both sexes and that adopted children were rated lower in social competence and school achievement. In contrast to the decrease in problems with increasing age in the study by Bohman and Sigvardsson (1980), Brodzinsky *et al.* (1984) did not find age differences. In a comparison of 41 adopted versus 2991 non-adopted children, Lindholm and Touliatos (1980) found that adopted children, especially adopted boys, exceeded non-adopted children in frequency of teacher-reported problem behavior, although the differences were rather small.

The studies discussed so far pertained mainly to intraracially adopted children. Several, mainly American, studies have pertained to the adjustment of internationally adopted children. These were mainly transracial adoptions by white parents (Rathbun *et al.* 1965, Kim 1977, Kim *et al.* 1979). However, conclusions are limited owing to small or selected samples, lack of standardized assessment procedures, and lack of comparison groups. In general, the conclusions of these studies are rather favorable.

Outcome studies pertaining to adolescents and young adults

A number of studies have investigated the functioning of adopted children through adolescence. Two longitudinal studies, the Swedish one mentioned above (Bohman 1970, 1972, Bohman and Sigvardsson 1978, 1979, 1980, 1985) and a British one (Tizard and Rees 1974, 1975, Tizard and Hodges 1978, Hodges and Tizard 1989a,b), contrasted the long-term behavioral adjustment of adopted children with that of two groups:

- a group of children who were brought up by their biological mothers who at first had given up their child but had changed their decision and reclaimed the child
- a group of children raised in permanent foster homes (Swedish study), or a group of children who were in residential care (British study).

The Swedish study demonstrated that the adopted children were well adjusted and differed little from normal control groups in their functioning at the age of 15. In both studies the adopted children had shown increased levels of teacher-reported problem behaviors at school age, but these problems had disappeared by the time they were adolescents. However, in the British study the adopted adolescents continued to have teacher-reported difficulties in their peer relationships, and showed increased levels of anxiety.

A third, prospective study (Maughan and Pickles 1990) compared the behavioral development of

- illegitimate children who were adopted
- illegitimate children who were raised by their mothers
- legitimate children derived from a large birth cohort of British children.

Subjects were assessed at ages 7, 11, 16, and 23 years. In adolescence (at age 16), adopted subjects showed high levels of teacher-reported unhappy and anxious behaviors and had problems in their relationships with peers. The adopted adolescents did not differ from legitimate adolescents on restless or antisocial behaviors. These findings were very similar to those of Hodges and Tizard (1989a,b).

An important aspect of the studies described so far is that the children in these studies are unlikely to have experienced the extreme adversities suffered by many children who are presently adopted in the US and Europe but who were born in developing countries or under poor political or socioeconomic circumstances. Also, the adopted children in the Swedish and British studies were mainly white, and intraracially adopted. At present, many children who are adopted have a racial and cultural background different from those of their adoptive parents.

So far, the results of the studies on adopted adolescents' functioning have depended on parents' or teachers' reports about the children's behavioral functioning. A number of studies also describe the behavioral functioning of adolescent adoptees based on self-reports. Hodges and Tizard (1989a,b) interviewed the 16 year olds in their longitudinal study. The interview covered problems in their relationships with their peers, parents, and teachers, as well as emotional problems such as depression, worries, fears, and self-depreciation and ideas of reference. The adopted adolescents had a significantly higher total problem score than their matched comparisons.

In the Swedish study by Bohman and Sigvardsson (1985), the male subjects were interviewed by a psychologist as part of the military enlistment procedure when they were 18 years old. The assessment included questions pertaining to education, occupational experience, social background, interests, personality, and social functioning. The adopted subjects showed no differences in adjustment compared to their non-adopted peer group.

In the British cohort study by Maughan and Pickles (1990), only teacher-reported problems are reported for 16 year olds. At age 23, information revealed from the adoptees themselves showed that adopted men but not adopted women had higher levels of job instability, unemployment, and relationship breakdowns. These results suggested that adopted men show increased vulnerabilities in the developmental transition from adolescence to adulthood.

Kühl (1985) assessed internationally adopted children and adolescents. In this study, from a sample of 145 children and adolescents mainly aged 13–18 years and adopted from Korea, Vietnam, and Latin America, self-reports were obtained to assess their self-concepts, educational achievement, and the extent to which they had positive and negative feelings towards themselves. The author found no difference between the adopted subjects and a comparison non-adopted group.

On the whole, the results of studies on the adjustment of adopted adolescents and young adults based on parents', teachers', and self-reports are somewhat conflicting; some findings suggest that adopted subjects have no more problems than non-adopted subjects, but others suggest higher levels of malfunctioning in adopted subjects.

Factors elevating the risk in adopted children

Adopted children are at elevated risk for maladjustment because a number of factors known to be disadvantageous (Rutter and Garmezy 1983) may exert their influence. These factors include:

- pre- and perinatal factors
    - maternal stress during pregnancy
    - inadequate pre- and perinatal medical care
    - malnutrition and infectious diseases of the mother during pregnancy
- factors operating after birth
    - malnutrition and medical conditions
    - discontinuous care-giving and poor adult–child relationships
    - deprivation, abuse
    - acquisition of behaviors that have a survival function but are maladaptive in the adoptive family
    - influences from the adoptive family, school, and social environment

The biological mothers are often subjected to personal and social stress during and after pregnancy. These factors may be especially prevalent in women in developing countries who live under great economic and social stress. There may have been a lack of antenatal care, and the children may have been subjected to birth hazards such as low birthweight. The lack of medical care for mother and child may have been further complicated by malnourishment.

Children often are subjected to negative environmental influences, such as separation from the natural mother, poor parent–child relationships, inharmonious family relationships, and discontinuous care-giving before adoption. Children may have been deprived from influences that are crucial for a healthy development, such as adequate stimulation (especially linguistic), affection, and opportunities for developing enduring attachments to others. Some children have been subjected to abuse. Furthermore, children who have been institutionalized are prone to show disturbed social relationships and may have acquired interaction styles that are appropriate for surviving in the institution but maladaptive outside it. There is also the possibility of interactions between effects of biological vulnerabilities, such as physical disabilities or disease, and parental frustration and rejection leading to abuse and neglect.

Lastly, there are factors operating after placement in the adoptive family. Relationships and expectations in the adoptive family, as well as psychosocial stress on the family, may enlarge the child's vulnerability to problem behavior. Adopted children in adolescence may have concerns about their biological parentage and, if they are of different ethnic background, their appearance may make them feel excluded from other family members or peers.

The factors listed above make adopted children at increased risk for developing problem behaviors. This is acknowledged by a number of authors including Bohman and Sigvardsson (1980), and Brodzinsky (1990). However, most knowledge concerning the development of adopted children is not based on much empirical evidence. Most studies rest on casework and clinical observation (Brodzinsky 1990).

From a theoretical point of view it is important to study the situation in which children with early deprivation are raised by usually highly motivated parents: a situation which can be regarded a 'natural experiment' concerning the vulnerability and resiliency of children subjected to early negative environmental influences. Not only in developing countries, but also in wealthy western societies, a substantial proportion of children are deprived or abused. Unless they are adopted, most of these children are chronically subjected to negative environmental influences, either in their own homes, or because they are institutionalized. In case of adoption, however, an inadequate or damaging environment is replaced by an environment that usually provides sufficient care and stimulation. This situation makes it possible to investigate to what extent the damaging effects of negative early experiences can be mitigated by a much more favorable environment.

Several authors have argued that the earlier the placement of the child in the adoptive home, the better (e.g. Bohman 1970, Hersov 1985). However, it is not clear which factors make children adopted at a later age more at risk of deviant development. One explanation is that the older the child at placement, the longer the child may have been subjected to negative environmental influences. Another factor may be that older children who have formed strong attachments to their care-givers have to cope with the trauma of loss, which may influence their development. Also, it may be that adoptive parents have more difficulty in adjusting to an older child with habits and behaviors that are unfamiliar to them. Lastly, the older the child, the greater the adjustments the child has to make such as learning a new language, or adapting to new demands.

The Dutch international adoption study: method and design

From the existing literature, it is clear that a number of issues concerning the adaptation of adopted children from childhood into adulthood, and factors influencing their development, remain unsolved. We assessed the behavioral development of 2148 adoptees originally aged

10–15 years and born in countries such as Korea, Colombia, India, Indonesia, and Bangladesh. This survey was motivated by increasing concern over the overrepresentation of foreign adopted children in residential treatment. The results of this survey facilitated the study of the development of children who may have been born and raised under adverse circumstances, and who, after being adopted, had to cope with adaptation to a new environment and with successive developmental tasks (see also Verhulst *et al.* 1990a–c, 1992, and Versluis-den Bieman and Verhulst 1995)

Time 1 sample

The Time 1 sample consisted of all children (N = 3519) adopted by non-relatives in the Netherlands and born outside the Netherlands between 1 January 1972 and 31 December 1975. (For a detailed description of the sample, see Verhulst *et al.* 1990a.) Parents were requested to complete the Child Behavior Checklist (CBCL; Achenbach 1991), a parent questionnaire for obtaining standardized parents' reports of children's competence and problem behaviors. In addition, parents were asked to provide information on a number of variables reflecting adverse environmental influences in the country of origin. Usable information was obtained from the parents of 64.9% (N = 2148) children. Children were aged 10–15 years (with the majority aged 11–14 years). Age of the adopted child at placement ranged from a few days to 10 years, with the majority being adopted before the fourth birthday. The distribution across native countries was: Korea, 32.0%; Colombia, 14.6%; India, 9.5%; Indonesia, 7.9%; Bangladesh, 6.7%; Lebanon, 4.9%; Austria, 5.0%; other European countries, 4.2%; other non-European countries, 15.2%. As in most adoption studies, the mean occupational level of parents of the adoption sample was much higher than that for the general population.

Time 2 sample

At follow-up, with a mean interval of 3.2 years, parents of 2071 subjects were requested to complete the CBCL, and a questionnaire with various questions about the general functioning of their adopted children. Parents were sent the questionnaires by mail. We received usable information on 1538 subjects (74%). Ages were 14–18 years. An analysis of some characteristics of the dropouts revealed that there was a slight underrepresentation of older and problematic children in the sample. Subjects on whom parent reports but no self-reports were available were slightly older, and functioned somewhat less well according to their parents, than subjects who cooperated.

Findings

Overview of Time 1 cross-sectional results

Prevalence

The prevalence of problem behaviors in the Time 1 sample of 2148 10–15 year old intercountry adoptees was determined by comparing the CBCL scores for adopted children with those of 933 same-aged non-adopted children from the general population (Verhulst *et al.* 1990a). Parents reported more problem behaviors, especially externalizing behaviors, for adopted

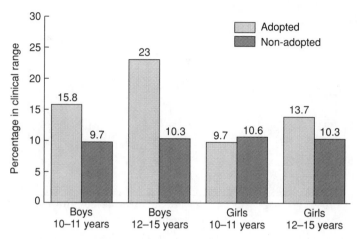

Fig. 6.1   Percentage of adopted and non-adopted children scoring in the clinical range of CBCL total problem scores by sex and age group.

than non-adopted children. More problems were reported for boys than for girls, and for 12–15 year olds tahn for 10–11 year olds. The largest proportion of deviant children was found among 12–15 year old boys, with more than twice as many boys with considerable problem behaviors in the adopted than in the non-adopted sample. Figure 6.1 shows the percentages of adopted versus non-adopted children scoring in the clinical range of the CBCL total problem score. The cutoff for the clinical range was set at the 90th percentile of the cumulative frequency distribution of CBCL total problem scores obtained for Dutch normative samples. For the syndrome scores the cutoff demarcating the clinical range was set at the 98th percentile. At the syndrome level, the largest differences were found for delinquent and hyperactive behavior in 12–15 year old boys, with adopted boys showing more problem behavior than non-adopted boys.

The sex difference in CBCL problem scores in the adoption sample was similar to that found for non-adopted children, with higher problem scores for boys versus girls. Adopted boys showed especially elevated problem scores over non-adopted boys, although the scores for adopted 12–15 year old girls were also higher than the scores for non-adopted girls (Verhulst *et al.* 1990a).

Unlike the sex difference, which was similar for adopted and non-adopted subjects, the higher CBCL problem scores for older versus younger children in the adoption sample contrasted with the slight decrease in CBCL problem scores with increasing age found for non-adopted children (Verhulst *et al.* 1985). It was not clear from the cross-sectional findings whether the increase of problems with increasing age in the adoption sample was truly developmental, or due to selection factors. Changing policies of governments in countries of origin, and variations in local selection procedures across time, may affect the characteristics of adopted children from year to year in unknown ways.

Age of the child at placement

Age of the child at placement was significantly associated with an increased risk for later maladjustment, although the relationship was not fully linear. Children who were adopted

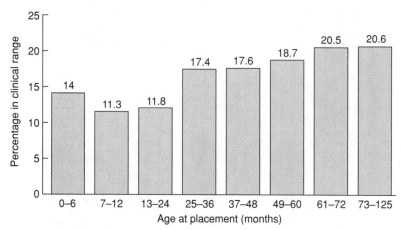

Fig. 6.2 Percentage of adopted children scoring in the clinical range of CBCL total problem scores by age of the child at placement.

within the first 6 months of their lives were at somewhat greater risk for later maladjustment than children who were adopted between 7 and 24 months of age. However, this difference was not significant. After the age of 24 months, there was a gradual increase of the risk for later maladjustment with increasing age at placement (see Fig. 6.2).

Early adversity

A large proportion of the study sample for whom there was information on their early backgrounds had been subjected to adverse influences. Parents reported that in the country of origin, children had been subjected to neglect in 45% of the sample, to abuse in 13%, and to changes of care-givers in 54%. Nearly 6% of the children in the sample underwent three or more changes of care-giving environments. According to their parents, more than 43% of the children in the sample were in poor physical condition on arrival in the adoptive family. Although physical condition cannot be regarded as merely a negative environmental influence, being also a consequence of adversity, this variable was included in our analyses. As expected, the probability that a child showed maladaptive behaviors at a later age increased strongly when the child had been subjected to early serious environmental adversity. Figure 6.3 shows the percentages of children who scored in the clinical range of the CBCL for different levels of early adverse influences. For example, half the children who experienced five or more changes in care-giving environment showed later maladjustment. Problem behaviors were shown by 24% of the children who had been severely neglected and by 31% of the severely abused children.

Children who have experienced early negative environmental influences thus run a greater risk of developing problem behaviors than children with relatively favorable backgrounds. Early adverse experiences—neglect, abuse, and number of changes of care-giving environment—were all positively associated with the age of the child at placement. Age of the child at placement was so strongly associated with each of these variables that it did not add to the contribution of the early background variables in the distribution of children across the two categories of deviant and non-deviant behavioral functioning. In other words, the increased risk of developing later problem behaviors in children adopted at a later age could be ascribed

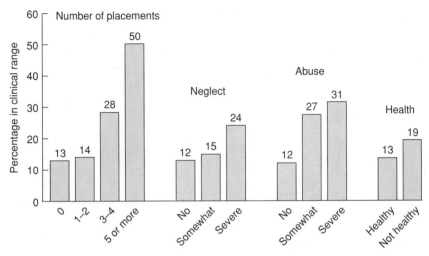

Fig. 6.3 Percentage of adopted children scoring in the clinical range of CBCL total problem scores for different levels of early adverse influences.

sufficiently by their having been subjected more to early adverse circumstances. In particular, knowing that a child had been abused was a potent predictor of later maladjustment. When these early influences are taken into account, the age of the child at placement as such is of lesser significance. It was hypothesized that raising a child from its first months onward is easier than raising an older child who speaks a foreign language and has already acquired skills and habits and has a history of its own. However, the findings of the present study could not support this hypothesis. Children adopted at a relatively greater age seem to run a greater risk for later maladjustment not so much because they were taken into their new family when they were older, but because they run a greater risk of having been subjected to early adverse experiences.

Of the early adverse factors examined, abuse was found to contribute most strongly to the prediction of later maladjustment. The effect of abuse in children's early histories was so strongly associated with later maladjustment that neglect and number of changes in care-giving environment had no significant additional value in predicting poor outcome. In other words, if a child was known to have been abused, this was sufficient information to expect a greater likelihood of later maladjustment.

More boys than girls showed high levels of problem behavior. However, although boys run a greater risk for maladjustment than girls, this greater risk could not be attributed to a greater vulnerability to early adverse factors.

Age at placement was associated with a higher risk of developing delinquent behavior and depressive symptoms. The strong associations between age at placement and the early adverse factors indicate that early adversities put the children in the present sample at greater risk for developing conduct problems and depression. This finding is informative with respect to the link between depression and early loss and other environmental adversities.

The results also demonstrated that the majority of children who had backgrounds known to be damaging seemed to function quite well. Apparently, the negative effects of early adverse

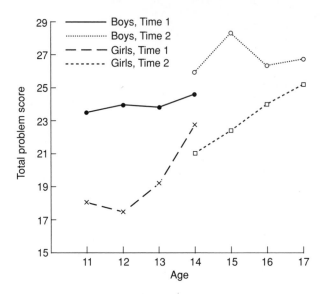

Fig. 6.4   Mean CBCL total problem scores at time 1 and time 2 for adopted children by age and sex.

influences can fade away under the positive influence of the adoptive family. Some children were able to escape the influences of early adverse experiences.

Although the results indicated that adverse preadoption influences increased the risk of later maladjustment, developmental aspects later in the children's lives may also play an important role in the development of problem behaviors. The cross-sectional findings did not indicate the direction in which later environmental influences will guide the adopted child's development. Problem behaviors resulting from early negative experiences may be ameliorated by later positive influences, but if they are resistant to these positive influences, they may remain. It is also possible that certain developmental strains will exacerbate maladjustment. Especially adolescence, characterized by the developmental increase of cognitive abilities, independence, identity formation, and sexual maturation, may be more stressful for adopted than for non-adopted children.

This was the starting point for the 3 year follow-up of adopted children's functioning into adolescence.

Results of the 3 year follow-up

Longitudinal course

Figure 6.4 shows the mean total problem scores at initial assessment and at follow-up for both sexes and four age groups separately.

As can be seen, there was an developmental increase in problem scores. The mean total problem scores and the mean scores for each of the eight CBCL syndrome scales and the Externalizing and Internalizing scales at Time 1 and Time 2, were compared using multivariate analysis of variance (MANOVA). Table 6.1 shows the results of these analyses. The size of significant differences is listed as percentage of variance accounted for. Table 6.1 also shows

Table 6.1 Percentage of variance accounted for by significant effects of MANOVAs of mean CBCL problem scores at Time 1 and Time 2, and correlation (*r*) between Time 1 and Time 2 CBCL problem scores

Scale	Percentage of variance	*r*
Withdrawn	6.5	0.60
Somatic Complaints	3.0	0.37
Anxious/Depressed	3.4	0.57
Social Problems	–	0.67
Thought Problems	0.8	0.34
Attention Problems	1.6	0.69
Delinquent Behavior	8.5	0.59
Aggressive Behavior	1.0	0.70
Internalizing	6.3	0.60
Externalizing	3.6	0.69
Total Problems	3.8	0.69

Only effects significant at $p < 0.001$ are reported; all effects indicate higher scores at Time 2 than at Time 1.

the stability coefficients for each of the CBCL scales indicating the extent to which the individuals' scores preserved their rank order across time. The correlations were considerable, with only two correlations (for Somatic Complaints and Thought Problems) lower than 0.50 and all other correlations greater than 0.50.

Scores on each of the 11 scales, except the Social Problems scale, showed a significant increase across time. The largest increase was for the Delinquent Behavior syndrome, followed by the syndrome designated Withdrawn. Apparently, withdrawal from contact and covert antisocial behaviors are of increasing concern to parents of internationally adopted children as they enter adolescence.

The increase in CBCL problem scores with increasing age contrasted with the results from our longitudinal general population studies (Verhulst *et al.* 1990d), which demonstrated a slight decrease of CBCL problem scores with increasing age. From our 4 year epidemiological follow-up we selected a sample ($N = 312$) which proportionally matched the present study's adoption sample as far as age at follow-up and sex was concerned. From our longitudinal, epidemiological database, the follow-up interval of 4.2 years came closest to the 3.2 years in the present study. We compared the CBCL total problem scores with *t*-tests. The CBCL total problem score in the adoption sample showed a significant *increase* (from 21.4 to 24.8) whereas it showed a significant *decrease* in the comparison group of non-adopted children (from 20.8 to 16.3). Figure 6.5 shows the results.

Effect of early environmental influences

To test the effects of preadoption environmental factors on the developmental increase of CBCL problem scores, the following variables reflecting adverse environmental influences in the country of origin were assessed:

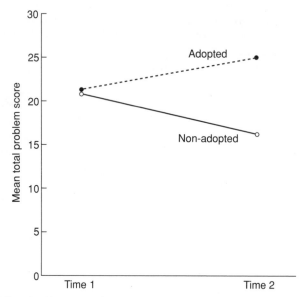

Fig. 6.5 Mean CBCL total problem scores at time 1 and time 2 for adopted versus non-adopted children.

- age of the child at placement
- medical conditions at the time of placement
- neglect/abuse; any of the following three conditions in the past scored as present:
  - at least three changes of care-giving environment
  - physical neglect
  - physical abuse.

 The effects of these preadoption variables on CBCL mean total problem scores were determined in three separate MANOVAs with time of assessment as within-factor, and the three preadoption environmental factors as between-factors. No significant two-way inter-actions were found between time of assessment and age at placement, between time of assessment and medical condition, and between time of assessment and neglect/abuse. The lack of interactions between the increase in mean total problem scores across time and the three preadoption variables indicates that early negative environmental influences, as measured in the present study, were not responsible for the increase in problems in our sample across time.

Effect of ethnicity

For the majority of European children, the adopted child was of similar ethnic background to the adoptive parents. This was not the case in the majority of children born in non-European, developing countries. The sample was divided into interracially adopted children born in non-European countries ($N = 1410$), and intraracially adopted children from European countries ($N = 128$). To test the possible effect of ethnicity on the increase of problem scores across time, a MANOVA was performed with time of assessment as within-factor, and intraracial versus interracial adoption as between-factor. No significant interaction was found between time of assessment and problem scores for intraracial versus interracial groups. From our results we could not conclude that differences in ethnicity between the parent and their adopted youngster were responsible for the longitudinal increase in problems.

Conclusions

We must conclude that a substantial number of internationally adopted children become increasingly maladjusted as their development progresses into adolescence. These findings do not confirm the much more favorable reports of the functioning of adopted adolescents by Bohman and Sigvardsson (1978, 1979, 1980) Tizard and Rees (1974, 1975), and Tizard and Hodges (1978). Although these studies demonstrated the beneficial effect of adoption, the mainly white and intraracially adopted children in these studies are unlikely to have experienced the extreme deprivation that many children in our Dutch survey of intercountry adopted children had suffered.

The adverse influences early in the lives of many of the children in the present study may have made them more vulnerable to the developmental stresses of adolescence The decline in adolescence of protective and supervisory influences exerted by the family (Larson and Richards 1991) and school may have a stronger effect on adopted children who have experienced early loss than on non-adopted children. The prolonged preadoption exposure of many children in our sample to other environmental adversities such as weak and often disrupted adult–child relationships, deviant adult and peer models of behavior, and poor discipline and supervision, may have made them more vulnerable to problem behaviors in adolescence with its decrease in environmental support and supervision. Although early environmental adversities were found to be associated with higher levels of later problems, the preadoption influences were *not* significantly related to the longitudinal increase in problem behaviors across time.

A factor that may influence the adolescent functioning of most intercountry adoptees is their ethnic background, which gives them a different physical appearance from that of their adoptive parents and their non-adopted siblings and peers. Adoption of children from developing countries by white parents from rich western countries has been a source of debate. Some are strongly opposed to adoption of non-white children by white parents, arguing that transracial adoption is a new form of colonialism, or that it can be seen as a form of cultural genocide (see Silverman and Feigelman 1990). Racial differences may put the adopted adolescent under undue stress with respect to establishing a satisfactory ethnocultural identity and sufficient self-esteem. Racism may also hamper the formation of adequate self-esteem and social adjustment. However, our comparison of intraracially versus interracially adopted adolescents suggest that transracial adoption is not related to later maladjustment. This does not imply that racism may not cause considerable suffering for non-white adopted adolescents. Our results showed merely that the role of possible racism does not affect the adopted adolescent's functioning to a degree that it can be regarded deviant.

It must be concluded that factors other than the effects of childhood deprivation or racial antagonism are responsible for the majority of problems in adopted adolescents. It is possible that with increasing age, adolescent adoptees become more and more prone to develop problem behaviors as a result of their increasing concerns over their biological parentage. Their increased cognitive abilities enable them to reflect on the meaning of being adopted. They are able to evaluate the lack of connectedness with their adoptive parents as well as with their biological parents. Their sense of loss of having once been abandoned, and their awareness of the lack of genealogical connectedness, are evaluated in adolescence in terms of their developing identity (Brodzinsky 1990). Emotional and behavioral reactions may result from this sense of loss, which is exacerbated by a loosening of the ties between the adolescent and his or her adoptive family, and by the adolescent's striving towards independence.

The internationally adopted adolescents in our sample deviated more and more from their peer group from the general population. This finding is a source of concern with respect to the adopted individuals' future functioning. The adolescent's development towards adulthood with its greater independence, greater responsibilities, greater emphasis on stable sexual relationships, and even parenthood may cause undue stresses, with still unknown consequences. It is important to evaluate how these adolescents do in the future and to determine which factors influence their development, in both negative and positive ways. It also needs to be stressed that the majority of adopted children, despite the many preadoption adversities and, once they were adopted, the many later stresses, seem to function well as adolescents. Our results supported the view that transracial adoption may be a viable means of providing stable homes for children who would otherwise have had to endure many adversities.

References

Achenbach, T.M. (1991). *Manual for the CBCL/4–18 and 1991 Profile*. University of Vermont Department of Psychiatry, Burlington, VT.

Bohman, M.S. (1970). *Adopted children and their families. A follow-up study of adopted children, their background, environment and adjustment*. Proprius, Stockholm.

Bohman, M. (1972). A study of adopted children, their background, environment and adjustment. *Acta Paediatrica Scandinavica*, **61**, 90–97.

Bohman, M. and Sigvardsson, S. (1978). An 18-year, prospective, longitudinal study of adopted boys. In: *The child in his family: vulnerable children*, ed. J. Anthony, C. Koupernik and, C. Chiland. Wiley, London.

Bohman, M. and Sigvardsson, S. (1979). Long term effects of early institutional care: a prospective longitudinal study. *Journal of Child Psychology and Psychiatry*, **20**, 111–117.

Bohman, M.S. and Sigvardsson, S. (1980). A prospective, longitudinal study of children registered for adoption. *Acta Psychiatrica Scandinavica*, **61**, 339–355.

Bohman, M. and Sigvardsson, S. (1985). A prospective longitudinal study of adoption. In *Longitudinal studies in child psychology and psychiatry*, ed. A.R. Nicol, pp. 137–155. Wiley, London.

Brodzinsky, D.M. (1990). A stress and coping model of adoption adjustment. In *The psychology of adoption*, ed. D.M. Brodzinsky and, M.D. Schechter, pp. 3–24). Oxford University Press, New York.

Brodzinsky, D.M., Schechter, D.E., Braff, A.M., and Singer, L.M. (1984). Psychological and academic adjustment in adopted children. *Journal of Consulting and Clinical Psychology*, **52**, 582–590.

Hersov, L. (1985). Adoption and fostering. In *Child and adolescent psychiatry: modern approaches*, ed. M. Rutter and L.Hersov, pp. 101–117. Blackwell Scientific Publications, Oxford.

Hodges, J. and Tizard, B. (1989a). IQ and behavioural adjustment of ex-institutional adolescents. *Journal of Child Psychology and Psychiatry*, **30**, 52–75.

Hodges, J. and Tizard, B. (1989b). Social and family relations of ex-institutional adolescents. *Journal of Child Psychology and Psychiatry*, **30**, 77–97.

Jerome, L. (1986). Overrepresentation of adopted children attending a childrens mental health centre. *Canadian Journal of Psychology*, **31**, 526–531.

Kim, D.S. (1977). How they fared in American homes. *Children Today*, **31**, 2–6.

Kim, S.P., Hong, S., and Kim, B.S. (1979). Adoption of Korean children by New York area couples. *Child Welfare*, **63**, 419–427.

Kühl, W. (1985). *When adopted children of foreign origin grow up: adoption succes and the psychosocial integration of teenagers. First results of a survey*. Terre des Hommes Germany e.V., Osnabrück.

Larson, R. and Richards, M.H. (1991). Daily companionship in late childhood and early adolescence: changing developmental contexts. *Child Development*, **62**, 284–300.

Lindholm, B.W. and Touliatos, J. (1980). Psychological adjustment of adopted and nonadopted children. *Psychological Reports*, **46**, 307–310.

Lipman, E.L., Offord, D.R., Boyle, M.H., and Racine, Y.A. (1993). Follow-up of psychiatric and educational morbidity among adopted children. *Journal of the American Academy of Child and Adolescent Psychiatry*, **32**, 1007–1012.

Maughan, B. and Pickles, A. (1990). Adopted and illegitimate children growing up. In *Straight and devious pathways from childhood to adulthood*, ed. L. Robins and M. Rutter, pp. 36–61). Cambridge University Press, Cambridge.

Plomin, R., DeFries, J.C., and McClearn, G.E. (1990). *Behavioral genetics: a primer*, 2nd edn. W.H. Freeman, New York.

Rathbun, C., McLaughlin, H., Bennett, C., and Garland, J.A. (1965). Later adjustment of children following radical separation from family and culture. *American Journal of Orthopsychiatry*, **35**, 604–609.

Rutter, M. and Garmezy, N. (1983). Developmental psychopathology. In *Handbook of child psychology*, vol. 4, ed. P.H. Mussen, pp. 775–911. Wiley, New York.

Seglow, J., Kellmer Pringle, M., and Wedge, P. (1972). *Growing up adopted: a long term study of adopted children and their families*. National Foundation for Educational Research in England and Wales, Windsor, U.K.

Silverman, A.R. and Feigelman, W. (1990). Adjustment in interracial adoptees: an overview. In *The psychology of adoption*, ed. D.M. Brodzinsky and, M.D. Schechter, pp. 187–200. Oxford University Press, New York.

Tizard, B. and Hodges, J. (1978). The effects of early institutional rearing on the development of eight-year-old children. *Journal of Child Psychology and Psychiatry*, **19**, 99–118.

Tizard, B. and Rees, J. (1974). A comparison of the effects of adoptions, restoration to the natural mother, and continued institutionalisation on the cognitive development of four-year-old children. *Child Development*, **45**, 92–99.

Tizard, B. and Rees, J. (1975). The effects of early institutional rearing on the behaviour problems and affectional relationships of four-year-old children. *Journal of Child Psychology and Psychiatry*, **16**, 61–73.

Van den Oord, E.J.C., Boomsma, D.I., and Verhulst, F.C. (1994). A study of problem behaviors related and unrelated international adoptees. *Behavior Genetics*, **24**, 193–205.

Verhulst, F.C., Akkerhuis, G.W., and Althaus, M. (1985). Mental health in Dutch children, I. A cross-cultural comparison. *Acta Psychiatrica Scandinavica*, **2**, suppl. 323.

Verhulst, F.C., Althaus, M., and Versluis-den Bieman, H.J.M. (1990a). Problem behavior in international adoptees I: an epidemiological study. *Journal of the American Academy of Child and Adolescent Psychiatry*, **29**, 94–103.

Verhulst, F.C., Althaus, M., and Versluis-den Bieman, H.J.M. (1990b). Problem behavior in international adoptees II. Age at placement. *Journal of the American Academy of Child and Adolescent Psychiatry*, **29**, 104–111.

Verhulst, F.C., Versluis-den Bieman, H.J.M., Van der Ende, J., Berden, G.F.M.G., and Sanders-Woudstra, J.A.R. (1990c). Problem behavior in international adoptees III. Diagnosis of child psychiatric disorders. *Journal of the American Academy of Child and Adolescent Psychiatry*, **29**, 420–428.

Verhulst, F.C., Koot, J.M., and Berden, G.F.M.G. (1990d). Four-year follow-up of an epidemiological sample. *Journal of the American Academy of Child and Adolescent Psychiatry*, **29**, 440–448.

Verhulst, F.C., Althaus, M., and Versluis-den Bieman, H.J.M. (1992). Damaging backgrounds: later adjustment of international adoptees. *Journal of the American Academy of Child and Adolescent Psychiatry*, **33**, 518–524.

Verhulst, F.C. and Versluis-den Bieman, H.J.M. (1995). Developmental course of problem behaviors in adolescent adoptees. *Journal of the American Academy of Child and Adolescent Psychiatry*, **34**, 151–159

Versluis-den Bieman, H.J.M. and Verhulst, F.C. (1995). Self-reported and parent-reported problems in adolescent international adoptees. *Journal of Child Psychology and Psychiatry*, **36**, 1411–1428

Warren, S.B. (1992). Lower threshold for referral for psychiatric treatment for adopted adolescents. *Journal of the American Academy of Child and Adolescent Psychiatry*, **31**, 512–527.

11   Clinical outcomes

7 Anxiety disorders

L. D. Seligman and T. H. Ollendick

Clinical picture

The anxiety disorders comprise a broad spectrum of syndromes ranging from very circumscribed anxiety to pervasive, sometimes 'free-floating' anxiety or worry. With the most recent edition of the *Diagnostic and Statistical Manual of Mental Disorders* (DSM-IV; APA 1994) and, similarly, the *International Classification of Diseases and Related Health Problems* (ICD-10; WHO 1992) children, adolescents, and adults can be categorized by eight major but separate diagnostic categories associated with anxiety:

- panic disorder with agoraphobia
- panic disorder without agoraphobia
- agoraphobia without history of panic
- specific phobia
- social phobia
- obsessive–compulsive disorder
- post-traumatic stress disorder
- generalized anxiety disorder.

Additionally, the DSM-IV and ICD-10 specify one anxiety diagnosis specific to childhood:

- separation anxiety disorder.

Earlier versions of the DSM (APA 1980, 1987) included two additional anxiety diagnoses specific to childhood, namely avoidant disorder and overanxious disorder. However, considerable evidence suggests that these are not distinct syndromes nor sufficiently different from their adult counterparts to merit separate diagnostic categories (Beidel 1991, Francis *et al.* 1992). Therefore, in the most recent revision of the DSM, avoidant disorder and overanxious disorder have been subsumed under the categories of social phobia and generalized anxiety disorder, respectively..

Although diagnostic systems such as the DSM and ICD describe anxiety as falling into several distinct syndromes or categories, there is also a rich body of literature examining anxiety at the symptom level. Rather than defining categorical distinctions, this view embraces a dimensional approach, examining the number of anxiety symptoms experienced by children and adolescents and the frequency or severity of such symptoms. This tradition is perhaps best exemplified in the work of Achenbach and Verhulst and their colleagues (cf. Stanger *et al.* 1992, Verhulst and Van der Ende 1992) and furthered by the development of parent, teacher, and child checklists such as the Child Behavior Checklist, Teacher Report Form, and Youth Self-Report (Achenbach 1991).

As is evident from the above discussion, the heading of anxiety disorders in childhood covers a broad range of topics. We have chosen to delimit the more specific aspects of our discussion to that perspective which examines anxiety as syndromes or disorders and, more specifically, to the examination of separation anxiety disorder, generalized anxiety disorder/overanxious disorder, and panic disorder. Owing to space constraints the current chapter cannot address the remainder of the anxiety disorders in sufficient depth; however, several recent reviews provide excellent resources for the interested reader. For example, obsessive–compulsive disorders are considered separately in Chapter 9 of this volume. Furthermore, a recent review by Beidel and Randall (1994) discusses issues in the phenomenology, assessment, epidemiology, and correlates of social phobia in children. Similarly, Ollendick *et al.* (1997) provide a review of findings pertaining to simple/specific phobias in childhood and the reader is referred to Saylor (1993) for a recent review of childhood post-traumatic stress disorder.

Separation anxiety disorder

As noted above, separation anxiety disorder is the only anxiety disorder specific to childhood in the DSM-IV (APA 1994) and the diagnosis therefore requires age of onset prior to 18 years. The ICD-10 (WHO 1992) includes corresponding criteria. The core feature of this disorder as defined by both diagnostic systems is developmentally inappropriate and excessive levels of anxiety or worry regarding separation from an attachment figure (usually a parent or primary care-giver) or from the home, for a duration of at least 4 weeks (WHO 1992, APA 1994).

Symptoms of separation anxiety disorder include somatic complaints upon or in anticipation of separation from the attachment figure, worries regarding events that may occur to the attachment figure or the child him/herself that would result in separation (e.g. accident or kidnapping), and difficulty separating at night that may lead to the child's reluctance to go to sleep or inability to sleep away from home. In addition, school refusal is a particularly disruptive symptom that may be present in some cases of separation anxiety disorder and may interfere with both academic and social development. In fact, school refusal is the most common reason for referral of children with separation anxiety disorder (Black 1995). Typically, onset is prior to adolescence, although symptoms may continue into adolescence and early adulthood and interfere with activities such as getting married or leaving home to attend college, or result in their avoidance.

As noted in DSM-IV (APA 1994) there is a good deal of cultural variation in the degree to which separation is expected and valued. Consequently, the severity of anxiety regarding separation that engenders significant distress and impairment, required to merit a diagnosis of separation anxiety disorder, may vary depending upon the child's contextual environment. This is an important factor to consider when working with culturally diverse populations. Moreover, variation in symptom presentation may occur. For example, in comparison with Caucasian children, African-American children may present with more specific fears (Neal *et al.* 1993) and less often with school refusal (Last and Perrin 1993).

Epidemiological investigations estimate the prevalence of separation anxiety disorder to range from 0.1% (Fergusson *et al.* 1993, Lewinsohn *et al.* 1993) to 13.1% (Cohen *et al.* 1993).

Further, it appears that the prevalence of separation anxiety disorder decreases with age and is somewhat higher for girls than for boys. Turning to clinical samples, in their analysis of admissions to an outpatient anxiety disorders clinic, Last *et al.* (1987) found separation anxiety disorder to be the most frequent primary diagnosis assigned. Comorbidity of separation anxiety disorder with other anxiety disorders and depression is common (Last *et al.* 1987, Black 1995).

Generalized anxiety disorder/overanxious disorder

Excessive and uncontrollable worry or anxious apprehension related to a number of events or activities which lasts for a period of 6 months or more constitutes the core symptom of generalized anxiety disorder as defined by both the DSM-IV and the ICD-10 diagnostic criteria (WHO 1992, APA 1994). As noted above, overanxious disorder is now subsumed under the diagnosis of generalized anxiety disorder. The principal differences between generalized anxiety disorder and overanxious disorder include the heavier reliance on somatic complaints in generalized anxiety disorder, and its somewhat more forward focus (anxious apprehension) as compared to overanxious disorder (in which one criterion is specifically related to worry or concern regarding past behavior). However, modifications to the requisite number of somatic complaints required for diagnosis of generalized anxiety disorder in children are made in both the DSM-IV and ICD-10 criteria. To date, little evidence exists to support or refute the application of these criteria to children.

Although few studies have documented the prevalence of generalized anxiety disorder in youth, those that do suggest between 1.7% (Costello *et al.* 1996) and 4.2% (Fergusson *et al.* 1993) of children and adolescents are affected by this disorder. Again, as with separation anxiety disorder, it is not uncommon for individuals presenting with generalized anxiety disorder/overanxious disorder to evidence comorbid conditions. For example, in a clinical sample, Strauss *et al.* (1988c) found high rates of comorbidity between overanxious disorder and other anxiety disorders, particularly separation anxiety disorder, as well as major depression.

Panic disorder

The hallmark of panic disorder is the occurrence of repeated and unexpected panic attacks. A panic attack is a discrete period of fear or discomfort, often with a rapid onset, accompanied by at least four physical sensations (e.g. accelerated heart rate, nausea, dizziness) and/or cognitive or perceptual symptoms (e.g. fear of losing control or going crazy, fear of dying, derealization, depersonalization) (WHO 1992, APA 1994). Attacks which involve fewer than four symptoms are referred to as limited symptom attacks. Panic disorder must be diagnosed as either with or without agoraphobia (i.e. anxiety about being in places from which escape would be difficult or embarrassing or in which help would be unavailable should a panic attack occur, and avoidance of such situations).

The criteria for panic disorder have changed from DSM-III-R to DSM-IV such that cognitive symptoms are more critical to the diagnosis in the most recent revision. In DSM-III-R, criteria for panic disorder could be met without the presence of cognitive symptomatology if the individual had four or more attacks within a 4 week period. However, in DSM-IV, frequent attacks are no longer sufficient to meet criteria; rather, the individual must experience

- persistent concern about having additional attacks, and/or
- worry about the implications of the attack or its consequences (e.g. losing control, having a heart attack, going crazy), and/or
- a significant change in behavior related to the attacks (APA 1994, p. 402).

Such a modification has important bearing on issues in the diagnosis of panic disorder in children and adolescents. Much controversy has surrounded the existence of panic attacks and panic disorder in youth, particularly prior to adolescence (see Moreau and Weissman 1992, King *et al.* 1994, Ollendick *et al.* 1994, for reviews). Specifically, some investigators have questioned whether children have the cognitive ability to make the necessary internal and catastrophic cognitions associated with the somatic symptoms of panic (Nelles and Barlow 1988). However, to our knowledge, the only investigation to directly test this hypothesis suggests children do have this ability (Mattis and Ollendick 1997). Nevertheless, although panic attacks and panic disorder may be common among adolescents they are less frequent in children and typically both adolescents and children report more physiological than cognitive symptoms in the context of their attacks (Ollendick *et al.* 1994).

Owing to the rarity of this disorder in childhood, few general community surveys provide estimates of panic disorder; however, Lewinsohn *et al.* (1993) found a prevalence rate of 0.4% in adolescents. Panic attacks appear to occur more frequently in girls than boys (King *et al.* 1994), although it should be noted that panic attacks may occur within the context of other disorders as well (e.g. separation anxiety disorder, specific phobias) and are not specific to panic disorder. Affective disorders are commonly comorbid with panic disorder (Black and Robbins 1990).

Intervention studies and their effects

Interventions: group outcome studies

Despite the prevalence of anxiety disorders in childhood and adolescence, few studies have examined the efficacy of psychotherapy for treating anxiety in youth. In fact, to date only four controlled group trials have been conducted and all of these investigations have used a cognitive-behavioral therapy (CBT) approach (Dadds *et al.* 1992, Kendall 1994, Barrett *et al.* 1996, Kendall *et al.* in press). In spite of the limited approaches that have been used, several characteristics of these research programs call for optimism. First, in addition to treatment focused specifically on the child, the beginnings of a systematic investigation of the effects of a parent component of treatment have been examined. Second, although treatment outcome research has been criticized for its lack of external validity (e.g. participants in treatment studies are often recruited for the study and are not help-seekers and excluded if presenting with comorbid conditions), children in all four of these investigations were referred by community resources (e.g. schools, mental health professional, medical practitioners). Additionally, limited exclusionary criteria were employed and, in line with actual clinical practice, children evincing comorbid conditions were included. Furthermore, preliminary attempts were made in these studies to look at the effects of the quality of the therapeutic relationship and degree of parental involvement, as well as the possibility of moderating effects of age, sex, and comorbidity on treatment efficacy.

For example, Kendall (1994) investigated the effectiveness of CBT for treating children between the ages of 9 and 13 with primary anxiety disorders (i.e. overanxious disorder, separation anxiety disorder, and avoidant disorder) as compared to a wait-list control condition. Kendall reported the CBT treatment significantly lowered children's self-reported state and trait anxiety, manifest anxiety, fears, depression, and negative self-statements and increased children's ratings of their ability to cope with anxiety provoking situations. In addition, parents also reported significant reduction in children's internalizing behaviors, anxiety, and externalizing behaviors and significant increases in social involvement. Overall, changes were both statistically and clinically (i.e. children scoring in the deviant range on parent/self-reports were returned to within the normal range) significant. Additionally, these effects were not moderated by the quality of the therapeutic relationship or degree of parental involvement in treatment.

More recently Kendall *et al.* (in press) conducted a second randomized clinical trial employing the same CBT program and again found support for the effectiveness of CBT treatment as compared to a no treatment control group. With this trial including a total of 94 participants aged 9–13 years with primary diagnoses of overanxious disorder, separation anxiety disorder, and avoidant disorder, Kendall and his colleagues were able to conduct preliminary analyses examining the effects of comorbidity on treatment outcome. Results indicated that children with one or more comorbid diagnoses were not different from the non-comorbid youth in their post-treatment levels of internalizing symptomatology or distress. However, it should be noted that the comorbid group was a heterogeneous one; thus, definitive conclusions regarding the effects of comorbidity on treatment outcome await more refined investigations.

Dadds *et al.* (1992) and Barrett *et al.* (1996) investigated the effects of parent treatment in conjunction with CBT treatment for children with anxiety disorders. In a preliminary examination, employing a small sample of 14 children between 7 and 14 years of age with primary diagnoses of either overanxious disorder or separation anxiety disorder, support was found for the effectiveness of the CBT plus parent treatment as compared to a no treatment control condition (Dadds *et al.* 1992). In a more extensive investigation, comparing CBT for the child alone with the CBT plus parent treatment (Barrett *et al.* 1996), support was found for the superiority of CBT plus parent treatment over CBT for the child alone. However, it should be noted that child self-reports did not support the effectiveness of either treatment as compared to a no treatment condition, nor the superiority of one method of treatment over the other. On the other hand, parent reports did suggest the superiority of treatment over non-treatment and, on some outcome measures, of CBT plus parent treatment over CBT for the child alone. The discrepancy in parent and child perceptions, however, calls into question the degree to which parent reports were affected by their involvement in treatment and whether the observed trends were influenced by parents' biases or true changes in their children's symptomatology. This caveat notwithstanding, girls and younger children (7–10 years as compared to 11–14 years) had better results with the CBT plus parent treatment as compared to the CBT treatment for the child alone. However, for boys and the older children the treatments were comparable.

In summary, group treatment outcome studies have demonstrated the effectiveness of CBT for anxious children. In addition, investigations have recognized the importance of considering parental involvement, comorbidity, the therapeutic relationship, and children's age and sex. However, we have little information about the effectiveness of other modes of therapy, such as psychodynamic therapy, play therapy, and client-centered therapy for treating childhood anxiety disorders. Furthermore, group studies provide no information about treatment for disorders that are relatively rare in childhood, such as panic disorder, because the rarity of these disorders makes it impractical to study them using group designs. Additionally, group studies typically investigate fairly heterogeneous samples of anxiety disordered children. That is, different diagnostic groups must be considered together. Therefore, we turn to several examples of single case designs that are able to address these issues.

Interventions: single case designs

Again, as with group treatment studies, few single case treatment studies have been conducted to investigate treatment effects on anxiety disorders in childhood and adolescence. Moreover, again similar to group studies, the single case design investigations evaluate solely CBT. For example, Ollendick *et al.* (1991), using a multiple baseline design across subjects, employed CBT to treat the nighttime fears of two young girls with separation anxiety disorder. Treatment consisted of two phases:

- 6 sessions of self-control training
- 8 sessions for one child and 12 sessions for the other of contingency management.

Nighttime fears were targeted specifically because of the prominence of such fears and the girls' inability to sleep in their own beds at the time they presented for treatment. Although self-control training had some impact on the girls' self-reports of anxiety, little evidence of behavioral change (i.e. nights slept in own bed) was shown until the contingency management component was added. Moreover, with the implementation of contingency management strategies, behavioral changes were marked and persistent. Additionally, treatment gains generalized to other aspects of the girls' separation anxiety. Similar effects were demonstrated by Hagopian *et al.* (1990) in the CBT treatment of an 11 year old girl who presented with excessive fears and worries and who was diagnosed with overanxious disorder. Although self-control training ameliorated her symptoms somewhat, the institution of a contingency management system resulted in rapid reduction of the symptoms.

In a similar vein, Hagopian and Slifer (1993) treated a 6 year old girl diagnosed with separation anxiety disorder (with no concurrent diagnoses) using graduated exposure and reinforcement. In this case, the girl's school avoidance was selected as the primary target of treatment because of interference in terms of the negative impact on the girl's academic performance and her mother's absence from work in order to accompany her in school. When exposure was coupled with reinforcement, the girl was successful in remaining in class. Additionally, treatment gains generalized to the girl's ability to cope with other separation situations (e.g. summer camp). At post-treatment the girl no longer met criteria for separation anxiety disorder or any other disorder. Therefore, although reinforcement strategies have not been used in isolation to treat separation anxiety disorder or overanxious disorder, these investigations begin to suggest that reinforcement may be a key component in treating separation anxiety disorder and overanxious disorder. Further investigations are, however, needed to confirm such a hypothesis.

Eisen and Silverman (1993) investigated the utility of CBT and, more specifically, compared the relative efficacy of relaxation training, cognitive therapy, and their combination in the treatment of four children and adolescents between the ages of 6 and 15 years with a primary diagnosis of overanxious disorder. Using a multiple baseline design across subjects they found some evidence for the superiority of cognitive therapy over relaxation training.

Similarly, using a multiple baseline design across subjects, the efficacy of CBT in the treatment of overanxious disorder was demonstrated by Kane and Kendall (1989). Similar to the findings of Hagopian and Slifer (1993), Hagopian *et al.* (1990), and Ollendick *et al.* (1991), treatment gains were most pronounced with the introduction of exposure and positive reinforcement.

Not surprisingly, given the rarity in child and adolescent populations, to our knowledge only one study has investigated treatment outcome in youth with panic disorder and this study was limited to adolescents (Ollendick 1995). Specifically, the adolescents, diagnosed with panic disorder with agoraphobia, were treated using a combination of relaxation training, breathing retraining, self-instruction training, development of positive self-statements and coping strategies, and *in vivo* exposure. Treatment was shown to successfully decrease the frequency of the youths' panic attacks as well as their agoraphobic avoidance. Additionally, the adolescents reported increased feelings of self-efficacy to cope with agoraphobic situations and decreased levels of manifest anxiety, depression, and anxiety sensitivity.

Pharmacological interventions

Tricyclic antidepressants, benzodiazepines, serotonin reuptake inhibitors, β-blockers, buspirone, and monoamine oxidase inhibitors have all been hypothesized as effective pharmacological treatments for anxiety symptomatology (Bernstein *et al.* 1996). However, as with psychotherapy interventions, few studies have investigated the efficacy of pharmacological interventions in treating youth with anxiety disorders. Of these studies, many have not selected participants on the basis of the presence of an anxiety disorder *per se*, rather children were included because of the presence of a specific behavior such as school refusal (e.g. Bernstein *et al.* 1990). Further, although some case studies suggest positive effects for drug interventions (Bernstein 1994), as do open trials (e.g. Kutcher and MacKenzie 1988), controlled, double-blind group studies suggest less optimizm. For example, a comparison of imipramine and placebo for use with children with separation anxiety disorder who did not respond to 1 month of behavioral treatment found no evidence for the superiority of imipramine treatment (Klein *et al.* 1992). Similarly, Simeon *et al.* (1992) did not find alprazolam to be superior to placebo in treating overanxious disorder and avoidant disorder in children between 8 and 16 years of age. These investigations therefore show little support for use of pharmacological interventions in childhood anxiety disorders. However, as noted by Bernstein (1994) these results must be interpreted with caution given methodological limitations in drug research with youth. For example, placebo response rates can be high in children, thus necessitating large sample sizes to detect positive response to drug treatment; however, the studies cited employed relatively small samples. Therefore, although current knowledge suggests weak support for the use of pharmacological treatment for children with anxiety disorders, this conclusion must be tempered by the fact that the studies that would be able to definitively address this issue have yet to be conducted.

Short-term and long-term outcome

Untreated outcomes

Several investigations have examined anxiety disorders in children and adolescents long-itudinally, affording the opportunity to examine the naturally occurring outcomes of anxiety in youth. Evidence from these investigations has suggested that one outcome of anxiety disorders in youth is later psychopathology. For example, McGee *et al.* (1992) examined a sample of youth enrolled in the Dunedin Multidisciplinary Health and Development study at ages 11 and 15 and found that presence of an internalizing disorder (i.e. anxiety or depression) at age 11 was predictive of later psychopathology. However, the specific nature of outcome was moderated by sex. That is, for boys internalizing disorder at age 11 did not predict the presence of an internalizing disorder at age 15. It did, however, predict the presence of an *externalizing disorder* at age 15. In fact, boys with an internalizing disorder at age 11 were almost 6 times as likely as those boys without an internalizing disorder at age 11 to develop an externalizing disorder at age 15. For girls, the opposite was true: girls with an internalizing disorder at age 11 were not more likely than girls without an internalizing disorder at 11 to be diagnosed with an externalizing disorder at age 15; however, they were over 6 times as likely to have an internalizing disorder at age 15. Feehan *et al.* (1993), again examining a group of adolescents from the Dunedin Multidisciplinary Health and Development project sample (partially distinct from the foregoing sample), this time at ages 15 and 18, found that of those with multiple anxiety disorders at age 15, 66.7% had a diagnosable disorder at age 18. Of the 15 adolescents diagnosed with multiple anxiety disorders at 15 years of age, 3 were diagnosed with an anxiety disorder, 3 with depression and anxiety, and 4 with oppositional defiant disorder and/or conduct disorder in conjunction with anxiety and/or affective disorder disorders at age 18. For those with one anxiety disorder (overanxious disorder, separation anxiety disorder, or social phobia) at age 15, 65.9% had a diagnosable disorder again at age 18. Specifically, of the 44 adolescents who had 1 anxiety disorder at age 15, 4 were depressed, 11 were anxious, 6 were anxious and depressed, 1 had conduct disorder, 2 were diagnosed with substance dependence, 1 with substance dependence and conduct disorder and, 4 evidenced oppositional defiant disorder and/or conduct disorder in conjunction with an anxiety and/or affective disorder at age 18. Therefore, it can be seen that one likely outcome of anxiety in youth is continued psychopathology. In fact, although it is commonly believed that anxiety disorders in youth are transient and of little consequence for later development, Feehan *et al.* (1993) found that anxiety comorbid with depression at age 15 was associated with one of the highest rates of later disorder (72.7%).

Additionally, anxiety has been demonstrated to have consequences for academic and social functioning. For example, Ialongo *et al.* (1994) found that children's self-reports of anxiety in the fall of first grade predicted low reading and mathematical achievement in the spring of first grade. In terms of social sequelae, Strauss *et al.* (1988a; 1989) have found that children with anxiety disorders are often socially neglected and that relative to normal controls, they demonstrate less appropriate social skills, are more awkward, shy, and lonely and are viewed as less socially competent.

Treated outcomes

In general, the immediate outcomes (i.e. post-treatment) of children treated for an anxiety disorder are fairly positive both in terms of anxiety and related symptomatology. Additionally, of the group studies reviewed, three included a follow-up assessment and these data too are suggestive of positive outcomes for treated children. For example, Kendall (1994) found that at 1 year post-treatment, most of the children originally diagnosed with overanxious disorder, separation anxiety disorder, or avoidant disorder were diagnosis free. In accordance with this finding, results revealed that treatment gains were maintained, including reductions in anxiety, fears, and depression and increases in coping skills. Recently, Kendall and Southam-Gerow (1996) reported a 3–4 year follow-up of these treated youth. Self- and parent reports, as well as structured diagnostic interviews, revealed maintenance of treatment gains. Similarly, Kendall *et al.* (1997) report maintenance of treatment effects in their most recent study at 1 year follow-up. Moreover, they found that mothers' perceptions of their children's internalizing behavior problems showed a significant decrease from post-treatment to follow-up.

Examining the comparability of outcome for children treated with individual CBT for the child only and CBT plus parent treatment at 6 and 12 months, Barrett *et al.* (1996) found that at 6 months there was no difference between the two groups in terms of number of children free of diagnosis (71.4% for the CBT for the child only group and 84.0% for the CBT plus parent treatment group). However, while the number of children who remained diagnosis free at 12 months decreased slightly in the CBT for child only treatment (70.3%), the number of children in the CBT plus parent treatment group who were diagnosis free at 12 months increased to 95.6%, suggesting significantly better long-term outcome for those children whose parents also received treatment. Moreover, this finding is supported in that at both 6 and 12 month follow-up clinician ratings of improvement were higher for the CBT plus parent treatment group than for the CBT only group.

Single case designs raise the question of impact of life stress and comorbidity on outcome. At 1 year follow-up Ollendick *et al.* (1991) found that their treatment addressing nighttime fears for a child with separation anxiety disorder comorbid with major depression affected both anxious and depressive symptomatology, whereas Kane and Kendall (1989) found differential outcome for the two children they treated with overanxious disorder who were comorbid with a simple phobia compared to the two children diagnosed solely with overanxious disorder. For the two children free of comorbid diagnoses, unqualified positive outcomes were reported at follow-up; however, for the two children with comorbid simple phobias, parent reports suggested some return of anxious symptomatology. For one child it was also noted that medical problems and a death in the family may have played some role in precipitating the return of symptoms. Hence it may be that even children with positive treatment outcomes may retain an increased vulnerability to anxiety.

Unfortunately, little data is available on outcomes other than diagnosis. That is, quality of life issues (e.g. long-term social sequelae, educational and occupational attainment) for anxiety disordered youth have been largely ignored. However, outcomes of treated children are significantly better than those of untreated children. In the absence of treatment, many anxiety-disordered children continue to display ongoing anxiety disorder and others develop depressive and/or disruptive/behavior disorders. Limited information also suggests that treatment effects may be less persistent and durable with comorbid children and adolescents.

Furthermore, optimal treatment outcome may be dependent upon matching of treatment with developmental and contextual factors (Shirk and Russell 1996). Both Kane and Kendall (1989) and Eisen and Silverman (1993) reported that the younger children they treated experienced difficulty with cognitive techniques or required developmentally sensitive modifications to use the techniques effectively. Similarly, the findings of Barrett *et al.* (1996) suggest parental involvement in treatment may enhance outcome for younger children and girls but have less affect on outcome for boys and older children and adolescents. Additionally, treatment may be most effective in producing positive outcome when matched to symptoms (Eisen and Silverman 1993).

Continuity versus discontinuity

Although it has been commonly assumed that anxiety disorders in childhood are transient in nature, current evidence is beginning to dispute this notion. Reviewing epidemiological studies in which multiple waves of data were collected, Costello and Angold (1995) found 20–30% of children having an anxiety disorder at later assessment also had an anxiety disorder at an earlier assessment. Furthermore, they note these estimates of continuity are close to the ceiling set by the reliability of the instruments used to diagnose disorder. In addition, Verhulst and Van der Ende (1992) reported no differences in stability and persistence of internalizing disorders versus externalizing disorders over a 6 year investigation period, whereas Feehan *et al.* (1993) found internalizing disorders to show a somewhat higher degree of specificity than externalizing disorders. Furthermore, as seen in the discussion above regarding the outcomes of anxiety disorders, the most widely documented outcome is subsequent disorder, including anxiety disorders although not limited to them. However, the continuity of internalizing disorders has been found to be more stable for girls than for boys (McGee *et al.* 1992).

Additionally, continuity may be different among the anxiety disorders. For example, Cantwell and Baker (1989) examined the continuity of overanxious disorder, avoidant disorder, separation anxiety disorder, and depressive–dysthymic disorder in a sample of 151 young people between 2 and 15 years. At 4–5 year follow-up, they found 24% of the children and adolescents to have the same disorder as at intake. An additional 42% had an internalizing disorder that differed from their original diagnosis at intake. A total of 66% therefore had either an anxiety disorder or an affective disorder at follow-up 4–5 years later. Specifically, and somewhat ironically inasmuch as the disorder has been dropped for DSM nomenclature, they found avoidant disorder to be the most stable of the anxiety disorders. On the other hand, children diagnosed with separation anxiety disorder showed the greatest rate of recovery and lowest stability. Overanxious disorder was associated with low rates of recovery but also little stability. In other words, children diagnosed with overanxious disorder were likely to continue to evidence difficulties but frequently their symptoms at later ages were reflective of other disorders (e.g. depression).

Similarly, Keller *et al.* (1992) investigated the continuity of disorder in children and adolescents between 6 and 19 years of age with overanxious disorder (some of whom also had a comorbid diagnosis of avoidant disorder) and separation anxiety disorder. They found that the mean duration of disorder for these children, to the point of the interview, was 4 years and that the probability of remaining ill after 8 years was 46%. Furthermore, they reported that of the children who recovered from an anxiety disorder, 31% experienced a subsequent episode of an anxiety disorder. On the other hand, Last *et al.* (1996) followed a group of anxiety disordered children over a 3–4 year period and found that at the end of follow-up, 82% no longer retained their intake diagnosis. Furthermore, they reported relapse for an anxiety disorder to be only 8%.

Offord *et al.* (1992) presented 4 year follow-up data from the Ontario Child Health Study, an epidemiological study of children between the ages of 4 and 12 years. Emotional (i.e. anxiety or depression) disorders were the most common both at the initial assessment (10.8%) and again at the 4 year follow-up (9.7%). Moreover, of the children diagnosed with an emotional disorder at the initial assessment, 26.2% continued to evidence an emotional disorder at follow-up, whereas 14.0% were diagnosed with hyperactivity, and 18.2% were diagnosed as conduct disordered.

Additionally, there is some evidence to suggest continuity between childhood anxiety disorders and anxiety in adulthood. For example, research based on retrospective reports suggest a developmental link between separation anxiety disorder in childhood and panic disorder with agoraphobia in adulthood (Laraia *et al.* 1994, Silove *et al.* 1995). However, it is questionable whether separation anxiety disorder is related specifically to later panic disorder with agoraphobia or if it is associated with adult anxiety disorder in general (Lipsitz *et al.* 1994) or any adult psychopathology (Van der Molen *et al.* 1989).

Risks and prognostic factors

Several areas of investigation, including temperamental factors, parent psychopathology, comorbidity with other disorders, and a host of other environmental and familial factors have been investigated as possible risk and prognostic factors for development and long-term course of anxiety disorders. In many cases the lack of prospective data precludes definitive conclusions regarding whether the characteristics associated with anxiety disorder in childhood are risk factors or correlates of anxiety disorder. In addition, there appears to be a lack of specificity in risk factors such that risks can differentiate between children with and without psychopathology but are not specific to any one disorder (Williams *et al.* 1990).

Temperament

Kagan *et al.* (1984, 1987) have undertaken the examination of one aspect of temperament that has been examined prospectively and linked to development of anxiety disorder, which they describe as behavioral inhibition to the unfamiliar. When exposed to unfamiliar stimuli, behaviorally inhibited children tend to be shy and cautious, withdraw from the unfamiliar, and evidence physiological arousal. Several investigations have linked behavioral inhibition, which can be identified in infancy, to anxiety disorder. Rosenbaum *et al.* (1988) for example, examined rates of behavioral inhibition in children of parents with panic disorder with agoraphobia. Reasoning that these children may be considered at high risk for anxiety disorder, the authors hypothesized that they would evidence higher rates of behavioral inhibition. Findings supported this hypothesis (76% of children of parents with panic disorder with agoraphobia evidenced the characteristics of behavioral inhibition). Although this study provides limited support for the link between behavioral inhibition and anxiety disorders, it should be noted that these children were only at risk for anxiety disorder; no data about actual rate of disorder was reported. However, a subsequent report showed some support for the link between actual anxiety disorder and behavioral inhibition status (Biederman *et al.* 1990). Although the only statistically significant difference between behaviorally inhibited children and their uninhibited counterparts was that the behaviorally inhibited children had higher rates of phobic disorders, a trend was noted for the inhibited children to have two or more anxiety disorders.

In a similar vein of research, Rende (1993) examined the relationship between temperament, measured prospectively for 164 children annually at ages 1–4 years, and behavioral and emotional problems at 7 years. Specifically, he measured three dimensions of temperament— emotionality, activity, and sociability. He found that emotionality but not activity or sociability were positively related to anxiety/depression in boys. For girls, both emotionality and sociability were correlated with girls' level of anxiety/depression, with emotionality being positively related and sociability negatively related.

Parental psychopathology

In general, studies investigating parental psychopathology have found that both anxiety and affective disorders in parents place a child at increased risk for anxiety disorder. For example, Turner *et al.* (1987) investigated psychopathology in offspring of parents with agoraphobia or obsessive–compulsive disorder, parents with dysthymic disorder, and parents without a disorder. They found that children of the anxious probands were seven times as likely to have an anxiety diagnosis as compared to children of the non-disordered probands, and that the risk for anxiety disorder was not significantly different for children of anxiety disordered parents and children of dysthymic parents.

Likewise, Weissman *et al.* (1984) found significantly higher rates of disorder in children of parents with major depression than in children of normal controls. Although major depression was the most prevalent (13.1%) diagnosis, attention deficit disorder and avoidant disorder were found to have the second highest prevalence, with 10.3% of the children of depressed parents evidencing each of these disorders. Similarly, comparing children of normal controls with children of parents with recurrent depression, Orvaschel *et al.* (1988) reported a nonsignificant trend for the children of the depressed parents to have an anxiety disorder. Lastly, Biederman *et al.* (1991) compared children of psychiatrically disordered parents (i.e. children of parents with panic disorder with agoraphobia only, children of parents with panic disorder with agoraphobia and major depression, and children of parents with major depression) to investigate the risk for anxiety and depression. They found that children of the panic disorder with agoraphobia probands, both with and without comorbid depression, were at increased risk for anxiety disorder, but contrary to the results reported above, children of the depressed probands were not at increased risk for an anxiety disorder.

Comorbidity

Children manifesting multiple anxiety disorders or an anxiety disorder comorbid with depression typically present with a more severe symptom presentation than those with only one anxiety disorder. For example, Strauss *et al.* (1988b) examined the effects of comorbidity of anxiety disorders with depression in a sample of 140 children and adolescents between the ages of 5 and 17 presenting to an outpatient anxiety disorders clinic. They found that anxious and depressed youth reported significantly more state and trait anxiety, more physiological anxiety, more worry and oversensitivity, and a greater number of fears than those youth who were anxious only. Additionally, Strauss *et al.* (1988a) reported less positive social outcomes for children with anxiety and depression than for children with anxiety alone. Furthermore, anxiety comorbid with depression has been found to be related to a high rate of later psychopathology (Feehan *et al.* 1993).

The effects of comorbidity of anxiety disorders with externalizing or disruptive behavior disorders are less clear. Moreover, studies investigating comorbid anxiety and externalizing disorders typically focus on prognosis in terms of externalizing symptomatology and not internalizing symptomatology (e.g. Walker *et al.* 1991).

Treatment effects for children with multiple diagnoses are also still unclear. Although some studies have suggested poorer outcome for those with comorbid disorders (Kane and Kendall 1989, Eisen and Silverman 1993), the one group outcome study to investigate the effect of comorbidity on treatment outcome suggested no differences between children with comorbid diagnoses and their anxious only counterparts (Kendall *et al.*, 1997). Nonetheless, comorbidity serves as a negative prognostic factor and is in need of additional inquiry.

Environmental factors, and family and child characteristics

Examining a number of potential risk factors in the Dunedin, New Zealand cohort, including socioeconomic status, children's cognitive ability, child sex, and family relations, Williams *et al.* (1990) found only child's sex and history of maternal depression to distinguish children with internalizing disorders from those with externalizing disorders and multiple disorders. Specifically, girls and children with a mother with a history of depression were at increased risk for internalizing disorder. Similarly, Jensen *et al.* (1990) examined risk factors in a clinic referred sample and non-referred comparison sample of children between the ages of 6 and 12 years whose fathers were in the military. Although they considered maternal/paternal psychopathology, number of children in the family, life stress (as reported by mothers), child's position in the family, and father's rank in the military, only life stress and father's rank were significant predictors of children's level of anxiety. Life stress was positively related to children's self-report of anxiety and father's rank was inversely related. However, together these factors explained only 5% of the variance in children's anxiety.

Finally, studying a cohort from the New York Longitudinal Study, Velez *et al.* (1989) found low socioeconomic status and more specifically, parent education level, and race to be a predictor for separation anxiety disorder, and paternal mental health problems and life events to be risk factors for overanxious disorder.

Conclusions

Recent years have witnessed considerable advances in the assessment, diagnosis, and treatment of anxiety disorders in youth. However, the extent to which current knowledge takes into consideration developmental and familial contextual issues is severely limited. The latest versions of the diagnostic nomenclature have considerably revised the anxiety disorders of childhood. As yet, it remains unclear whether these changes will have positive or negative effects.

Although epidemiological investigations have documented the prevalence rates of anxiety in children and adolescents from several countries, relatively little attention has been devoted to developing treatments for these youth and investigating their efficacy. Nevertheless, psychosocial treatments, and more specifically CBT, have been shown to be effective in ameliorating the effects of anxiety in childhood and adolescence. Moreover, although anxiety disorders in youth may have negative effects such as continued disorder, social maladjustment, and academic difficulties, treated children tend to fare better than those left untreated. Further investigation is needed however, to elucidate the ways in which treatment can be matched to developmental and familial context and to determine whether there are benefits in outcome when this is accomplished. So, too, further investigation is required to examine the cultural context and its role in the development, expression, and treatment of anxious youth.

Early behavioral inhibition, parental anxiety and depression, and life stress appear to be major risk factors for the development of anxiety. Additionally, comorbidity with other disorders may predict a poor prognosis. Many questions have yet to be answered in terms of the stability of anxiety disorders in youth and their relationship to adult anxiety. Continuity of disorder into adulthood has often been used as a marker of significant psychopathology; however, regardless of outcome, the phenomenon of anxiety in children and adolescents is characterized by significant distress and, as such, should not be discounted. The study of anxiety disorder in youth is in its own stage of adolescence; we know much but clearly there is much more to know.

References

Achenbach, T.M. (1991). *Integrative guide for the 1991 CBCL/ 4–18, YSR, and TRF profiles.* University of Vermont, Burlington, VT.

APA (1980). *Diagnostic and statistical manual of mental disorders*, 3rd edn. American Psychiatric Association, Washington, DC.

APA (1987). *Diagnostic and statistical manual of mental disorders*, 3rd edn, revised. American Psychiatric Association, Washington, DC.

APA (1994). *Diagnostic and statistical manual of mental disorders*, 4th edn. American Psychiatric Association, Washington, DC.

Barrett, P.M., Dadds, M.R., and Rapee, R.M. (1996). Family treatment of childhood anxiety: A controlled trial. *Journal of Consulting and Clinical Psychology*, **64**, 333–342.

Beidel, D.C. (1991). Social phobia and overanxious disorder in school-age children. *Journal of the American Academy of Child and Adolescent Psychiatry*, **30**, 545–552.

Beidel, D.C. and Randall, J. (1994). Social phobia. In International handbook of phobic and anxiety disorders in children and adolescents, ed. T.H. Ollendick, N.J. King, and W.Yule, pp. 111–129. Plenum Press, New York.

Bernstein, G.A. (1994). Psychopharmacological interventions. In International handbook of phobic and anxiety disorders in children and adolescents, ed. T.H. Ollendick, N.J. King, and W.Yule, pp. 439–452. Plenum Press, New York.

Bernstein, G.A., Garfinkel, B.D., and Borchardt, C.M. (1990). Comparative studies of pharmacotherapy for school refusal. *Journal of the American Academy of Child and Adolescent Psychiatry*, **29**, 773–781.

Bernstein, G.A., Borchardt, C.M., and Perwien, A.R. (1996). Anxiety disorders in children and adolescents: A review of the past 10 years. *Journal of the American Academy of Child and Adolescent Psychiatry*, **35**, 1110–1119.

Biederman, J., Rosenbaum, J.F., Hirshfeld, D.R., Faraone, S.V., Bolduc, E.A., Gersten, M., Meminger, S.R., Kagan, J., Snidman, N., and Reznick, J.S. (1990). Psychiatric correlates of behavioral inhibition in young children of parents with and without psychiatric disorders. *Archives of General Psychiatry*, **47**, 21–26.

Biederman, J., Rosenbaum, J.F., Bolduc, E.A., Faraone, S.V., and Hirshfeld, D.R. (1991). A high risk study of young children of parents with panic disorder and agoraphobia with and without comorbid major depression. *Psychiatry Research*, **37**, 333–348.

Black, B. (1995). Separation anxiety and panic disorder. In *Anxiety disorders in children and adolescents*, ed. J.S. March, pp. 212–234. Guilford Press, New York.

Black, B. and Robbins, D.R. (1990). Panic disorder in children and adolescents. *Journal of the American Academy of Child and Adolescent Psychiatry*, **29**, 36–44.

Cantwell, D.P. and Baker, L. (1989). Stability and natural history of DSM-III childhood diagnoses. *Journal of the American Academy of Child and Adolescent Psychiatry*, **28**, 691–700.

Cohen, P., Cohen, J., Kasen, S., Velez, C.N., Hartmark, C., Johnson, J., Rojas, M., and Streuning, E.L. (1993). An epidemiological study of disorders in late childhood and adolescence: I. Age- and gender-specific prevalence. *Journal of Child Psychology and Psychiatry and Allied Disciplines*, **34**, 851–867.

Costello, E.J. and Angold, A. (1995). Epidemiology. In *Anxiety disorders in children and adolescents*, ed. J.S. March, pp. 109–124. Guilford Press, New York.

Costello, E.J., Angold, A., Burns, B.J., Stangl, D.K., Tweed, D.L., Erkanli, A., and Worthman, C.M. (1996). The Great Smoky Mountain Study of Youth: Prevalence and correlates of DSM-III-R disorders. *Archives of General Psychiatry*, **53**, 1129–1136.

Dadds, M., Heard, P.M., and Rapee, R.M. (1992). The role of family intervention in the treatment of child anxiety disorders: Some preliminary findings. *Behaviour Change*, **9**, 171–177.

Eisen, A.R. and Silverman, W.K. (1993). Should I relax or change my thoughts? A preliminary examination of cognitive therapy, relaxation training, and their combination with overanxious children. *Journal of Cognitive Psychotherapy*, **7**, 265–279.

Feehan, M., McGee, R., and Williams, S. (1993). Mental health disorders from age 15 to age 18 years. *Journal of the American Academy of Child and Adolescent Psychiatry*, **32**, 1118–1126.

Fergusson, D.M., Horwood, J., and Lynskey, M.T. (1993). Prevalence and comorbidity of the DSM-III-R diagnoses in a birth cohort of 15 year olds. *Journal of the American Academy of Child and Adolescent Psychiatry*, **32**, 1127–1134.

Francis, G., Last, C.G., and Strauss, C.C. (1992). Avoidant disorder and social phobia in children and adolescents. *Journal of the American Academy of Child and Adolescent Psychiatry*, **31**, 1086–1089.

Hagopian, L.P. and Slifer, K.J. (1993). Treatment of separation anxiety disorder with graduated exposure and reinforcement targeting school attendance: A controlled case study. *Journal of Anxiety Disorders*, **7**, 271–280.

Hagopian, L.P., Weist, M.D., and Ollendick, T.H. (1990). Cognitive-behavior therapy with an 11-year-old girl fearful of AIDS infection, other diseases, and poisoning: A case study. *Journal of Anxiety Disorders*, **4**, 257–265.

Ialongo, N., Edelsohn, G., Werthamer-Larsson, L., Crockett, L., and Kellam, S. (1994). The significance of self-reported anxious symptoms in first-grade children. *Journal of Abnormal Child Psychology*, **22**, 441–455.

Jensen, P.S., Bloedau, L., Degroot, J., Ussery, T., and Davis, H. (1990). Children at risk: I. Risk factors and child symptomatology. *Journal of the American Academy of Child and Adolescent Psychiatry*, **29**, 51–59.

Kagan, J., Reznick, J.S., Clarke, C., and Snidman, N. (1984). Behavioral inhibition to the unfamiliar. *Child Development*, **55**, 2212–2225.

Kagan, J., Reznick, J.S., and Snidman, N. (1987). The physiology and psychology of behavioral inhibition in children. *Child Development*, **58**, 1459–1473.

Kane, M.T. and Kendall, P.C. (1989). Anxiety disorders in children: A multiple-baseline evaluation of a cognitive-behavioral treatment. *Behavior Therapy*, **20**, 499–508.

Keller, M.B., Lavori, P.W., Wunder, J., Beardslee, W.R., Schwartz, C.E., and Roth, J. (1992). Chronic course of anxiety disorders in children and adolescents. *Journal of the American Academy of Child and Adolescent Psychiatry*, **31**, 595–599.

Kendall, P.C. (1994). Treating anxiety disorders in children: Results of a randomized clinical trial. *Journal of Consulting and Clinical Psychology*, **62**, 100–110.

Kendall, P.C. and Southam-Gerow, M. (1996). Long-term follow-up of a cognitive-behavioral therapy for anxiety-disordered youth. *Journal of Consulting and Clinical Psychology*, **64**, 724–730.

Kendall, P.C., Flannery-Schroeder, E., Panichelli-Mindel, S.M., Southam-Gerow, M.A., Henin, A., and Warman, M. (1997). Therapy youths with anxiety disorders: A second randomized clinical trial. *Journal of Consulting and Clinical Psychology*, **65**, 366–380.

King, N.J., Ollendick, T.H., and Mattis, S.G. (1994). Panic in children and adolescents: Normative and clinical studies. *Australian Psychologist*, **29**, 14–17.

Klein, R.G., Koplewicz, H.S., and Kanner, A. (1992). Imipramine treatment of children with avoidant disorder. *Journal of the American Academy of Child and Adolescent Psychiatry*, **31**, 21–28.

Kutcher, S.P. and MacKenzie, S. (1988). Successful clonazepam treatment of adolescents with panic disorder. *Journal of Clinical Psychopharmacology*, **8**, 299–301.

Laraia, M.T., Stuart, G.W., Frye, L.H., Lydiard, R.B., and Ballenger, J. (1994). Childhood environment of women having panic disorder with agoraphobia. *Journal of Anxiety Disorders*, **8**, 1–17.

Last, C.G. and Perrin, S. (1993). Anxiety disorders in African-American and White children. *Journal of Abnormal Child Psychology*, **21**, 153–164.

Last, C.G., Strauss, C.C., and Francis, G. (1987). Comorbidity among childhood anxiety disorders. *Journal of Nervous and Mental Disease*, **175**, 726–730.

Last, C.G., Perrin, S., Hersen, M., and Kazdin, A.E. (1996). A prosective study of childhood anxiety disorders. *Journal of the American Academy of Child and Adolescent Psychiatry*, **35**, 1502–1510.

Lewinsohn, P.M., Hops, H., Roberts, R.E., Seeley, J.R., and Andrews, J.A. (1993). Adolescent psychopathology: I. Prevalence and incidence of depression and other DSM-III-R disorders in high school students. *Journal of Abnormal Psychology*, **102**, 133–144.

Lipsitz, J.D., Martin, L.Y., Mannuzza, S., Chapman, T.F., Liebowtiz, M.R., Klein, D., and Fyer, A. (1994). Childhood separation anxiety disorder in patients with adult anxiety disorders. *American Journal of Psychiatry*, **151**, 927–929.

Mattis, S.G. and Ollendick, T.H. (1997). Childrens cognitive responses to the somatic symptoms of panic. *Journal of Abnormal Child Psychology*, **25**, 47–57.

McGee, R., Feehan, M., Williams, S., and Anderson, J. (1992). DSM-II disorders from age 11 to age 15 years. *Journal of the American Academy of Child and Adolescent Psychiatry*, **31**, 50–59.

Moreau, D. and Weissman, M.M. (1992). Panic disorder in children and adolescents: A review. *American Journal of Psychiatry*, **149**, 1306–1314.

Neal, A.M., Lilly, R.S., and Zakis, S. (1993). What are African-American children afraid of? *Journal of Anxiety Disorders*, **7**, 129–139.

Nelles, W.B. and Barlow, D.H. (1988). Do children panic? *Clinical Psychology Review*, **8**, 259–272.

Offord, D.R., Boyle, M.H., Racine, Y.A., Fleming, J.E., Cadman, D.T., Munroe Blum, H., Byrne, C., Links, P.S., Lipman, W.L., MacMillan, H.L., Rae Grant, N.I., Sanford, M.N., Szatmari, P., Thomas, H., and Woodward, C.A. (1992). Outcome, prognosis, and risk in a longitudinal follow-up study. *Journal of the American Academy of Child and Adolescent Psychiatry*, **31**, 916–923.

Ollendick, T.H. (1995). Cognitive behavioral treatment of panic disorder with agoraphobia in adolescents: A multiple baseline design analysis. *Behavior Therapy*, **26**, 517–531.

Ollendick, T.H., Hagopian, L.P., and Huntzinger, R.M. (1991). Cognitive-behavior therapy with nighttime fearful children. *Journal of Behavior Therapy and Experimental Psychiatry*, **22**, 113–121.

Ollendick, T.H., Mattis, S.G., and King, N.J. (1994). Panic in children and adolescents: A review. *Journal of Child Psychology and Psychiatry*, **35**, 113–134.

Ollendick, T.H., Hagopian, L.P., and King, N.J. (1997). Specific phobias in childhood. In *Phobias: a handbook of description, treatment, and theory*, ed. G. Davey, pp. 201–224. Wiley, London.

Orvaschel, H., Walsh-Allis, G., and Ye, W. (1988). Psychopathology in children of parents with recurrent depression. *Journal of Abnormal Child Psychology*, **16**, 17–28.

Rende, R.D. (1993). Longitudinal relations between temperament traits and behavioral syndromes in middle childhood. *Journal of the American Academy of Child and Adolescent Psychiatry*, **32**, 287–290.

Rosenbaum, A.F., Biederman, J., Gersten, M., Hirshfeld, D.R., Meminger, S.R., Herman, J.B., Kagan, J., Reznick, S., and Snidman, N. (1988). Behavioral inhibition in children of parents with panic disorder and agoraphobia: A controlled study. *Archives of General Psychiatry*, **45**, 463–470.

Saylor, C.F. (ed.) (1993). *Children and disasters*. Plenum, New York.

Shirk, S.R. and Russell, R.L. (1996). *Change processes in child psychotherapy: revitalizing treatment and research*. Guilford Press, New York.

Silove, D., Harris, M., Morgan, A., Boyce, P., Manicavasagar, V., Hazdi-Pavlovic, D., and

Wilhelm, K. (1995). Is early separation anxiety a specific precursor of panic disorder-agoraphobia? A community study. *Psychological Medicine*, **25**, 405–411.

Simeon, J.G., Ferguson, B., Knott, V., Roberts, N., Gauthier, B., Dubois, C., and Wiggins, D. (1992). Clinical, cognitive, and neuropsychological effects of alprazolam in children and adolescents with overanxious and avoidant disorders. *Journal of the American Academy of Child and Adolescent Psychiatry*, **31**, 29–33.

Stanger, C., McConaughy, S.H., and Achenbach, T.M. (1992). Three year course of behavioral/emotional problems in a national sample of 4- to 16- year-olds: II. Predictors of syndromes. *Journal of the American Academy of Child and Adolescent Psychiatry*, **31**, 941–950.

Strauss, C.C., Lahey, B.B., Frick, P., Frame, C.L., and Hynd, G.W. (1988a). Peer social status of children with anxiety disorders. *Journal of Consulting and Clinical Psychology*, **56**, 137–141.

Strauss, C.C., Last, C.G., Hersen, M., and Kazdin, A.E. (1988b). Association between anxiety and depression in children and adolescents with anxiety disorders. *Journal of Abnormal Child Psychology*, **16**, 57–68.

Strauss, C.C., Lease, C.A., Last, C.G., and Francis, G. (1988c). Overanxious disorder: An examination of developmental differences. *Journal of Abnormal Child Psychology*, **16**, 433–443.

Strauss, C.C., Lease, C.A., Kazdin, A.E., Dulcan, M.K., Last, C.G. (1989). Multimethod assessment of the social competence of children with anxiety disorders. *Journal of Clinical Child Psychology*, **18**, 184–189.

Turner, S.M., Beidel, D.C., and Costello, A. (1987). Psychopathology in the offspring of anxiety disorders patients. *Journal of Consulting and Clinical Psychology*, **55**, 229–235.

Van der Molen, G.M., Van den Hout, M.A., Van Dieren, A.C., and Griez, E. (1989). Childhood separation anxiety and adult-onset panic disorders. *Journal of Anxiety Disorders*, **3**, 97–106.

Velez, C.N., Johnson, J., and Cohen, P. (1989). A longitudinal analysis of selected risk factors for childhood psychopathology. *Journal of the American Academy of Child and Adolescent Psychiatry*, **28**, 861–864.

Verhulst, F.C. and Van der Ende, J. (1992). Six-year developmental course of internalizing and externalizing problem behaviors. *Journal of the American Academy of Child and Adolescent Psychiatry*, **31**, 924–931.

Walker, J.L., Lahey, B.B., Russo, M.F., Frick, P.J., Christ, M.A., McBurnett, K., Loeber, R., Stouthamer-Loeber, M., and Green, S. (1991). Anxiety, inhibition, and conduct disorder in children: I. Relations to social impairment. *Journal of the American Academy of Child and Adolescent Psychiatry*, **30**, 187–191.

Weissman, M.M., Prusoff, B.A., Gammon, G.D., Merikangas, K.R., Leckman, J.F., and Kidd, K.K. (1984). Psychopathology in the children (ages 6–18) of depressed and normal parents. *Journal of the American Academy of Child Psychiatry*, **23**, 78–84.

WHO (1992). *International classification of diseases*, 10th edn. World Health Organization, Geneva.

Williams, S., Anderson, J., McGee, R., and Silva, P.A. (1990). Risk factors for behavioral and emotional disorder in preadolescent children. *Journal of the American Academy of Child and Adolescent Psychiatry*, **29**, 413–419.

8 Depressive disorders

Richard C. Harrington

Although childhood and adolescence have traditionally been considered times of great turmoil and emotionality, most young people are generally happy individuals and serious depression is infrequent. Nevertheless, over the past 15 years there has been growing concern about those adolescents who do develop major depressive conditions. The use of structured personal interviews, together with standardized diagnostic criteria, has shown that depressive syndromes resembling adult depressive disorders can and do occur among the young. Long-term follow-up studies suggest that severe cases have a high risk of recurrence extending into adult life (Harrington *et al.* 1990) and are at increased risk of both attempted (Myers *et al.* 1991) and completed suicide (Rao *et al.* 1993). The public health importance of depressive disorder in young people is further underlined by the finding that, over the past decade, rates of suicide among young men have increased steadily (Diekstra 1993). Many young suicides suffered from depressive disorders (Marttunen *et al.* 1993).

In this chapter, discussion of the clinical features and epidemiology of childhood-onset depressive conditions precedes a review of interventions, outcomes, and continuities with adult disorders. The general perspective to be presented is that depressive disorder in young people can be a serious problem, with strong continuities over time.

Clinical picture

Great progress has been made in the diagnosis of depressive disorder in children and adolescents. Nevertheless, several problems remain. The clinical assessment of depression depends to an important extent on the young person's verbal account of his or her subjective state. Children do not find it easy to provide an accurate description of how they are feeling, and may confuse emotions such as anger and sadness (Kovacs 1986). Adolescents are better able to describe their emotions, but there is concern that, in comparison with adults, they may overreport depressive symptoms (Allgood-Merten *et al.* 1990). Indeed, feelings such as self-dislike and transient thoughts of self-harm appear to be very common in the general population of adolescents. Presumably, then, adolescents are assigning a different meaning to such phenomena.

Research on depressive conditions in young people has tended to avoid these issues by assuming that adult criteria for depression can be applied unmodified to both children and adolescents. If the appropriate criteria are met, then it is assumed that a significant depressive disorder is present. However, it is becoming clear that, just because a patient meets the symptomatic criteria for a *Diagnostic and Statistical Manual* (DSM) diagnosis, it does not necessarily mean that that person has a clinically significant disorder. Early versions of the

DSM defined a case of major depressive disorder in terms of numbers of symptoms only, and did not require that suffering or social impairment were present. As a result, one adolescent with many minor symptoms causing no impairment came to be regarded as having major depression, whereas another whose few symptoms caused much suffering and social problems was not so regarded.

There is, then, a continuing uncertainty about when normal fluctuation in mood becomes clinical depression. Some investigators have defined major depressive disorder quite broadly, regarding it as present when only the symptom criteria are met. Others attempt to exclude mild, brief, or situational syndromes from the concept of depressive disorder. It is argued that they constitute no more than simple unhappiness, demoralization, or bereavement, and that the credibility of the concept of depressive disorder among the young is damaged by their inclusion (Coyne 1994).

In the present chapter, major depression will be defined using the criteria in the fourth revision of the *Diagnostic and Statistical Manual* (DSM-IV) (APA 1994). These criteria require that symptoms of depressed mood or loss of interest are accompanied by at least four associated symptoms for the same 2 week period, and that these symptoms cause clinically significant distress or impairment in social functioning.

Prevalence and incidence

Given the difficulties with definition, it is not surprising to find that rates of major depressive disorders have varied greatly from study to study. Epidemiological studies of preadolescents have found that the point prevalence of major depression (variously defined, but always in the year prior to interview) is in the 0.5–2.5% range. Epidemiological studies of adolescents have reported higher prevalences, with current rates of major depression ranging from 2 to 8% (Harrington 1994). Studies in clinical samples have found that depressive disorders may be quite common among children referred to mental health centres, occurring in around 25% of cases (Carlson and Cantwell 1980, Kolvin *et al.* 1991).

Early-onset depressive disorders show marked variations in rate with age. Both clinic (Zeitlin 1986, Kolvin *et al.* 1991) and general population studies (Rutter *et al.* 1970, 1976, Cohen *et al.* 1993) suggest that severe depressive conditions are relatively infrequent in early and middle childhood, probably reaching a peak in late adolescence or early adult life. These age trends are particularly marked for girls (Angold and Rutter 1992) so that by late adolescence there is a female preponderance.

It has been suggested that major depression is becoming more common among both adolescents and children. The evidence for this suggestion, however, comes mostly from retrospective accounts of age of onset that have been obtained from subjects who have been ascertained in cross-sectional studies. Probably most of the apparent increase is artefactual, but a small proportion is due to a real change in prevalence (Fombonne 1995).

Comorbidity

One of the most consistent findings from research in clinical populations has been that early onset depressive disorder frequently occurs in conjunction with other conditions, especially behavioural disorders (Harrington *et al.* 1991), and anxiety states (Brady and Kendall 1992). Apparent comorbidity between psychiatric diagnoses in clinical samples could be artefactual as a result of referral or Berksonian biases. However, the epidemiological data confirm that the co-occurrence of depression and other conditions far exceeds that expected by chance (Caron and Rutter 1991).

This high degree of co-occurrence of supposedly distinct psychiatric syndromes raises important questions about the validity of the diagnosis of major depression in this age group. There is some evidence that comorbidity with conduct disorder does signify a different kind of depressive disorder. Thus, in comparison with depressed children who do not have conduct problems, children who meet criteria for both depressive disorder and conduct disorder have been found to have lower rates of depressive disorder and suicidality when followed into adulthood (Harrington *et al.* 1991, 1994), lower rates of depression among relatives (Puig-Antich *et al.* 1989), and greater variability of mood (Costello *et al.* 1991). Depression seems to have a different meaning when it occurs in conjunction with conduct disorder. The converse, however, does not hold. Conduct disorder appears to have the same implications when it is comorbid with depression as when it occurs alone. For instance, young people with depression and behavioural problems are at a greater risk of subsequent antisocial behaviour (Harrington *et al.* 1991). Depressive conduct disorder should, then, be distinguished from other forms of depression.

The nosological implications of the overlap between depression and non-behavioural disorders are unclear. For instance, although anxiety may signal a more severe type of disorder and tends to precede the depression (Brady and Kendall 1992), on present evidence it is unlikely that it indicates a qualitatively different form of depressive condition.

Studies of natural course

Little is known about the natural history of untreated depression among the young. Most outcome studies have been based on clinical samples, who have usually had treatment of one kind or another. However, retrospective studies of untreated cases suggest that a high proportion will recover eventually (Keller *et al.* 1988).

Intervention studies

Individual psychological treatments

The best treatment for major depression in adolescence is not yet clearly established. However, in the absence of reliable evidence from controlled trials that antidepressant medications significantly improve the outcomes (see below), the treatments of first choice for many clinicians are psychological. By far the best evaluated of the psychological interventions is cognitive-behavioural therapy (CBT). Studies of clinically depressed adolescents have repeatedly shown that CBT is more effective than comparison interventions (Harrington *et al.* in press). For instance, Wood *et al.* (1996) found that CBT led to a significantly greater improvement than relaxation training in both depression and global functioning. These changes were clinically significant and, in many cases, persisted for 6 months.

A variety of slightly different CBT programmes have been developed for use with depressed adolescents; most of them have been published or are available as manuals. Training of therapists can, therefore, be accomplished with relative ease. Most CBT programmes last for no longer than 15 sessions and several are available that last for just 8.

Several other individual psychological treatments are available for use with depressed adolescents, of which probably the best-known is interpersonal psychotherapy. This has an emphasis on dealing with interpersonal issues and role transitions, and appears to be feasible in this age group (Moreau *et al.* 1991). It remains to be seen whether it will prove to be effective in randomized controlled designs.

Serotonin selective reuptake inhibitors

Concerns about both the efficacy and safety of the tricyclic antidepressants (see below) have meant that in many centres the serotonin selective reuptake inhibitors (SSRIs) have become the most commonly used antidepressants. Unfortunately, less is known about the effectiveness and side-effects of the SSRIs in this age group than about the tricyclics. However, on the basis of adult experience, drugs such as fluoxetine and paroxetine should be less toxic to the heart and nervous system than the tricyclics (TCAs).

The most commonly used SSRIs with adolescents are fluoxetine and paroxetine. Experience is also accumulating with sertraline and fluvoxamine. The evidence from open studies is that around 60–70% of cases will show some improvement, but there have thus far been only two published placebo-controlled trials, one with a negative result (Simeon *et al.* 1990) and one with a positive result (Emslie *et al.* 1997).

Tricyclic antidepressants

Controlled trials with tricyclic antidepressants (TCAs) have mostly shown no significant benefits over placebo (Harrington 1992). It is unclear why TCAs are less effective for depressive disorders in adolescents than they are for the apparently identical condition in adults. It has been suggested that there are developmental variations in the rate of metabolism of psychotropics, which make it harder to get the dosage right. It is also possible that adolescent depression, though phenotypically similar to adult depression, differs in some respect that might affect drug responsiveness. For instance, it may be that the patients admitted to drug trials have been more severely impaired. Alternatively, it is possible that adolescents differ from adults in the neurotransmitter systems on which TCAs are thought to act.

There are not only uncertainties about the efficacy of TCAs, but also concerns about their toxicity. Many depressed adolescents are suicidal and the TCAs are very toxic in overdose. Moreover, even in therapeutic doses, the TCAs have been associated with electrocardiographic changes, and in vulnerable individuals there may be untoward effects on the central nervous system, such as drowsiness or confusion. There are large interindividual variations in steady-state plasma levels of TCAs, so one-off plasma levels are not a reliable guide to toxicity. It can, therefore, be very difficult to get the dosage right.

It should be borne in mind, however, that there have still been only a handful of properly conducted randomized controlled trials of the TCAs in this age group (Hazell *et al.* 1995). The evidence that TCAs are effective in adult depressive disorders is so strong that there is still a case for using them as second-line treatments with older adolescents who have typical depressive disorders and in whom the risk of attempted suicide is low.

Prevention of relapse

Many studies have shown that young people who remit from major depression have a high risk of relapse (see later). In clinical samples, this is probably as high as 50% within the year after remission. Relapse seems to be particularly high within the first few months of remission. Factors that have been shown to predict relapse include comorbidity with non-depressive disorders, greater severity, and higher levels of adversity.

A similarly high rate of relapse after remission from the acute episode has been found in studies of adult depressed cases. However, controlled studies with depressed adults suggest that this relapse risk can be significantly reduced by continuing either pharmacological or psychological treatments for several months after apparent remission (Kupfer 1992). The theory underlying these continuation treatments is that suppression of symptoms by the acute phase of the treatment does not necessarily mean that the individual has completely recovered from the index episode. He or she may remain vulnerable to a relapse for several months. Continuation of treatment aims to stop symptoms returning.

Research on the prevention of depression in young people is at an early stage. Preliminary findings from community studies of children and adolescents designated as at risk because of depressive symptoms have shown that CBT is associated with a reduced risk of subsequent depressive disorder (Clarke *et al.* 1995). In clinical samples, a non-randomized study suggests that continuation of CBT for 6 months after apparent remission is both feasible and associated with an apparent lower risk of recurrence (Kroll *et al.* 1996). It remains to be seen whether efficacy will be demonstrated in randomized controlled trials. In the meantime, it is sensible to continue the treatments that have led to remission for several months. Alternatively, cases at low risk for relapse should be seen regularly for check-ups during which the adolescent's mental state should be assessed. Depressive disorders in adolescents require long-term approaches to treatment.

Family interventions

There is a strong association between depressive disorder in adolescence and mental problems in parents. We shall see later that this association almost certainly arises in part from environmental processes, such as exposure to parental criticism or from other problems in parenting. However, present evidence from controlled trials suggests that family therapy is not as effective as individual CBT with the child (Brent *et al.* 1997).

Short-term outcomes

Issues in the definition of outcome

A review (Frank *et al.* 1991) has highlighted the problems involved in defining change-points in the course of depressive disorder in adults. For example, when does partial remission become recovery? How should an episode of depression be defined? Much the same kinds of questions have been raised in research on the course of depression in young people. Definitions have been very heterogeneous. For instance, in the study of Kovacs *et al.* (1984a, b) the definition of 'recovery' included mental states in which there was persistence of some subclinical symptoms, whereas in the study by Goodyer and Altham (1991) recovery was defined as no mental state abnormalities whatsoever.

These problems of defining and measuring recovery and relapse are formidable enough, but a further problem in the interpretation of follow-ups of depressed children arises from the fact that these children often have other psychiatric problems, such as conduct disorder. The problem is that few follow-ups of depressed young people have used a comparison group who were closely matched according to the *presence* of non-depressive symptomatology. It is therefore often unclear whether the risk for adverse outcomes is a function of the earlier depression or whether, in fact, it stems from these associated psychiatric problems.

Recovery from the index episode

The available data suggest that many children with major depression will recover from their initial episode within a year or two. Probably the best data on recovery come from the studies of Kovacs and her colleagues. These investigators reported that the cumulative probability of recovery from major depression by 1 year after onset was 74%, and 2 years it was 92% (Kovacs *et al.* 1984b). This study included many subjects who had previous emotional–behavioral problems and some form of treatment. However, very similar results were reported by Keller *et al.* (1988) in a retrospective study of time to recovery from first episode of major depression in young people who had mostly not received treatment. Goodyer and Altham (1991) found that one-half of depressed children were free of symptoms within a year of their first assessment. Similarly, it seems that most adolescents with major depression usually recover within a year (Strober *et al.* 1993).

Unfortunately, in some cases depression in young people can become chronic and unremitting. Different definitions of chronicity have been used and therefore it is difficult to be confident about the exact rates of chronicity. Ryan *et al.* (1987) for example, defined chronicity as a duration of depression of more than 2 years, whereas Shain *et al.* (1991) defined it as a duration of just 1 year. In the study of Ryan and colleagues nearly one-half of subjects had either chronic major depression or fluctuating dysthymia with major depression. Roughly the same proportion turned out to be chronic cases in the study of Shain *et al.* (1991): chronicity seemed to be associated with increased suicidality but not, surprisingly, with an increased length of stay in hospital.

Outcome

Even when they recover, young people with depressive disorders are at increased short-term risk of subsequent episodes of depression. Thus, many early uncontrolled studies reported that children who had had one episode of depression were at risk of another. For instance, Poznanski *et al.* (1976) found that 5 out of 10 depressed children who were re-evaluated on average 6 years later were depressed. Controlled studies have, by and large, confirmed that the risk of subsequent depression among depressed young people is more than would be expected by chance. In one of the most systematic studies conducted so far, Kovacs *et al.* (1984a; Kovacsb) undertook a follow-up of child patients with a major depressive disorder, a dysthymic disorder, an adjustment disorder with depressed mood, and some other psychiatric disorder. The development of subsequent episodes of depression was virtually confined to children with major depressive disorders and dysthymic disorders. Within the first year at risk, 26% of children who had recovered from major depression experienced another episode; by 2 years this figure had risen to 40%; and by 5 years the cohort ran a 72% risk of another episode. Similarly, Asarnow *et al.* (1988) found that children who had been hospitalized with major depression were at increased risk of rehospitalization during the year after discharge because of suicidal behaviour or increasing depression.

Studies of the short-term stability of depressive symptoms in community samples of adolescents have also found significant correlations over time. Larsson *et al.* (1991) found a correlation over a period of 4–6 weeks on the Beck Inventory of 0.66. Garrison *et al.* (1990) reported that stability of adolescents' scores on the Centre for Epidemiological Studies Depression Scale was 0.53 at one year, and 0.36 at 2 years after the initial assessment.

Continuities versus discontinuities

None of the studies discussed above has yet extended beyond mid-adolescence, but a similarly high rate of subsequent psychiatric morbidity has been reported in follow-up studies of depressed adolescents that have extended into late adolescence or early adult life. These studies have suggested both that self-ratings of depression in adolescent community samples predict similar problems in early adulthood (Kandel and Davies 1986) and that adolescent patients with depressive disorders are at high risk of subsequent major affective disorder (Strober and Carlson 1982, Garber *et al.* 1988). Although the findings of these studies are limited by issues such as the uncertainty regarding the connection between depression questionnaire scores and clinical depressive disorder and high rates of sample attrition, they clearly suggest that adolescents with depression are at increased risk of depression in early adulthood.

Moving still further into adult life, Harrington *et al.* (1990) followed up 63 depressed children and adolescents, on average 18 years after their initial contact. The depressed group had a significantly greater risk of depression in adulthood than a control group who had been carefully matched for a large number of variables, including non-depressive symptoms. Depressed children were no more likely than control children to suffer non-depressive disorders in adulthood, suggesting that the risk for adult major depression was specific and unrelated to comorbidity with other psychiatric problems. Rao *et al.* (1995) have also found that the risk of depressive disorder in adulthood was significantly higher in childhood depressed cases that in controls. Zeitlin (1986), in his study of child psychiatric patients who attended the same hospital as adults, also found strong child- to-adult continuities for depression.

Several studies have examined the long-term social impact of depression in young people. Puig-Antich *et al.* (1993, 1985a,b) found impairment of peer relationships persisted for months or even years after recovery from depression. Kandel and Davies (1986) reported that self-ratings of dysphoria in adolescence were associated with heavy cigarette smoking, greater involvement in delinquent activities, and impairment of intimate relationships as young adults. Garber *et al.* (1988) found that depressed adolescent in-patients reported more marital and relationship problems when they were followed up 8 years after discharge than non-depressed psychiatric control subjects.

Association with suicidal behaviour and suicide

Depressed young people very commonly have suicidal thoughts and some of them make suicidal attempts. For instance, Ryan *et al.* (1987) found that about 60% of children and adolescents with major depression had suicidal thinking. Mitchell *et al.* (1988) reported that around two-thirds of depressed children and adolescents had suicidal ideation, and 39% had made an attempt. Conversely, it seems that suicidal children are at increased risk of depression. For example, Kerfoot *et al.* (1996) found that around one-half of adolescents who had taken an overdose met criteria for major depression. It may be, however, that depression has a different meaning when it occurs in the context of an overdose. Follow-up of the sample of Kerfoot *et al.* showed that so-called major depression remitted very rapidly in the majority of cases. It seemed that adolescent self-reports of depression were relatively unstable in that sample.

Little is known about the risk of completed suicide in depressed children and adolescents, but the available data suggest that there is a significant risk of subsequent completed suicide. In a preliminary communication from a longitudinal study of the depressed children and adolescents initially studied by Puig-Antich and coworkers, Rao *et al.* (1993) reported that seven (4.4%) had committed suicide in adulthood. There were no suicides in the psychiatric control group. This rate of suicide is far in excess of that expected in the general population of young adults. It is important to note, however, that three of the seven suicides were by TCA overdoses. Clearly, physicians need to be careful not to contribute to their patients' adverse outcomes.

Psychological autopsy studies of suicide in young people have generally found high rates of affective disorders. Around 50% of young people who kill themselves have suffered from a significant depressive condition (Marttunen *et al.* 1993). Other mental disorders are, however, also relevant to juvenile suicide. A significant proportion of young suicides suffer from conduct disorders or antisocial personality, and around a quarter abuse alcohol or drugs (Marttunen *et al.* 1993). It seems likely that it is the combination of depression and certain personality characteristics, such as risk-taking behaviour, that is especially likely to lead to suicide in young people. There seems to be an important relationship between comorbid disorders and depression in respect of suicidal risk.

Risks and prognostic factors

The characteristics of the index depressive episode appear to be important to the extent that children with 'double depression' (DSM major depression and dysthymia) have a worse short-term outcome than children with major depression alone (Kovacs *et al.* 1984a,b, Asarnow *et al.* 1988). Continuity to adulthood seems best predicted by a severe 'adult-like depressive presentation' and, interestingly, by the absence of conduct disorder (Harrington *et al.* 1990, 1991). Two studies have found that older depressed children have a worse prognosis than younger depressed children (Kovacs *et al.* 1989, Harrington *et al.* 1990).

There is evidence that certain kinds of stressors, particularly those occurring within the family, may be important in predicting the outcome in depressed young people. Asarnow *et al.* (1993) found that relapse of major depression was strongly linked with high maternal expressed emotion. Hammen and her colleagues (Hammen *et al.* 1988, Hammen 1991) examined the influence of initial depression in the child, stressful events, maternal depressive symptoms, and the interaction between events and symptoms in predicting depression at 6 month follow-up. The level of initial depression in the child was the strongest predictor of subsequent depression, but maternal symptoms were also a strong independent predictor of subsequent depression. Of course, it could be that this association is simply a reflection of the fact that both maternal depression and depression in the child are the result of genetic predisposition. However, Hammen *et al.* (1991) also found a close *temporal* relationship between maternal and child depression, suggesting that the links may have been a reflection of some kind of environmental factor, such as chronic intrafamilial stress.

Longitudinal studies suggest that extrafamilial adversities, such as problems in peer relationships (Goodyer *et al.* 1991) or adverse life events can also predict continuity. It is likely that there is an interaction between family variables and these adversities, such that one increases the risk of the other. Thus, Goodyer *et al.* (1993) reported that the families of depressed girls seemed to become life event prone as a result of parental psychopathology. Perhaps, then, young people become depressed when depressed parents are no longer able to protect them from, or support them through, adversity.

Conclusions

What, then, can be concluded from this research? The most important point is that both researchers and clinicians need to take a long-term view of the management of juvenile depressive disorders. It is sometimes assumed that the rapid recovery of depressed children means that treatment endeavours need only focus on the short-term. This is clearly not the case. It is apparent that both assessment and treatment need to be viewed as extending over a prolonged period of time. Young people with depressive disorders are likely to have another episode and it is important that we develop effective maintenance and/or prophylactic treatments. Thus, for example, studies are urgently needed on continuation or maintenance treatments. Preliminary findings indicate that such treatments are feasible, but it remains to be seen whether they will be effective in preventing relapse.

The second point is that, although early-onset depressive conditions often have substantial self-perpetuating qualities, the course is much influenced by environmental circumstances, especially family difficulties. It may be possible to intervene therapeutically to improve patterns of family relationships, although it has to be said that the evidence available so far suggests family therapies are not as effective as individual treatments.

The final point concerns the extent of the continuities between child and adolescent depressive disorders and depression in adulthood. The evidence reviewed here suggests that there are substantial temporal continuities between early-onset depression and depression in adult-life. The implication is that, at least in some instances, depression in young people represents the same condition as depression in adulthood. It is puzzling, then, that is does not respond to one of the best established treatments for adult depression, TCAs. These contradictory findings suggest that there are *both* similarities and differences between child and adult depression. A better understanding of this pattern of continuities and discontinuities should lead to better treatments and, eventually, to improved outcomes.

Acknowledgements

The author's recent research on depressive disorders has been supported by the MacArthur Foundation Network on Psychopathology and Development and by the Mental Health Foundation.

References

Allgood-Merten, B., Lewinsohn, P.M., and Hops, H. (1990). Sex differences and adolescent depression. *Journal of Abnormal Psychology*, **99**, 55–63.

Angold, A. and Rutter, M. (1992). Effects of age and pubertal status on depression in a large clinical sample. *Development and Psychopathology*, 4, 5–28.

APA (1994). *Diagnostic and statistical manual of mental disorders*, 4th edn. American Psychiatric Association, Washington DC.

Asarnow, J.R., Goldstein, M.J., Carlson, G.A., Perdue, S., Bates, S., and Keller, J. (1988). Childhood-onset depressive disorders. A follow-up study of rates of rehospitalization and out-of-home placement among child psychiatric inpatients. *Journal of Affective Disorders*, **15**, 245–253.

Asarnow, J.R., Goldstein, M.J., Tompson, M., and Guthrie, D. (1993). One-year outcomes of depressive disorders in child psychiatric inpatients: evaluation of the prognostic power of a brief measure of expressed emotion. *Journal of Child Psychology and Psychiatry*, **34**, 129–137.

Brady, E.U. and Kendall, P.C. (1992). Comorbidity of anxiety and depression in children and adolescents. *Psychological Bulletin*, **111**, 244–255.

Brent, D., Holder, D., Kolko, D., Birmaher, B., Baugher, M., Roth, C., Iyengar, S., and Johnson, B. (1997). A clinical psychotherapy trial for adolescent depression comparing cognitive, family, and supportive treatments. *Archives of General Psychiatry*, **54**, 877–885.

Carlson, G.A. and Cantwell, D.P. (1980). A survey of depressive symptoms, syndrome and disorder in a child psychiatric population. *Journal of Child Psychology and Psychiatry*, **21**, 19–25.

Caron, C. and Rutter, M. (1991). Comorbidity in child psychopathology: concepts, issues and research strategies. *Journal of Child Psychology and Psychiatry*, **32**, 1063–1080.

Clarke, G.N., Hawkins, W., Murphy, M., Sheeber, L.B., Lewinsohn, P.M., and Seeley, J.R. (1995). Targeted prevention of unipolar depressive disorder in an at-risk sample of high school adolescents: a randomized trial of a group cognitive intervention. *Journal of the American Academy of Child and Adolescent Psychiatry*, **34**, 312–321.

Cohen, P., Cohen, J., Kasen, S., Velez, C.N., Hartmark, C., Johnson, J., Rojas, M., Brook, J., and Streuning, E.L. (1993). An epidemiological study of disorders in late childhood and adolescence—I. Age- and gender-specific prevalence. *Journal of Child Psychology and Psychiatry*, **34**, 851–867.

Costello, E.J., Benjamin, R., Angold, A., and Silver, D. (1991). Mood variability in adolescents: a study of depressed, nondepressed and comorbid patients. *Journal of Affective Disorders*, **23**, 199–212.

Coyne, J.C. (1994). Self-reported distress: Analog or ersatz depression? . *Psychological Bulletin*, **116**, 29–45.

Diekstra, R.F.W. (1993). The epidemiology of suicide and parasuicide. *Acta Psychiatrica Scandinavica, Suppl* **371**, 9–20.

Emslie, G., Rush, A., Weinberg, W., Kowatch, R., Hughes, C., Carmody, T. and Rintelmann, J. (1997). A double-blind, randomized placebo-controlled trial of fluo–xetine in depressed children and adolescents. *Archives of General Psychiatry*, **54**, 1031–1037.

Fombonne, E. (1995). Depressive disorders: time trends and putative explanatory mechanisms. In *Psychosocial disorders in young people: time trends and their origins*, ed. M.Rutter and D.Smith, pp. 544–615. Wiley, Chichester.

Frank, E., Prien, R.F., Jarrett, R.B., Keller, M.B., Kupfer, D.J., Lavori, P.W., Rush, A.J., and Weissman, M.M. (1991). Conceptualization and rationale for consensus definitions of terms in major depressive disorder. Remission, recovery, relapse, and recurrence. *Archives of General Psychiatry*, **48**, 851–855.

Garber, J., Kriss, M.R., Koch, M., and Lindholm, L. (1988). Recurrent depression in adolescents: a follow-up study. *Journal of the American Academy of Child Psychiatry*, **27**, 49–54.

Garrison, C.Z., Jackson, K.L., Marsteller, F., McKeown, R., and Addy, C. (1990). A longitudinal study of depressive symptomatology in young adolescents. *Journal of the American Academy of Child Psychiatry*, **29**, 581–585.

Goodyer, I.M., and Altham, P.M. E. (1991). Lifetime exit events and recent social and family adversities in anxious and depressed school-age children and adolescents—I. *Journal of Affective Disorders*, **21**, 219–228.

Goodyer, I.M., Germany, E., Gowrusankur, J., and Altham, P. (1991). Social influences on the course of anxious and depressive disorders in school-age children. *British Journal of Psychiatry*, **158**, 676–684.

Goodyer, I.M., Cooper, P.J., Vize, C., and Ashby, L. (1993). Depression in 11 to 16 year old girls: the role of past parental psychopathology and exposure to recent life events. *Journal of Child Psychology and Psychiatry*, **34**, 1103–1115.

Hammen, C. (1991). *Depression runs in families. the social context of risk and resilience in children of depressed mothers*. Springer-Verlag, New York.

Hammen, C., Adrian, C., and Hiroto, D. (1988). A longitudinal test of the attributional vulnerability model in children at risk for depression. *British Journal of Clinical Psychology*, **27**, 37–46.

Hammen, C., Burge, D., and Adrian, C. (1991). Timing of mother and child depression in a longitudinal study of children at risk. *Journal of Consulting and Clinical Psychology*, **59**, 341–345.

Harrington, R.C. (1992). Annotation: the natural history and treatment of child and adolescent affective disorders. *Journal of Child Psychology and Psychiatry*, **33**, 1287–1302.

Harrington, R.C. (1994). Affective disorders. in, *Child and adolescent psychiatry: modern approaches*, 3rd edn, ed. M.Rutter, E. Taylor and L. Hersov, pp. 330–350. Blackwell Scientific, Oxford.

Harrington, R.C., Fudge, H., Rutter, M., Pickles, A., and Hill, J. (1990). Adult outcomes of childhood and adolescent depression: I. Psychiatric status. *Archives of General Psychiatry*, *47*, pp. 465–473.

Harrington, R.C., Fudge, H., Rutter, M., Pickles, A., and Hill, J. (1991). Adult outcomes of childhood and adolescent depression: II. Risk for antisocial disorders. *Journal of the American Academy of Child Psychiatry*, *30*, pp. 434–439.

Harrington, R.C., Bredenkamp, D., Groothues, C., Rutter, M., Fudge, H., and Pickles, A. (1994). Adult outcomes of childhood and adolescent depression. III. Links with suicidal behaviours. *Journal of Child Psychology and Psychiatry*, **35**, 1380–1391.

Harrington, R.C., Wood, A., and Verduyn, C. (1998) Principles and practice of cognitive-behaviour therapy in clinically depressed adolescents. In *Cognitive behaviour therapy for children and their families*, ed. P.Graham, pp. 156–93. Cambridge University Press, Cambridge.

Hazell, P., OConnell, D., Heathcote, D., Robertson, J., and Henry, D. (1995). Efficacy of tricyclic drugs in treating child and adolescent depression: a meta-analysis. *British Medical Journal*, **310**, 897–901.

Kandel, D.B. and Davies, M. (1986). Adult sequelae of adolescent depressive symptoms. *Archives of General Psychiatry*, **43**, 255–262.

Keller, M.B., Beardslee, W., Lavori, P.W., Wunder, J., Drs, D.L., and Samuelson, H. (1988). Course of major depression in non-referred adolescents: a retrospective study. *Journal of Affective Disorders*, **15**, 235–243.

Kerfoot, M., Dyer, E., Harrington, V., Woodham, A., and Harrington, R.C. (1996). Correlates and short-term course of self-poisoning in adolescents. *British Journal of Psychiatry*, **168**, 38–42.

Kolvin, I., Barrett, M.L., Bhate, S.R., Berney, T.P., Famuyiwa, O.O., Fundudis, T., and Tyrer, S. (1991). The Newcastle Child Depression Project: diagnosis and classification of depression. *British Journal of Psychiatry*, **159** (suppl. 11), 9–21.

Kovacs, M. (1986). A developmental perspective on methods and measures in the assessment of depressive disorders: the clinical interview. In, *Depression in young people: developmental and clinical perspectives*, ed. M. Rutter, C.E. Izard, and R.B. Read, pp. 435–465. Guilford Press, New York.

Kovacs, M., Feinberg, T.L., Crouse-Novak, M., Paulauskas, S.L., Pollock, M., and Finkelstein, R. (1984a) Depressive disorders in childhood. II. A longitudinal study of the risk for a subsequent major depression. *Archives of General Psychiatry*, **41**, 643–649.

Kovacs, M., Feinberg, T.L., Crouse-Novak, M.A., Paulauskas, S.L., and Finkelstein, R. (1984b) Depressive disorders in childhood. I. A longitudinal prospective study of characteristics and recovery. *Archives of General Psychiatry*, **41**, 229–237.

Kovacs, M., Gatsonis, C., Paulauskas, S., and Richards, C. (1989). Depressive disorders in childhood. IV. A longitudinal study of comorbidity with and risk for anxiety disorders. *Archives of General Psychiatry*, **46**, 776–782.

Kroll, L., Harrington, R.C., Gowers, S., Frazer, J., and Jayson, D. (1996). Continuation of cognitive-behavioural treatment in adolescent patients who have remitted from major depression. Feasibility and comparison with historical controls. *Journal of the American Academy of Child and Adolescent Psychiatry*, **35**, 1156–1161.

Kupfer, D. (1992). Maintenance treatment in recurrent depression: current and future directions. *British Journal of Psychiatry*, **161**, 309–316.

Larsson, B., Melin, L., Breitholtz, E., and Andersson, G. (1991). Short-term stability of depressive symptoms and suicide attempts in Swedish adolescents. *Acta Psychiatrica Scandinavica*, **83**, 385–390.

Marttunen, M.J., Aro, H.M., and Lonnqvist, J.K. (1993). Adolescence and suicide: a review of psychological autopsy studies. *European Child and Adolescent Psychiatry*, **2**, 10–18.

Mitchell, J., McCauley, E., Burke, P.M., and Moss, S.J. (1988). Phenomenology of depression in children and adolescents. *Journal of the American Academy of Child Psychiatry*, **27**, 12–20.

Moreau, D., Mufson, L., Weissman, M.M., and Klerman, G.L. (1991). Interpersonal psychotherapy for adolescent depression: description of modification and preliminary application. *Journal of the American Academy of Child Psychiatry*, **30**, 642–651.

Myers, K., McCauley, E., Calderon, R., and Treder, R. (1991). The 3-year longitudinal course of suicidality and predictive factors for subsequent suicidality in youths with major depressive disorder. *Journal of the American Academy of Child Psychiatry*, **30**, 804–810.

Poznanski, E.O., Kraheneuhl, V., and Zrull, J.P. (1976). Childhood depression—a longitudinal perspective. *Journal of the American Academy of Child Psychiatry*, **15**, 491–501.

Puig-Antich, J., Lukens, E., Davies, M., Goetz, D., Brennan-Quattrock, J., and Todak, G. (1985a) Psychosocial functioning in prepubertal major depressive disorders. II. Interpersonal relationships after sustained recovery from affective episode. *Archives of General Psychiatry*, **42**, 511–517.

Puig-Antich, J., Lukens, E., Davies, M., Goetz, D., Brennan-Quattrock, J., and Todak, G. (1985b) Psychosocial functioning in prepubertal major depressive disorders. I. Interpersonal relationships during the depressive episode. *Archives of General Psychiatry*, **42**, 500–507.

Puig-Antich, J., Goetz, D., Davies, M., Kaplan, T., Davies, S., Ostrow, L., Asnis, L., Twomey, J., Iyengar, S., and Ryan, N.D. (1989). A controlled family history study of prepubertal major depressive disorder. *Archives of General Psychiatry*, **46**, 406–418.

Puig-Antich, J., Kaufman, J., Ryan, N.D., Williamson, D.E., Dahl, R.E., Lukens, E., Todak, G., Ambrosini, P., Rabinovich, H., and Nelson, B. (1993). The psychosocial functioning and family environment of depressed adolescents. *Journal of the American Academy of Child and Adolescent Psychiatry*, **32**, 244–253.

Rao, U., Weissman, M.M., Martin, J.A., and Hammond, R.W. (1993). Childhood depression and risk of suicide: preliminary report of a longitudinal study. *Journal of the American Academy of Child Psychiatry*, **32**, 21–27.

Rao, U., Ryan, N.D., Birmaher, B., Dahl, R.E., Williamson, D.E., Kaufman, J., Rao, R., and Nelson, B. (1995). Unipolar depression in adolescence: clinical outcome in adulthood. *Journal of the American Academy of Child and Adolescent Psychiatry*, **34**, 566–578.

Rutter, M., Tizard, J., and Whitmore, K. (ed.). (1970). *Education, health and behaviour*. Longmans, London.

Rutter, M., Graham, P., Chadwick, O.F., and Yule, W. (1976). Adolescent turmoil: fact or fiction? *Journal of Child Psychology and Psychiatry*, **17**, 35–56.

Ryan, N.D., Puig-Antich, J., Ambrosini, P., Rabinovich, H., Robinson, D., Nelson, B., Iyengar, S., and Twomey, J. (1987). The clinical picture of major depression in children and adolescents. *Archives of General Psychiatry*, **44**, 854–861.

Shain, B.N., King, C.A., Naylor, M., and Alessi, N. (1991). Chronic depression and hospital course in adolescents. *Journal of the American Academy of Child Psychiatry*, **30**, 428–433.

Simeon, J.G., Dinicola, V.F., Ferguson, H.B., and Copping, W. (1990). Adolescent depression: a placebo-controlled fluoxetine treatment study and follow-up. *Progress in Neuro-Psychopharmacology and Biological Psychiatry*, **14**, 791–795.

Strober, M. and Carlson, G. (1982). Bipolar illness in adolescents with major depression: clinical, genetic and psychopharmocologic predictors in a three- to four-year prospective follow-up investigation. *Archives of General Psychiatry*, **39**, 549–555.

Strober, M., Lampert, C., Schmidt, S., and Morrell, W. (1993). The course of major depressive disorder in adolescents: I. Recovery and risk of manic switching in a 24-month prospective, naturalistic follow-up of psychotic and nonpsychotic subtypes. *Journal of the American Academy of Child Psychiatry*, **32**, 34–42.

Wood, A.J., Harrington, R.C., and Moore, A. (1996). Controlled trial of a brief cognitive-behavioural intervention in adolescent patients with depressive disorders. *Journal of Child Psychology and Psychiatry*, **37**, 737–746.

Zeitlin, H. (1986). *The natural history of psychiatric disorder in children*. Oxford University Press, Oxford.

9   Obsessive–compulsive disorder

Martine F. Flament

When childhood obsessive–compulsive disorder (OCD) was still considered to be a rare disorder, retrospective studies with adult obsessive–compulsive patients suggested that 30–50% had experienced their first symptoms during childhood or adolescence (Black 1974). Over the last decade, a number of systematic studies conducted on children and adolescents with OCD, both in clinical settings and in the community, have greatly increased our knowledge of the disorder in its early stage and shown that, in contrast to other forms of psychopathology, the specific features of OCD are essentially identical in children, adolescents, and adults.

Clinical picture

Symptoms of OCD in children are clearly distinct from developmentally normal childhood rituals. Normal rituals (Leonard *et al.* 1990) include bedtime rituals, not stepping on cracks, counting, having lucky and unlucky numbers, and wanting things in their right place. They are most intense in 4–8 year olds; they stress rules about daily life, help the child master anxiety, and enhance the socializing process. In contrast, obsessive–compulsive rituals are perceived —even by young children—as unwanted and irrational, they are incapacitating and painful, promoting social isolation and regressive behaviour.

The clinical presentation of OCD during childhood and adolescent years has been documented in various cultures. In a series of 70 young patients examined at the National Institute of Mental Health (NIMH) in the US (Swedo *et al.* 1989), obsessions dealt primarily with fear of dirt or germs (40%), danger to self or a loved one (24%), symmetry (17%), or scrupulous religiosity (13%); the major presenting ritual symptoms included, in order of decreasing frequency, washing rituals (85%), repeating (51%), checking (46%), touching (20%), ordering (17%), counting (18%), and hoarding (11%). Toro *et al.* (1992) described a series of 72 children and adolescents with OCD in Barcelona, for whom the most common compulsions were repetitions (74%) and cleaning rituals (56%). For Khanna and Srinath (1989), in India, obsessions were less frequently reported by obsessive–compulsive children than by adults, fear of harm being the single theme which occurred most often, and, in a group of 61 obsessive–compulsive children in Japan (Honjo *et al.* 1989), the most common obsession was dirt phobia and the most common compulsions were washing rituals. All these reports argue for the isomorphism between childhood and adult presentations of OCD. For comparison, we can refer to a population of 250 adult OCD patients from a speciality clinic in the US (Rasmussen and Eisen 1992): the most common obsessions were fear of contamination

(45%), pathological doubt (42%), somatic obsessions (36%), and the need for symmetry (31%), whereas the most frequent compulsions consisted of checking (63%), washing (50%), counting (36%), and the need to ask or confess (31%).

Typically, children and adolescents with OCD have both obsessions and compulsions (Swedo *et al.* 1979, Flament *et al.* 1988, Riddle *et al.* 1990). Generally, compulsions are carried out to dispell anxiety and/or in response to an obsession (e.g. to ward off harm to someone). Some of the obsessions and rituals involve an internal sense that 'it does not feel right' until the thought or action is completed. In DSM-IV (APA 1994), OCD is characterized, regardless of age, by recurrent obsessions and/or compulsions (criterion A), that are severe enough to cause marked distress or to interfere significantly with the person's normal routine, occupational (or academic) functioning, or usual social activities or relationships (criterion C). The specific content of the obsessions or compulsions cannot be restricted to another Axis I diagnosis, such as preoccupations about food resulting from an eating disorder, or guilty thoughts from a major depressive disorder (criterion D). The only difference in diagnostic criteria between children and adults regards criterion B stating that, at some point during the course of the disorder, the person must recognize that obsessions are not simply excessive worries about real-life problems, and that compulsions are excessive or unreasonable. Though most children and adolescents acknowledge the senselessness of their obsessions and compulsions, the requirement that insight is preversed (criterion B) is waived for children. However, the difference with adult patients is minimal, since persons of all ages who lack insight receive the designation 'poor insight type'.

Comorbidity

In children and adolescents, the pattern of associated disorders follow that reported for adults. In the NIMH sample (Swedo *et al.* 1989), only 26% had uncomplicated OCD. Depression and anxiety disorders were most common, occurring in 35% and 40% of the group, respectively; in approximately half of the cases the anxiety or affective disorder had predated OCD, but in the rest of the subjects it appeared that the symptoms were secondary. Although occurring less frequently, associated diagnoses of disruptive behavior disorder or substance abuse were seen in 33% of the sample; in virtually all cases, the disruptive disorder had predated the OCD. In the Toro *et al.* (1992) study, 77% of the children or adolescents had one or more associated lifetime disorders, most commonly an anxiety (42%) or affective (37%) disorder, and anorexia nervosa was seen in 8%; anxiety disorders and anorexia nervosa tended to precede the onset of OCD, and affective disorders to parallel or follow the onset of OCD. Of particular importance in juvenile OCD is the high rate of comorbid tic disorders (Tourette syndrome or other tic disorders), which has been reported in 17% (Toro *et al.* 1992) to 40% (Geller *et al.* 1996) of referred OCD patients.

Epidemiology

The first epidemiological study on juvenile OCD was conducted in a US population of 5596 high school students (Flament *et al.* 1988). Using a two-stage procedure whereby students with questionnaire scores suggestive of obsessive–compulsive symptomatology and controls were blindly reinterviewed by clinicians, the current prevalence rate of OCD in adolescence (by DSM-III criteria) was estimated to 1 (± 0.5)%, and the lifetime prevalence to 1.9 (± 0.7)%. There was a lifetime comorbidity rate of 75% for other psychiatric disorders, including major depression, dysthymia, bulimia nervosa, overanxious disorder, and phobias. Nevertheless, only 20% of the OCD cases had ever been under professional care. The study demonstrated that OCD in adolescence was clearly underdiagnosed and undertreated. In a later study (Zohar et al. 1992), examining 562 consecutive inductees into the Israeli Army aged 16 and 17 years, the point prevalence of OCD (using DSM-III-R criteria) was 3.6 (± 0.7)%, but dropped to 1.8% when subjects with obsessions only were excluded; among the OCD individuals, there was a significant elevation of tic disorders, including Tourette syndrome. Reinherz et al. (1993) examined, with a structured clinical interview, 386 adolescents included in an ongoing 14 year longitudinal panel study that began when these youth entered kindergarten in a working class community, in the northeastern US: at a mean age of 17.9 years, 2.1% met DSM-III-R criteria for OCD. In New Zealand, Douglass et al. (1995) interviewed an unselected birth cohort of 930 males and females, when aged 18 years; they found an overall 1 year prevalence rate of OCD of 4%, decreasing to 1.2% when exluding subjects with obsessions only.

Thus, it appears that OCD might be as frequent in adolescents as it is in adults: in the NIMH Epidemiological Catchment Area (ECA) study, the lifetime prevalence rate of OCD among adults ranged from 1.9 to 3.3% across five different metropolitan sites in the US (Robins et al. 1984, Karno et al. 1988), and in the Cross National Epidemiological Study, lifetime prevalence rates were consistent among the different countries (except Taiwan), ranging from 1.9% to 2.5% (Weissman et al. 1994).

Age of onset

Reports of the mean age at onset of OCD in referred children and adolescents have ranged from 9.0 years (Riddle et al. 1990) to 11.6 years (Honjo et al. 1989). In the NIMH series (Swedo et al. 1989), the modal age at onset was 7 years, and the mean ($\pm$SD) age at onset was 10.1 (± 3.5) years, implying an early-onset group and a group with onset in adolescence. Seven of the patients had become ill before 7 years of age. Boys tended to have an earlier (prepubertal) onset, usually around age 9, whereas girls were more likely to have a later (pubertal) illness onset, around age 11. Other studies have found either no difference (Hanna 1995) or an earlier onset for girls (Honjo et al. 1989). In a community-based sample of adolescents, the age at onset of OCD varied from 7 to 18 years, with a mean of 12.8 years (Flament et al. 1988).

Sex ratio

In community-based samples of adolescents with OCD, there are approximately equal numbers of males and females (Flament et al. 1988, Zohar et al. 1992), whereas in most studies of referred children and adolescents, males outnumber females 2 : 1 or 3 : 2 (Despert 1955, Flament et al. 1985, Last and Strauss 1989, Swedo et al. 1989, Thomsen et al. 1991). The relative overrepresentation of boys in clinical samples may reflect a greater severity of the

Table 9.1 Percentage improvement from baseline on obsessive compulsive symptoms measures during short-term (5–12 weeks) pharmacological treatment of children and adolescents with OCD

Study	Flament et al. (1987)	Leonard et al. (1989)	DeVeaugh-Geiss et al. (1992)	Riddle et al. (1992)	Apter et al. (1994)	Wolkow et al. (1997)
N	19	47	60	14	14	187
Age (years)	6–18	7–19	10–17	8–15	13–18	6–17
Drug	clomipramine	clomipramine	clomipramine	fluoxetine	fluvoxamine	sertraline
Daily dose (mg)	100–200	Mean 150	15075–200	20	100–300	Maximum 200
Study design	Vs placebo	Vs desipraminevs	Vs placebo	Vs placebo	open study	Vs placebo
% improvement on active drug across measures	22–44	19–29	34–37	33–44	28	21–28

disorder, and an earlier age of onset (Flament *et al.* 1985, Last and Strauss 1989, Swedo *et al.* 1989); in addition, boys are more likely than girls to have a comorbid tic disorder (Leonard *et al.* 1992). In contrast, OCD appears to be more common in adult females than in adult males (Weissman 1994), this being probably related to the later onset in women.

Intervention studies

The literature on childhood and adolescent OCD over the last decade has brought evidence of the efficacy of two types of therapeutic interventions, previously documented in adult OCD patients: psychopharmacological agents which are potent serotonin specific reuptake inhibitors (SSRIs), and specific cognitive behavioral treatment (CBT).

Psychopharmacological treatment

Clomipramine hydrochloride was the first known antiobsessional agent. Its efficacy for children and adolescents with OCD has been demonstrated in three controlled studies (see Table 9.1). In the first one by Flament *et al.* (1985) at the NIMH, clomipramine was significantly superior to placebo, after 5 weeks of treatment, for improvement of both observed and self-reported obsessions and compulsions; this was independent of the presence of depressive symptoms at baseline. Improvement of OC symptoms was closely correlated with pretreatment platelet serotonin concentration, as well as with decrease of this measure during clomipramine administration (Flament *et al.* 1987). A subsequent study by Leonard *et al.* (1989), also at the NIMH, further documented the specificity of the antiobsessional effect of clomipramine, which was clearly superior to desipramine, after 5 weeks, in significantly reducing OC symptoms. Of patients who received clomipramine as their first active treatment, 64% showed at least some sign of relapse during subsequent desipramine treatment. De

Veaugh-Geiss *et al.* (1992) reported on 60 children and adolescents with OCD included in an 8 week, multicenter, double-blind, parallel groups trial of clomipramine versus placebo. At the end of 8 weeks, 53% of patients receiving active drug rated themselves as very much improved or much improved, versus 8% receiving placebo. In a 1 year open label maintenance treatment for 47 patients, clomipramine continued to be effective and well tolerated.

Fluoxetine was investigated by Riddle *et al.* (1992) in a 8 week, placebo-controlled, crossover study involving 14 children and adolescents with OCD. The degree of symptomatic improvement on fluoxetine was comparable with that observed in similar trials of clomipramine. In a 8 week open-label trial by Apter *et al.* (1994) in Israel, fluvoxamine, in addition to standard in-patient treatment, also induced significant decrease in the severity of OC symptoms. The largest of the studies completed to date is a double-blind, multicentre, 12 week placebo-controlled trial of sertraline in 187 children and adolescents with OCD: compared with placebo, sertraline was associated with a significantly greater improvement in OC symptoms on all clinical scales (Wolkow *et al.* 1997).

The selective efficacy of SSRIs is also supported by a desipramine substitution study during long-term clomipramine maintenance treatment of a group of 26 children and adolescents with severe primary OCD (Leonard *et al.* 1991). In this study 8 (89%) of 9 of the substituted, and only 2 of 11 of the nonsubstituted group subjects relapsed during the 2 month comparison period. All 8 patients who relapsed with desipramine regained their clinical response within 1 month of clomipramine reinstallment.

Overall, there is now clear evidence (Table 9.1) that pharmacological treatment with an SSRI—at doses comparable to those used for adults—induces a clinically substantial reduction of OC symptoms for most children and adolescents with the disorder. However, improvement is often incomplete, few patients become asymptomatic, and long-term maintenance treatment may be required.

Cognitive-behavioral therapy (CBT)

A few open studies have shown beneficial effects of CBT, alone or in addition to pharmacotherapy, for children and adolescents with OCD. Graded exposure and response prevention form the core of treatment, anxiety management training and OCD-specific family interventions playing an adjunctive role. Bolton *et al.* (1983) reported the outcome of CBT (generally combined with other treatment approachs) for a series of 15 adolescents: in most cases, symptoms were relieved entirely (47%) or reduced to a mildly incapacitating level (40%). March *et al.* (1994) presented an open trial of CBT for 15 children and adolescents with OCD, most of whom were also receiving medication: 9 patients experienced at least a 50% reduction in symptoms at post-treatment, and 6 were asymptomatic. No patients relapsed at follow-up intervals as long as 18 months. Booster behavioral treatment allowed medication discontinuation in 6 patients.

Short-term and long-term outcomes

Follow-up studies of adult patients with OCD have stressed the chronic course and relative 'purity' of outcome of the disorder (Goodwin *et al.* 1969, Kringlen 1985). In these studies, the

Table 9.2 Retrospective follow-up studies of children and adolescents with OCD

Study	Hollingsworth *et al.* (1980)	Allsop and Verduyn (1988)	Thomsen and Mikkelsen (1995a)
Place	UCLA, USA	Oxford, UK	Denmark
Sample size	10/17 (13M, 4F)	20/26(14 M, 12 F)	47 (28 M, 19 F)/55 + 49 control patients
Diagnostic criteria	Judd's criteria	CD-9 + Judd's criteria	DSM-III
Mean age (range) (years)	at F/U 19.9 (12–30)	at admission 15.3 (12.5–18.4) at F/U: 25.1 (20.1–28.5)	at admission 11.8 for boys 12.4 for girls at F/U: 27.4 (18–36)
Mean F/U period (range) (years)	6.5 (1.5–14)		15.6 (6–22)
Initial treatment	intensive psychotherapy	behavioral response prevention + family work	diverse (SRIs, psychotherapy, family therapy)
Outcome	3 (30%) recovered 7 (70%) some degree of OC symptoms	10 (50%) recovered 6 (30%) persistent OCD 2 (10%) schizophrenia 2 (10%) depressive disorder	13 (28%) recovered 12 (25%) subclinical OCD 10 (21%) phasic OCD 12 (25%) chronic OCD

M, male; F, female; F/U, follow-up; SRIs, serotonin reuptake inhibitors.

prognosis of obsessional states was considered more severe than that of other neurotic disorders, complete recovery was rare (12–32%), but spontaneous improvement was reported in 14–50% of the patients. More recently, prospective epidemiological studies in adult subjects from the community, with repeated interviews at lenghty intervals, have found considerable spontaneous fluctuation in OCD symptoms (Degonda *et al.* 1993).

Retrospective follow-up studies

In retrospective studies (see Table 9.2), patients are selected based on chart review, and fluctuations in the severity of psychiatric symptoms and their impact on functioning over time are ascertained based on subjects' recall. In addition, diagnosis and symptomatology at first admission are generally not documented with standardized assessment procedures.

Hollingsworth *et al.* (1980) identified 17 cases of severe obsessive–compulsive neurosis from a retrospective chart review of all children treated as in- or outpatients at the UCLA Neuropsychiatric Institute for a 16 year period. All obsessive–compulsive children had been treated with intensive psychotherapy (for an average of 17.7 months), and one of them also received behavior therapy. The authors interviewed 10 of these cases, 1.5–14 years after their first admission, at ages ranging from 12 to 30 years. Only 3 of the 10 (30%) denied any obsessive thoughts or compulsions, whereas 7 (70%) reported that obsessive–compulsive behavior still continued to some degree but was less than pretreatment level. One had decompensated during adolescence in an acute schizophrenic reaction, which had resolved without recurrence. On follow-up, all 10 subjects reported problems with social life and peer relationships, and none was married.

Allsopp and Verduyn (1988) reported on 26 patients identified by a retrospective chart review at a regional adolescent psychiatry unit in Oxford (UK), who had been admitted between 1974 and 1979 and had received a diagnosis of OCD. Behavioral response prevention programmes combined with family work had been the management strategy of choice during the admission period. The mean age of the group was 15.25 years at first assessment, and 25.1 years at follow-up. Of the 20 subjects for whom follow-up information was obtained, 10 had remained psychiatrically ill, 6 with persistent OCD.

A first Danish study by Thomsen and Mikkelsen (1993, 1995a) examined the clinical course of childhood OCD in 47 subjects re-evaluated 6–22 years after initial referral; they were compared with a control group of 49 age- and sex-matched control patients with former admissions for other non-psychotic disorders during the same period (mainly emotional disorders or conduct disorders). Of the childhood OCD patients, 34 (72%) had at least one Axis I diagnosis at follow-up, 22 (47%) with OCD. In the control group, rates of psychiatric diagnoses at follow-up ranged from 17% to 40% according to initial diagnostic group (except for 2 anorectic patients who both still had an eating disorder). Education and employment were comparable in the two groups, but OCD patients were more socially isolated: more still lived with their parents (30% versus 4% of the controls) and fewer had partnerships (32% versus 59%). At follow-up, 68% of the OCD probands, like 61% of the psychiatric controls, had at least one personality disorder. Among OCD probands, the most common personality disorder was avoidant personality disorder (23% vs 8% of the controls), whereas obsessive–compulsive personality disorder (OCPD) was not found more often than among controls (17% versus 10%). However, in the OCD group, 7 of the 8 subjects with OCDP had continued OCD at follow-up. Generally, most personality disorders were found in the group of patients with chronic OCD at follow-up, and fewest (only 3) in the group without OCD or subclinical OCD.

Prospective follow-up studies

The design and the results of five prospective follow-up studies of children and adolescents with OCD, in the US and in Europe, are summarized in Table 9.3.

An early study by Warren (1960) described 15 adolescents admitted to the Maudsley Hospital in London with obsessive–compulsive states, between 12 and 17 years of age, and re-examined when aged 19–24 years. No treatment was specified, except for one patient who had been leucotomized. At follow-up, only 2 subjects were considered completely recovered, 4 had a tendency to mild OC symptoms under stress, 4 were somewhat handicapped by obsessional symptoms, and the remaining 5 still had severe symptomatology, 1 being hospitalized.

Two prospective longitudinal studies of children and adolescents with OCD have been successively conducted at the NIMH Child Psychiatry Branch. Flament *et al.* (1990) reported outcome for 25 of 27 patients (93%) admitted between 1977 and 1983 for a 5 week treatment trial with clomipramine. At first evaluation, patients aged 10–18 years were matched for sex, age, and IQ with normal controls from the local community. Following the initial drug trial, only 7 patients were maintained on clomipramine (not available in the US at the time), for

Table 9.3 Prospective follow-up studies of children and adolescents with OCD

Study	Warren (1960)	Flament et al. (1990)	Leonard et al. (1993)	Thomsen and Mikkelsen (1995b)	Bolton et al. (1995)
Place	Maudsley, London, UK	NIMH, USA	NIMH, USA	Denmark	Maudsley, London, UK
Sample size	15	25 (16M, 4F)/27 + 23/29 normal controls	54/54 (36M, 18F)	23 (17M, 6F)/26 + 24 control patients	14/15 (8M, 7F)
Diagnostic criteria	No specific criteria	DSM-III	DSM-III	DSM-III-R	DSM-III-R
mean age (range) (years)	At admission: (12–17) At F/U: (19–24)	At admission: 14.4 (10–18) At F/U: 18.8 (13–24)	At admission: 14 (7–19) At F/U: 17.4 (10–24)	At admission: 14.1 (9–17) At F/U: 16.6 (12–22)	At admission: 14.1 (12–18) At F/U: 27 (23–31)
Interim treatment	No treatment specified (except 1 leucotomized)	Intermittent and non specific drug- or psychotherapy	96% SRIs 46% behavior therapy	57% SRIs behavior therapy (rate not specified)	50% SRIs and/or behavior therapy
Outcome	2 (13%) recovered 4 (27%) mild OC symptoms under stress 4 (27%) handicapping OC symptoms 5 (33%) severe OC symptoms	7 (28%) recovered 17 (60%) OCD 1 (4%) psychosis	6 (11%) recovered (3 on medication) 15 (28%) OC features 10 (18%) subclinical OCD 23 (43%) OCD	6 (26%) recovered 9 (39%) subclinical OCD 8 (35%) clinical OCD	8 (57%) recovered 6 (43%) OCD (2 unremitting, 4 with relapse)

M, male; F, female; F/U, follow-up; SRIs, serotonin reuptake inhibitors.

between a few months and 3 years. Others received non-specific drug (other tricyclic antidepressants, neuroleptics, anxiolytics) or psychological treatment (supportive psychotherapy, family or group therapy); these treatments had often been only briefly or irregularly administered. Patients and controls were reevaluated at 2–7 year follow-up. The patient group had marked psychosocial impairment and most often continued psychopathology. At the same age, more patients (74%) than controls (57%) were still living with their families, more controls (86%) than patients (59%) were still at school. Seventeen patients (68%) still met criteria for OCD, and comorbidity was common as 13 (52%) of the group had another Axis I psychiatric disorder, most commonly an anxiety and/or depressive disorder.

The second study, by Leonard et al. (1993), concerned children and adolescents who participated in the NIMH clomipramine treatment studies between 1984 and 1988. The objective of this later study was to assess the outcome of patients who had access to continued psychopharmacological treatments, to determine whether there had been any long-term gains and if there were any predictors of outcome. After discharge from the NIMH, 96% of the patients received additional pharmacological treatment with clomipramine or another SRI, 33% behavioral therapy, 54% individual therapy, and 20% family therapy. At the time of follow-up, 70% were still taking psychoactive medication. During the follow-up period, several interim contacts with most of the subjects showed that many patients met DSM-III-R criteria for OCD at some times but not at others, illustrating the waxing and waning pattern of the disorder. All subjects were assessed 2–7 years after first referral. Only 6 (11%) were free of any obsession or compulsion. Of those 6, 3 were still under medication, therefore only 3 (6% of the sample) could be considered in true remission. Although OC symptoms continued for most subjects, the group as a whole was significantly improved from endpoint of initial clomipramine treatment on measures of OCD, anxiety, depression, and global functioning, indicating significant gains over those of short-term treatment; only 10 subjects (19%) were rated as unchanged or worse. Comorbidity was extremely high: at follow-up, only 2 subjects (4%) had no current psychiatric diagnosis. Most common lifetime diagnoses were tic disorder (59%), major depression (56%), overanxious disorder (54%), and oppositional disorder (30%). Three patients (6%) had developed a psychotic disorder subsequent to baseline evaluation; this disorder resolved in 2 of the patients (one of whom had a brief reactive psychosis while receiving medication), but the third patient had comorbid schizoaffective disorder and severe OCD at follow-up.

In a second Danish study (Thomsen and Mikkelsen 1995b), 23 of 26 children and adolescents with OCD were prospectively evaluated every 6 months for OC symptomatology. The study was done when behavioral therapy and medication with SSRIs were available in Denmark. The duration of initial treatment ranged from 10 sessions of outpatient therapy to 1 year of in-patient treatment. After discharge, all children who had been in-patients had a shorter or longer outpatient program, including individual or family sessions with behavioral therapy and control of medication; 13 of the probands received medication (clomipramine or citalopram) for a period of 6 months to 2 years. At follow-up, 1½–5 years after referral, 8 subjects (35%) retained an OCD diagnosis, including 3 who were still receiving medication (with OC symptoms on a much less severe level than at baseline); 9 subjects (39%) had subclinical OCD, mostly with the same form and content as the clinical OCD presented at baseline, although they were neither distressed nor functionally or socially affected by these subclinical symptoms; the remaining 6 (26%) had no OCD at follow-up. Interim evaluations supported the theories of OCD as an illness of fluctuating severity.

Bolton *et al.* (1995) reported on 15 young adults treated for OCD in adolescence (Bolton *et al.* 1983), mainly by behavior therapy (response prevention with artificial exposure if necessary) and family task-setting therapy; 5 subjects had also received clomipramine. Betweeen 9 and 14 years later, data could be collected on 14 of the cases. Of the 15 patients, 13 had responded positively to treatment in adolescence, and follow-up information was obtained for 12 of them: 5 cases settled into a chronic course, 1 immediately after discharge, whereas the other 4 relapsed between 3 and 6 years later, with only partial relief from subsequent and temporary pharmacological or behavioral treatment. The other 7 adolescent responders stayed well (despite, in one case, a fluctuating course for a short time after discharge), they were all treatment-free at follow-up. As to the 2 patients with no response to protracted treatment in adolescence, 1 case (with obsessional slowness) remained chronic, whereas the other responded well to further behavior therapy a year later. Recovered participants (57%) were all treatment-free, and long-lasting recovery was associated with good social adjustment. Chronic course was not attributable to lack of subsequent treatment.

In addition, we can also cite a 2 year prospective follow-up study of OCD cases identified in a community study (Flament *et al.* 1988). At follow-up (Berg *et al.* 1989), 74% of adolescents previously diagnosed as having OCD or 'obsessive–compulsive spectrum' disorders and a control sample were reinterviewed by clinicians blind to prior diagnosis. Of 16 subjects initially diagnosed with OCD, 5 (31%) still met full criteria for the disorder, 4 (25%) had subclinical OCD, 2 (12%) OCPD, 5 (31%) subclinical OCPD, 6 (37%) other disorders with OC features, and only 2 (12%) had no diagnosis. Of the 10 students who had subclinical OCD at baseline, only 1 (10%) had developed full OCD, 4 (40%) still had subclinical OCD, and 3 (30%) other disorders with OC features. The study showed the relative stability of the diagnosis of OCD in a natural setting, with variations in intensity. Contrary to the authors expectations, subjects initially diagnosed with subclinical OCD did not progress into true cases of OCD, reinforcing the importance of using a high diagnostic threshold of severity.

Continuity versus discontinuity

Some research has focused on the type of symptoms in relation to age, and their changes over time. Minichiello *et al.* (1990) reported that patients who were predominantly cleaners had a later age of onset than those who checked or had mixed symptoms; additionally, cleaning rituals were more prominent among females, whereas primarily obsessional patients tended to be males. Honjo *et al.* (1989) noted that compulsions were more apt to appear earlier than were obsessions. Other studies have not reported any differences between patients with different types of symptoms. Thomsen (1991) found no relation between age and the number of OCD symptoms. Rasmussen and Eisler (1990) found no differences between symptom groups in age of onset, sex, course of illness, or comorbid Axis I disorders. Typically, there seems to be a high degree of overlap within patients between symptom groups of obsessions and compulsions (Hafner and Miller 1990).

One study at the NIMH (Rettew *et al.* 1992) tried to determine the types of symptoms in childhood onset OCD patients, their relationship to age, and their changes over time. The authors studied the individual symptoms of 79 children and adolescents with severe OCD over an average of 7.9 years (range 2–16 years). Symptoms were obtained from chart review and obsessive–compulsive checklists, and grouped according to the categories of the Yale–Brown Symptom Checklist (Goodman *et al.* 1989). The vast majority of patients reported having many different symptoms that spanned several symptom categories. Of 7 possible divisions of obsessions, and 8 possible divisions of compulsions, at baseline the mean number of obsessions was 2.1 ± 1.3 (range 0–5), and the mean number of compulsions was 2.5 ± 1.4 (range 0–6). At follow-up, the means were 1.7 ± 1.4 and 2.3 ± 1.7, respectively. On cross-sectional analysis, no significant age-related trends were found with either the number or the type of OCD symptoms. As in the Honjo study, there was some evidence that compulsions appear before obsessions, particularly for patients with very early onset (before age 6). Early symptoms were sometimes unusul (such as blinking and breathing rituals, arm flapping, or other repetitive movement) but also included classical obsessive–compulsive symptoms (washing, walking, touching). Besides this finding, no relationship was found between the number or type of symptoms and developmental phases. Across the follow-up study period, no patient maintained the same constellation of symptoms from presentation to follow-up. Despite this, there were no discernable patterns with regard to any specific symptoms and age.

Patients reported symptoms from many different categories, with 47% of the subjects displaying both washing and checking compulsions at some time during their illness. With many exceptions, the typical progression of symptoms noted for this group was a gradual increase in the number of symptoms followed by a decrease as the patient reached late adolescence and early adulthood. In 30 patients (38%), family members or the patients themselves believed a specific event had precipitated onset of their obsessive–compulsive behavior. The most common events involved stressful family events or fears developing from television shows, that is, usually not a particularly traumatic event, or one not commonly encountered by children. If the initial OCD symptoms often reflected the content of the reported event, in no case was the symptom specificity preserved at follow-up.

As described in details under the section on short-term and long-term outcomes, all follow-up studies of subjects with pediatric-onset OCD clearly demonstrate the continuity of the diagnosis of OCD from childhood to adulthood, with a relative intraindividual stability for the content of symptoms. Spontaneous course is most often marked by a waxing and waning severity of the disorder, whereas remissions under treatment may be followed by relapses, even after long periods of time.

Risks and prognostic factors

Several studies, both on the natural course of OCD and on clinical response to treatment interventions, have attempted to identify demographic or clinical features that may influence outcome or course of illness in OCD, with mainly negative or inconsistent results.

Because of the possible biases and uncertainties mentioned above, results from retrospective studies are limited. Allsopp and Verduyn (1988) found that all patients who were asymptomatic at discharge had remained well with no further psychiatric help, whereas a family history of psychiatric illness was associated with further treatment of the probands for psychiatric disorders. In the Thomsen and Mikkelsen study (1995a), a number of baseline variables were examined, using bivariate or multivariate analysis, as possible predictors of OCD outcome: sex, age at onset of OCD and at first admission, type of OCD or comorbid symptoms during childhood, neurological soft signs and organic traits, parental mental disorder, social background, and IQ level. None seemed to predict outcome, except OCD severity in childhood, as measured by the number of hours spent on symptoms, which predicted presence of OCD (episodic or chronic) at follow-up. The course of OCD was predicted by gender, as more women than men had an episodic course, and more males (32%) than females (5%) belonged to the poorest outcome group (Global Assessment of Functioning score < 50). However, just as many females than males had OCD. No significant predictive factors from childhood were found for presence of OCDP or any personality disorder at follow-up.

In one-short term pharmacological study male subjects responded significantly better than did female subjects (Flament *et al.* 1985), but in the other studies, treatment response could not be predicted by sex, age of onset, duration or severity of illness, or type of symptoms (Leonard *et al.* 1989, De Vaugh-Geiss *et al.* 1992). In no study were the plasma concentrations of clomipramine or metabolites during treatment associated to clinical response.

As for long-term course, inconsistent results have been reported regarding the predictive value of baseline characteristics or initial treatment response. In the Flament *et al.* (1990)

study, there was difficulty in prediction of outcome as so few subjects were considered well at follow-up. What was most striking, however, was that an initial good response to clomipramine treatment conveyed no long-term prognostic benefit. In the Leonard *et al.* (1993) study, a stepwise regression analysis was performed with representative baseline and week 5 variables. A worse OCD outcome score at follow-up (NIMH–OCD severity scale) was predicted, in a stepwise multiple regression, by (1) more severe OCD symptoms score after 5 weeks of clomipramine therapy (31% of the variance), followed by (2) presence of parental Axis I psychiatric diagnosis (16%), and (3) lifetime history of tics at baseline (15%). In a similar fashion, the Global Assessment of Functioning score at follow-up was predicted by the severity of OCD symptoms at week 5, then by the number of parents with a high Expressed Emotions score. In the Bolton *et al.* (1995) study, no risk or protective factors were detected, but the authors aknowledge that this was possibly due to the small number of subjects. Good treatment outcome in adolescence predicted medium-term prognosis (1–4 years) fairly well, but it failed to predict long-term prognosis (9–14 years), reflecting the fact that some patients relapsed into a chronic course even after several years of remission following treatment.

Conclusions

Childhood OCD may represent the disorder in child psychiatry whose clinical picture most closely resembles its adult counterpart. Despite a relative diversity, the symptom 'pool' is remarquably finite and very similar to that seen in older individuals. Prevalence of OCD, comorbidity, and response to pharmacological and behavioural treatment also appear continuous across the life span.

Children and adolescents with OCD often suffer from a wide range of symptoms simultaneously, which may change over time. Most subjects have both obsessions and compulsions, and there do not seem to be age-related patterns in the prevalence of specific types of symptoms, except that patients with very early onset are found to have more compulsions than obsessions. For reasons still unknown, the onset of OCD generally occurs earlier in life for males than for females.

A chronic, fluctuating course appears to be supported both retrospectively and in follow-up after treatment. Studies using prospective design and standardized criteria have shown that episodicity in this disorder (with distinct periods of complete remission off medication, similar to major depressive disorder) is uncommon. Once established, obsessions and compulsions usually persist, although the content, intensity, and frequency of these symptoms change over time. Although comorbidity with other disorders (anxiety and depressive disorders, tics) is common, the development of schizophrenia is rare if that diagnosis has been adequately excluded at baseline.

One might infer from the results of the longitudinal studies that multiple treatment interventions can improve long-term prognosis of childhood onset OCD and reduce impairment from the condition. Recent studies suggest that appropriate pharmacological treatment substantially improves outcome, but that patients might need to pursue the treatment for long periods of time. CBT interventions might have more durable benefits. One of the main problems we still face with childhood OCD is the difficulty in predicting the long-term outcome of the disorder. According to both course and treatment literature on predictors of follow-up outcome for OCD, surprisingly few demographic and clinical features, including age of onset, type, severity and duration of symptoms, seem apt to predict long-term course. Invaluable benefits can now be obtained from available pharmacological and behavioral treatments, but complete remission remains uncertain, and long-term management may be required for pediatric-onset OCD.

References

Allsopp, M. and Verduyn, C. (1988). A follow-up of adolescents with obsessive-compulsive disorder. *British Journal of Psychiatry*, **154**, 829–834.

APA (1994) *Diagnostic and Statistical Manual of Mental Disorders*, 4th edn. American Psychiatric Association, Washington, D.C.

Apter, A., Ratzoni, G., King, R.A. *et al.* (1994). Fluvoxamine open-label treatment of adolescent inpatients with obsessive-compulsive disorder or depression. *Journal of the American Academy of Child and Adolescent Psychiatry*, **33**, 342–348.

Berg, C.Z., Rapoport, J.L., Whitaker, A., Davies, M., Leonard, H., Swedo, S.E., Braiman, S., and Lenane, M. (1989). Childhood obsessive compulsive disorder: A two-year prospective follow-up study of a community sample. *Journal of the American Academy of Child and Adolescent Psychiatry*, **28**, 528–533.

Black, A. (1974) The natural history of obsessional neurosis. In *Obsessional states*, ed. H.R. Beech. Methuen, London.

Bolton, D., Collins, S., and Steinberg, D. (1983). The treatment of obsessive-compulsive disorder in adolescence. A report of fifteen cases. *British Journal of Psychiatry*, **142**, 456–464.

Bolton, D., Luckie, M., and Steinberg, D. (1995). Long-term course of obsessive-compulsive disorder treated in adolescence. *Journal of the American Academy of Child and Adolescent Psychiatry*, **34**, 1441–1450.

Degonda, M., Wyss, M., Angst, J. (1993). Obsessive-compulsive disorders and syndromes in the general population. *European Archives of Psychiatry and Clinical Neuroscience*, **243**, 16–22.

Despert, L. (1955). Differential diagnosis between obsessive-compulsive neurosis and schizophrenia in children. In *Psychopathology of childhood*, ed. P.H. Hoch and J. Zubin, Grune and Stratton, New York.

DeVeaugh-Geiss, J., Moroz, G., Biederman, J., Cantwell, D., Fontaine, R., Greist, J.H., Reichler, R., Katz, R., Landau, P. (1992). Clomipramine hydrochloride in childhood and adolescent obsessive-compulsive disorder: A multicenter trial. *Journal of the American Academy of Child and Adolescent Psychiatry*, **31**, 45–49.

Douglass, H.M., Moffitt, T.E., Reuven, D. *et al.* (1995). Obsessive-compulsive disorder in a birth cohort of 18-year-olds: prevalence and predictors. *Journal of the American Academy of Child and Adolescent Psychiatry*, **34**, 1424–1431.

Flament, M.F., Rapoport, J.L., Berg, C.J., Sceery, W., Kilts, C., Mellström, B., Linnoila, M. (1985). Clomipramine treatment of childhood obsessive-compulsive disorder. A double-blind controlled study. *Archives of General Psychiatry*, **42**, 977–983.

Flament, M.F., Rapoport, J.L., Murphy, D.L. Lake, C.R., and Berg C.J. (1987).

Biochemical changes during clomipramine treatment of childhood obsessive compulsive disorder. *Archives of General Psychiatry*, **44**, 219–225.

Flament, M.F., Whitaker, A., Rapoport, J.L., Davies, M., Berg, C.Z., Kalikow, K., Sceery, W., and Schaffer, D. (1988). Obsessive compulsive disorder in adolescence: An epidemiological study. *Journal of the American Academy of Child and Adolescent Psychiatry*, **27**, 764–771.

Flament, M.F., Koby, E., Rapoport, J.L., Berg, C.J., Zahn, T., Cox, C., Denckla, M., Lenane, M. (1990). Childhood obsessive-compulsive disorder: A prospective follow-up study. *Journal of Child Psychology and Psychiatry*, **31**, 363–380.

Geller, D.A., Biederman, J., Griffin S. *et al.* (1996). Comorbidity of obsessive-compulsive disorder with disruptive behavior disorders. *Journal of the American Academy of Child and Adolescent Psychiatry*, **35**, 1637–1646.

Goodman, W.K., Price, L.H., Rasmussen, S.A., Mazure, C., Rleischmann, R.L., Hill, C.L., Heninger, G.R., and Charney, D.S. (1989). The Yale-Brown Obsessive Compulsive Scale: I. Development, use and reliability. *Archives of General Psychiatry*, **46**, 1006–1011.

Goodwin, D.W., Guze, S.B., and Robins, E. (1969). Follow-up studies in obsessional neurosis. *Archives of General Psychiatry*, **20**, 182–187.

Hafner, R.J. and Miller, R.J. (1990). Obsessive-compulsive disorder: an exploration of some unresolved clinical issues. *Australian and New Zealand Journal of Psychiatry*, **24**, 480–485.

Hanna, G.L. (1995). Demographic and clinical features of obsessive-compulsive disorder in children and adolescents. *Journal of the American Academy of Child and Adolescent Psychiatry*, **34**, 19–27.

Hollingsworth, C.E., Tanguay, P.E., Grossman, L., Pabst, P. (1980). Long-term outcome of obsessive-compulsive disorder in childhood. *Journal of the American Academy of Child and Adolescent Psychiatry*, **19**, 134–144.

Honjo, S., Hirano, C., Murase, S., Kaneko, T., Sugiyama, T., Othaka, K., Ayoma, T., Takei, T., Inoko, K., and Wakabayashi, S. (1989). Obsessive-compulsive symptoms in childhood and adolescence. *Acta Psychiatrica Scandinavica*, **80**, 83–91.

Karno, M., Golding, J.M., Sorenson, S.B., and Burnam, M.A. (1988). The epidemiology of obsessive-compulsive disorder in five US communities. *Archives of General Psychiatry*, **45**, 1094–1099.

Khanna, S. and Srinath, S. (1989). Childhood obsessive compulsive disorder. I. Psychopathology. *Psychopathology*, **32**, 47–54.

Kringlen, E. (1985). Obsessional neurotics: a long-term follow-up. *British Jounral of Psychiatry*, **111**, 709–722.

Last, C.G. and Strauss C.C. (1989). Obsessive-compulsive disorder in childhood. *Journal of Anxiety Disorders*, **3**, 295–302.

Leonard, H.L., Swedo, S.E., Rapoport, J.L., Koby, E.V., Lenane, M.C., Cheslow, D.L., and Hamburger, S.D. (1989). Treatment of obsessive-compulsive disorder with clomipramine and desipramine in children and adolescents. *Archives of General Psychiatry*, **46**, 1088–1092.

Leonard, H.L., Goldberger, E.L., Rapoport, J.L., Cheslow, D.L., and Swedo, S.E. (1990). Childhood rituals: Normal development or obsessive-compulsive symptoms? *Journal of the American Academy of Child and Adolescent Psychiatry*, **29**, 17–23.

Leonard, H.L., Swedo, S.E., Lenane, M.C., Rettew, D.C., Cheslow, D.L., Hamburger, S.D., and Rapoport, J.L. (1991). A double-blind desipramine substitution during long-term clomipramine treatment in children and adolescents with obsessive-compulsive disorder. *Archives of General Psychiatry*, **48**, 922–927.

Leonard, H.L., Lenane, M.C., Swedo, S.E., Rettew, D.C., Gershon, E.S., and Rapoport, J.L. (1992). Tics and Tourettes disorder. A 2- to 7- year follow-up study of 54 obsessive-compulsive children. *American Journal of Psychiatry*, **149**, 1244–1251.

Leonard, H.L., Swedo, S.E., Lenane, M.C., Rettew, D., Hamburger, S.D., Bartko, J.J., and Rapoport, J.L. (1993). A 2- to 7- year follow-up study of 54 obsessive-compulsive children and adolescents. *Archives of General Psychiatry*, **50**, 429–439.

March, J.S., Mulle, K., and Herbel, B. (1994). Behavioral psychotherapy for children and adolescents with obsessive-compulsive disorder: an open trial of a new protocol-driven treatment package. *Journal of the American Academy of Child and Adolescent Psychiatry*, **33**, 333–341.

Minichiello, W.E., Baer, L., Jenike, M.A., and Holland, A. (1990). Age of onset of major subtypes of obsessive-compulsive disorder. *Journal of Anxiety Disorders*, **4**, 147–150.

Rasmussen, S.A. and Eisen, J.L. (1990). Epidemiology of obsessive compulsive disorder. *Journal of Clinical Psychiatry*, **51** (Suppl2), 10–13.

Rasmussen, S.A. and Eisen, J.L. (1992). The epidemiology and differential diagnosis of obsessive compulsive disorder. *Journal of Clinical Psychiatry*, **53** (Suppl 4), 4–10.

Reinherz, H.Z., Giaconia, R.M., Lefkowitz, E.S., Pakiz, B., and Frost, A.K. (1993). Prevalence of psychiatric disorders in a community population of older adolescents. *Journal of the American Academy of Child and Adolescent Psychiatry*, **32**, 369–377.

Rettew, D.C., Swedo, S.E., Leonard, H.L., Lenane, M., Rapoport, J.L. (1992). Obsessions and compulsions across time in 79 children and adolescents with obsessive-compulsive disorder. *Journal of the American Academy of Child and Adolescent Psychiatry*, **31**, 1050–1056.

Riddle, M.A., Scahill, L., King, R. *et al.* (1990). Obsessive compulsive disorder in children and adolescents: Phenomenology and family history. *Journal of the American Academy of Child and Adolescent Psychiatry*, **29**, 766–772.

Riddle, M.A., Scahill, L., King, R.A., Hardin, M.T., Anderson, G.M., Ort, S.I., Smith, J.C., Leckman, J.F., and Cohen, D.J. (1992). Double-blind, crossover trial of fluoxetine and placebo in children and adolescents with obsessive-compulsive disorder. *Journal of the American Academy of Child and Adolescent Psychiatry*, **31**, 1062–1069.

Robins, L.N., Helzer, J.E., Weissman, M.M., Orvaschel, H., Gruenberg, E., Burke, J.D., and Regier, D.A. (1984). Lifetime prevalence of specific disorders in three sites. *Archives of General Psychiatry*, **41**, 949–958.

Swedo, S.E., Rapoport, J.L., Leonard, H., Lenane, M., and Cheslow, D. (1989). Obsessive-compulsive disorder in children and adolescents. Clinical phenomenology of 70 consecutive cases. *Archives of General Psychiatry*, **46**, 335–340.

Thomsen, P.H. (1991). Obsessive-compulsive symptoms in children and adolescents. A phenomenological analysis of 61 Danish cases. *Psychopathology*, **24**, 12–18.

Thomsen, P H. and Mikkelsen, H.U. (1993). Development of personality disorders in children and adolescents with obsessive-compulsive disorder. A 6- to 22- year follow-up study. *Acta Psychiatrica Scandinavica*, **87**, 456–462.

Thomsen, P H. and Mikkelsen, H.U. (1995a). Obsessive-compulsive disorder in children and adolescents: Predictors in childhood for long-term phenomenological course. *Acta Psychiatrica Scandinavica*, **92**, 255–259.

Thomsen, P H. and Mikkelsen, H.U. (1995b). Course of obsessive-compulsive disorder in children and adolescents: A prospective follow-up study of 23 Danish cases. *Journal of the American Academy of Child and Adolescent Psychiatry*, **34**, 1432–1440.

Toro, J., Cervera, M., Osjeo, E., and Salamero, M. (1992). Obsessive-compulsive disorder in childhood and adolescence: A clinical study. *Journal of Child Psychology and Psychiatry*, **33**, 1025–1037.

Warren, W. (1960). Some relationships between the psychiatry of children and adults. *J Mental Science*, **106**, 815–826.

Weissman, M.M., Bland, R.C., Canino, G.L., Greenwald, S., Hwu, H.G., Lee, C.K., Newman, S.C., Oakley-Browne, M.A., Rubio-Stipec, M., Wickramaratne, P.J., Wittchen, H.U., and Yeh, E.K. (1994). The cross national epidemiology of obsessive-compulsive disorder. *Journal of Clinical Psychology*, **55**, 5–10.

Wolkow, R., March, J., Safferman, A., and Biederman, J. (1997). A placebo-controlled trial of sertraline treatment for pediatric obsessive compulsive disorder. *6th World Congress of Biological Psychiatry*, Nice, France, 22–27 June,

Zohar, A.H., Ratzosin, G., Pauls, D.L., Apter, A., Bleich, A., Kron, S., Rappaport, M., Weizman, A., and Cohen D.J. (1992). An epidemiological study of obsessive-compulsive disorder and related disorders in Israeli adolescents. *Journal of the American Academy of Child and Adolescent Psychiatry*, **31**, 1057–1061.

10 Hyperkinetic disorders

Eric A. Taylor

Clinical picture

The core symptoms of hyperkinetic disorder are the behavioural problems of inattentiveness, overactivity, and impulsiveness. Several aspects of this simple definition need elaborating.

- Firstly, they are *behavioural* problems. The widespread use of the phrase 'attention deficit disorder' to describe the problems is clear and popular; but it does mislead some people into imagining that the core problem is a deficit in the cognitive processes of attention. This may or may not be true. Probably it is not the case: cognitive impairments are common, but they are not universal. Experimental analysis of the cognitive impairments has in fact suggested that attention is not the problem. The difficulties reside in response organization, selection and inhibition rather than in anything involving competition between inputs or maintenance of readiness: 'attention deficit' is therefore something of a misnomer (Taylor 1995). Inattentiveness is still a very helpful idea in accounting for the psychopathology, but it refers to inattentiveness in behavioural senses and is measured by behavioural observation and detailed behavioural interview accounts.

- The second aspect of the definition to stress is that these are behavioural *problems*. Many children show the behaviours to a greater or lesser degree; they only become a diagnosable disorder if they are adversely affecting the development of the child and if they are out of keeping with the child's developmental level. Furthermore, there needs to be some pervasiveness of symptoms across different situations (such as home and school) and persistence over time before they are regarded as signs of a disorder in the child's development.

- The third necessary emphasis is that these are *core* problems. Children with hyperactivity show many other associated difficulties of non-specific type. They are more likely to be oppositional, aggressive, volatile, disruptive, unpopular with other children, and criticized intensely by adults. Many are prone to accidents, and some develop antisocial or even depressive problems. All these are real problems for the children and may be the key targets for therapy in an individual child. Accordingly, many checklists of symptoms include them. But these items have predictive validity, not discriminative validity. They can be features of other sorts of disorder as well, so they ought not to be part of the diagnosis of hyperkinetic disorders.

Definitions of disorder

Different diagnostic traditions have evolved rather different categories of disorder, and many words are used to refer to them. To avoid confusion, this article will adopt a convention for the main terms:

- *Hyperactivity* will refer to a trait continuously distributed in the population: an enduring disposition to behave in a restless, inattentive, impulsive and disorganized fashion.
- *Attention deficit-hyperactivity disorder* (ADHD) will refer to a category defined by the criteria of the American Psychiatric Association (APA 1994)—a common category, applicable to perhaps 5% of the child population.
- *Hyperkinetic disorder* (HKD) will refer to the category defined by the World Health Organization's (1990) *International Classification of Disease*—a subgroup of ADHD, applicable to perhaps 0.5% of the child population.

ADHD is the broader definition and the commoner diagnosis. Either inattentiveness or overactivity–impulsivity can on its own be sufficient for the diagnosis. Other disorders, such as anxiety states, are expected to be frequently comorbid with ADHD. They are only exclusion criteria if the ADHD symptoms are 'better accounted for by another mental disorder'.

The ICD-10 diagnosis of hyperkinetic disorder is the narrower category, and almost all cases of hyperkinetic disorder should be included within ADHD. The additional criteria for hyperkinetic disorder are that all three problems of attention, hyperactivity, and impulsiveness should be present; that more stringent criteria for pervasiveness across situations are met; and that the presence of another disorder such as anxiety state is in itself an exclusion criterion. The expectation is that most cases will have a single diagnosis.

Both these diagnostic schemes have their advantages and disadvantages and a narrower or a broader definition will be suitable for different purposes. ADHD has three subtypes: with predominant inattentiveness, predominant overactivity–impulsivity, or a mixture of the two. The mixed subtype of AD/HD, in the absence of comorbid conditions other than conduct or oppositional disorders, corresponds reasonably well to the ICD-10 definition of hyperkinetic disorder.

Clinical criteria

- *Inattentiveness* has been examined in several observational studies. The most characteristic aspects are a reduced length of time spent on a task or toy presented by the examiner; an increase in the number of orientations away from a centrally presented task; and more rapid changes between activities (Milich *et al.* 1982, Dienske *et al.* 1985, Taylor 1986)
- *Overactivity* means an excess of movements. Simple measures such as actometers strapped on to various parts of the body, stabilimeter chairs, and interruption of ultrasonic beams around the room have confirmed that there is indeed excessive activity in children with ADHD, which cannot be reduced to impulsiveness or inattentiveness (Porrino *et al.* 1983, Reichenbach *et al.* 1992).
- *Impulsiveness* means acting without reflecting, and this can be conceptualized in several ways: overrapid responsiveness, sensation seeking, excessive attraction to immediate reward, aversion to waiting and a failure to plan ahead can all be seen. The behavioural criteria, in both the ICD-10 and the DSM-IV, are somewhat different and consist of

    – often blurting out answers before questions have been completed

    – having difficulty in waiting for one's turn when this is appropriate

    – frequent interruption and intrusion upon the activities of other people.

In some studies these have appeared to be a non-specific behavioural problem. Further clinical research on the nature and specificity of behavioural impulsiveness will be needed.

Epidemiological studies of prevalence

Reported prevalence rates vary considerably, but much of the variation seems to come from the definitions employed in different studies rather than from true geographical differences in prevalence. Hyperkinetic disorder is, as indicated above, rather tightly defined and the few studies so far have given consistent results. Gillberg *et al.* (1983) reported a two-stage screening survey and found a rate of hyperkinetic disorder for about 1.3% in males at primary school. Taylor *et al.* (1991) used a similar design and found a rate of 1.7% for boys at the age of 6–8 years.

When a reasonably strict definition of ADHD is used, then again the results are consistent. It applies to about 1 child in 20 of the general population. For example, the Ontario Child Health study reported an overall rate between the ages of 4–16 years of 6.3% (males 9%, females 3.3%) (Offord *et al.* 1987). The Dunedin multidisciplinary child development study found a similar rate: 6.7% (males 10.8%, females 2.1%) (Anderson *et al.* 1987, McGee *et al.* 1990). A stricter definition still—requiring the combination of impairment evidenced by a detailed interview with the teacher and a high rating score 6 months previously—gave a point prevalence rate of 4% for 7 year old boys in London, England (Taylor *et al.* 1991). The same study indicated that hyperkinetic disorder is indeed a subset of ADHD.

Considerably higher rates are reported when the diagnosis of ADHD is based entirely on symptom counts at one point in time. Shekim *et al.* (1985), using structured interview techniques, found 16% of a 9 year old sample to show hyperactivity; Taylor *et al.* (1991) found a similar rate (17%) in boys, using a structured interview. Velez *et al.* (1989) also described a rate of about 17% in 9–12 year old children studied in New York State, USA. A study in Puerto Rico reported by Bird *et al.* (1988) found that 9.9% of 4–16 year old children showed ADHD. All these prevalence estimates have been based on children of school age. Estimates are not yet reliable for preschoolers, adolescents, or adults.

Studies of natural course

The natural course of untreated disorder can be inferred from longitudinal studies of epidemiologically ascertained groups. Fergusson *et al.* (1994) analysed a birth cohort studied at different points with parent and teacher rating scales. Hyperactive, inattentive behavior proved not to be a risk factor at all for later offending and antisocial activity. It appeared as a risk only because of its prior association with conduct disorder, which was the true risk. Hyperactivity was not trivial, for it did predict educational underachievement, but it was not the risk factor for social adjustment that had been supposed. Moffitt (1990) analysed another birth cohort, and came to different conclusions. Even when early aggressive behavior (at age 5) was statistically controlled, hyperactive behavior predicted antisocial behaviors in adolescence.

Birth cohorts are typically too small to contain adequate numbers of children who meet criteria for the presence of disorder. Their analyses therefore tend to be based on dimensional analyses of continuous measures in the general population of children. Their results may well be, in large part, determined by findings for children who are in the 'normal' range for hyperactivity, and it would be possible to mislead if one drew conclusions directly for those at the extreme of the distribution.

Only a few studies have been able to base their conclusions about natural history on cases of disorder. Schachar *et al.* (1981) reanalysed the Isle of Wight longitudinal epidemiological study, and concluded that hyperactivity—if it was pervasive across situations and informants—strongly predicted the persistence of psychological deviance between the ages of 9 and 14 years. However, the initial stratification of cases had been for other types of disorder, so their cases of hyperactivity were probably particularly likely to show comorbid disorder. It is therefore possible that their prediction resulted, not from hyperactivity being a specific risk, but from its being a marker to increased severity of psychological disturbance. Gillberg *et al.* (1988) concluded that childen with hyperkinetic disorder were at high risk for a range of adverse psychological outcomes. Here too there was a real possibility that comorbid problems might be the factors responsible for later psychosocial dysfunction. The initial identification of cases had been in part because they met criteria for problems in the domains of attention, motor and perceptual organization; and the outcome included a number of cases showing the features of pervasive developmental disorders, which would have been exclusion criteria in most investigations.

Taylor *et al.* (1996) described a follow-up study of children who were identified, by parent and teacher ratings in a large community survey of 7–8 year olds, because they met criteria for pervasive hyperactivity. At the age of 17, 9 years later, they were compared with controls using detailed interview techniques as well as parental ratings. Hyperactivity was a risk factor for later development, even after allowing for the coexistence of conduct disorder problems and excluding children who showed the problems of emotional disorder or autism. The affected children were at risk of a wide range of psychological problems, including violence and other conduct problems, and social and peer problems. A minority of the children with hyperactivity at age 7 seemed to escape complications and develop out of the disorder, so that their young adult outcome was not at all compromised.

More research is needed about the natural history of the disorder. Already, however, it seems clear that the untreated course in population samples includes a substantial risk of continuing hyperactivity and developing other problems of personality function. This is the main reason for concluding that it should be a prime target of treatment by child mental health services.

Intervention studies

There is a massive evidence base from controlled trials of a variety of treatments. The strongest evidence is for the effect of a sympathomimetic central nervous system stimulant, methylphenidate, over treatment periods up to a year and in doses up to 60 mg daily. Scores of random-allocation placebo-controlled trials have been reported—indeed, there is a large number of reviews and several quantitative reviews have appeared. The reader is therefore referred to a review of reviews (Swanson *et al.* 1993). Results have been unequivocal. Methylphenidate reduces hyperactive behaviour. The conclusion is replicated across different designs (e.g. crossover and parallel treatment comparisons), different definitions of disorder, and different measures of effect (such as rating scales by parent or teacher, interviews with parent, direct observation of child, and mechanical recordings of activity level). The effect size is large; in excess of 1 SD. There are also beneficial effects on tests of cognitive performance, academic productivity, oppositionality, and social interactions with parents and peers (Schachar *et al.* 1996). Adverse effects can include sleeplessness, headache, loss of appetite, abdominal pain, tics, tachycardia, social withdrawal, and hallucinations; but these problems are for the most part minor and can often be managed by attention to dosage level and timing of doses.

Two other stimulants, dexamphetamine and pemoline, have been shown to be more effective than placebo in a smaller number of short-term trials conducted some years ago (Swanson *et al.* 1993). Superiority to placebo in random-allocation, double-blind trials of varying methodology has also been reported for clonidine, tricyclic antidepressants such as imipramine and desipramine, and neuroleptic antidopaminergic drugs (thioridazine, haloperidol).

The longer-term effects of medication are not scientifically clear. On the one hand, some children are still helped by a stimulant drug even after years of continuous therapy (Sleator *et al.* 1974); some children lose all the benefit of medication if it is stopped after a few months (Brown *et al.* 1986). On the other hand, some children on long-term therapy show no worsening when it is stopped and are not deriving benefit from it (Charles and Schain 1981). These are not necessarily contradictions. Clinical experience suggests that both sides of the argument are true. Most children who obtain benefit will require a lengthy period of therapy for several years. At some point—which cannot yet be predicted in advance—many childen improve to the point where the drug is no longer needed. In practice, therefore, children on maintenance therapy need a regular trial off medication to assess whether there is a continuing need. The aim is to maintain medication until the child's maturation and learning of cognitive skills make medication unnecessary.

Stimulants are effective, but it does not follow that all children with ADHD require them. Many children will be helped by psychosocial interventions without medication. Opinions differ between clinical authorities as to exactly what the indications for the treatment should be. The use of stimulants therefore varies very greatly between different centres and different nations. Research has not yet established exactly what the indications should be: the action of the drugs is clear, but their superiority to other types of treatment is not yet clearly established, and the generalization from research trials to community practice has not been adequately addressed. Most published trials are based on well-characterized groups at a high level of severity. Cases have typically been diagnosed by explicit research criteria requiring that problems are shown both by parental account and by a rating scale completed by teachers; comorbid disorders have been excluded; and very often the problems are of sufficient severity to warrant a referral to a specialist centre. These aspects mean that most children in trials are likely to have met hyperkinetic disorder criteria as well as ADHD. By contrast, children treated in routine practice often have lesser degrees of hyperactivity and higher rates of other problems. There is little good information on the efficacy of medication in these children, with ADHD that falls short of the definition of hyperkinetic disorder. We need to know more about the costs and benefits of therapy for these children. Within one series of boys showing a wide range of disruptive behaviours, a good response to methylphenidate (by comparison with placebo) was predicted by severity and pervasiveness of hyperactive behaviour, poor scores on tests of attention, and an absence of emotional symptoms such as anxiety (Taylor *et al.* 1987). This group corresponds quite well to the narrower diagnosis of hyperkinetic disorder, and is probably the best indication for a trial of stimulants as a first line of management. In less severe cases, many European clinicians prefer to reserve medication for situations in which psychological approaches are insufficient by themselves.

A range of psychosocial interventions have also been shown to be effective, either by random allocation trials (Barkley 1990) or good studies of single cases (Yule 1986). Pelham (personal communication) has identified 7 strongly evidential group trials of behavioural parent training, 3 studies using waiting list controls, and 4 trials where the evidence is less good because either the numbers are rather small or there is only a pre–post-treatment comparison without a comparison untreated group. He has also identified 3 well-designed comparison trials of behaviour modification in classroom settings, together with 25 published reports using informative single-subject designs, 3 pre–post group trials, and some 20 group studies of classroom interventions that were not targeted specifically on children with ADHD but would have included many such children among their subjects. The cumulative weight of these investigations is to establish some forms of behaviour modification at school and at home as effective therapies. Long-term trials, however, are not available.

There is too little direct comparison between psychological and drug treatments for any scientific conclusions so far; but large-scale comparison trials of these therapies are in progress. Other forms of psychological treatment, such as cognitive therapy, have not yet shown their efficacy in controlled trials; and some treatments such as problem-solving training are promising but not yet sufficiently evaluated. Nevertheless, the multitude of problems often presented by hyperactive children and those who take care of them calls for multimodal intervention; responsive advice for parents, the children themselves, and their teachers or nurses is the base of any treatment plan.

Diet treatments have had a chequered history. For years the scientific trials were dominated by testing the Feingold hypothesis that certain synthetic dyes and preservatives added to food, together with naturally occurring salicylates, had a direct and harmful effect upon children with ADHD. Challenge studies showed that the treatment was not effective. More recently, the question has been reopened because four studies have found evidence in random-allocation placebo-controlled designs that some children with hyperactive behaviour can be helped by elimination diets (Carter *et al.* 1995). These diets were different from those based on the Feingold hypothesis. They identified for the individual child those foods to which he or she had developed an intolerance, and assessed the diet in designs where the incriminated food (and therefore the placebo and excipient) was different for each child but the outcome measures and design were constant. Results make it probable that the diet is helpful in selected cases, but leave open the questions of how many (and which) children can be helped in this way, whether there is any long-term effect, and the comparison with psychological and pharmacological treatments.

Short-term and long-term outcomes

The short-term outcomes for children with hyperkinetic disorders can be inferred from the intervention studies described above. Treatments can have a sizeable effect. Indeed, in the case of stimulant medication, the effect on behaviour can seem to be dramatically large. Nevertheless, problems are seldom abolished. There has been considerable debate about whether medication achieves 'normalization': at least two issues are involved. First, some authorities point encouragingly to the undoubted fact that many treated children are reduced in their hyperactivity to a score that lies within a 'normal' range—say, within 2 SD of the population mean. This is true, but it ignores the extent to which population studies have found that the developmental risk of hyperactivity is dimensional (e.g. Fergusson *et al.* 1994). Even within an arbitrarily defined normal range, the children may still be at increased risk. It is rare indeed for a child's hyperactivity to be reduced to the 'normal' level in the sense of being at or below the mean for the population.

The second reservation about the supposedly normalizing action of medication in the short term is that it refers only to hyperactive behaviour; and the problems of children with hyperactivity are often multiple. Some components of the clinical picture are relatively refractory to medication. The ability to acquire new academic or social skills, or indeed to defer gratification, is not necessarily helped much by medication. This restriction of efficacy of medication is likely to apply to other treatments too, and is all the more of a limitation for treatment given routinely by a generic service rather than with all the care that can be provided by a highly specialized service running a clinical trial.

In the longer term, it is clear that hyperactivity can be persistent over time and can impair development even though effective therapies are given. Several studies have followed clinically diagnosed schoolchildren with ADHD over periods of 4–14 years. All have found that they show, by comparison with normal controls, a much higher rate of disruptive behavior disorders at follow-up (Hoy *et al.* 1978, Satterfield *et al.* 1982, August *et al.* 1983, Loney *et al.* 1983, Hechtman *et al.* 1984, Gittelman *et al.* 1985, Wallander 1988, Barkley *et al.* 1990, Esser *et al.* 1990, Mannuzza *et al.* 1991).

One of the adverse outcomes is the persistence of hyperactive behaviour. In adolescence, the ability to concentrate improves and activity levels decrease, in normal subjects as well as in hyperactive cases, as demonstrated by longitudinal analyses of repeated measures (Fischer *et al.* 1993). Hill and Schoener (1996) reviewed the prospective studies that reported the persistence of the diagnosis of ADHD, and concluded that the rate fell with time: 7–10 year old children with ADHD had about a 40% chance of still showing a diagnosis at the age of 13, but by the age of 18 only 15–30% showed ADHD. This is still a high rate, and in the one study that originally identified the children with research criteria the outlook was much worse: 88% still had ADHD 8 years later (Barkley *et al.* 1990). When children with ADHD have reached their 20s, the rate has fallen considerably, to only 8% (still 8 times higher than that in normal controls) according to Mannuzza *et al.* (1993).

Other adverse outcomes include aggressive and antisocial behavior and delinquency, educational problems, and impairment in social relationships. In a follow-up of untreated community cases, 23 out of 51 children with hyperactivity had at least one DSM-III-R diagnosis 9 years later and for 10 of them the diagnosis was conduct disorder (Taylor *et al.* 1996). In clinic-referred cases the rate in adolescence is higher, and does not decrease with time: about three-quarters are likely to show antisocial behaviour (Satterfield *et al.* 1982, Barkley *et al.* 1990). Substance abuse, however, does not seem to be a specific outcome.

The literature is still dependent on case–control comparisons in which the cases have been referred to specialized clinics and the controls are from the general population; or in which the controls are non-referred brothers (Loney *et al.* 1983, Mannuzza *et al.* 1991). It seems likely that many other factors besides the presence of hyperactive behavior will determine referral to clinical services (Woodward *et al.* 1997). This makes it difficult to be clear about the exact nature of the developmental risk. What components of the disorder, or what associated adversities, or what complications account for the adverse outcome? The question matters greatly to clinicians, because it will determine how they intervene and with what therapeutic goals. Answering it will require new generations of study that address the questions of developmental mechanisms.

Continuity versus discontinuity

In one sense, the outcome studies reviewed above have shown clear evidence for continuity. Hyperactive behaviour is likely to lead on to psychological problems even when treatment is provided. The nature of this continuity raises further questions:

- Is the continuity of a single problem of hyperactivity, or does the nature of the problem change over time?
- Even when there is continuity of hyperactivity, does it mean the same thing at different ages?
- Is the continuity for the whole complex of hyperactivity or the individual components separately?
- Is the continuity that of a dimension or a category, i.e. is there continuity only at a high level of problems?

Continuity in type of problem

Longitudinal follow-up studies have emphasized that the adolescent outcome of hyperactivity includes many types of mental disturbance, especially conduct disorder. It was once taught that hyperactivity was only a risk if it set in motion a course of conduct disorder, and that the usual outcome of hyperactivity itself was one of steady maturation out of the problem so that it largely disappeared by the age of puberty. Unfortunately, this has turned out not to be the case. The follow-up studies of the last decade have demonstrated that hyperactivity itself persists (see above). In a longitudinal epidemiological study from London (Taylor *et al.* 1996), the strongest continuity found was from hyperactive behaviour at 7 to hyperactive behaviour at the age of 17. This pathway was not contingent upon the presence of conduct disorder. Hyperactive children without conduct disorder were at very nearly as much risk as those who showed a combination of both problems. When those with conduct disorder were excluded from the analysis, then hyperactivity at 7 remained a strong risk factor for social adjustment at the age of 17. We do not yet know whether persistence of hyperactivity is a necessary condition for the development of other types of problem, but a longitudinal study from New York has suggested just that (Gittelman *et al.* 1985).

Continuity over developmental stages

So far, the behavioural problems that comprise hyperactivity have been considered as though they were constant throughout development. This may well not be the case. It is far from clear, for instance, that inattentiveness will have the same significance at the age of 3 as at the age of

17. In general, it seems likely to do so. Even in the preschool period, severely hyperactive behaviour seems to carry the associations of developmental delays and high persistence that are seen in school age children. Even so, the possibility that different factors determine it at different stages should receive serious research attention. Developmentalists who have studied related fields have suggested that apparently similar behaviours may have rather different significance at different ages. An example comes from the study of habituation during the first years of life, relevant because it is quite likely that habituation is related to some aspects of attention deficit (McCall and Carriger 1993). It is not a stable trait, and the correlations between children's habituation over a period of 5 months is virtually zero. Nevertheless a measure of habituation taken between the age of 2 and 8 months is a moderately good predictor of later IQ. Rapid habituation predicts a higher IQ years later. There is an apparent paradox that measures of habituation should have a low stability but a very high predictive value. This paradox is resolved if one supposes that the determinants of habituation are different at different ages.

Another example of possible discontinuity comes from studies of gaze in infancy. There is a good deal of variation between infants in the length of time for which they fixate visual stimuli. These differences are stable over the first year of life, and predict cognitive ability later (Taylor 1995). Infants who look for short periods at visually presented objects at the age of 3 months, typically perform better than long-looking ones when they are cognitively tested in later childhood. Presumably therefore inspection time in infancy is a measure of the speed and efficiency with which children process visual stimuli, not of the duration of attention. Attending to objects has different determinants, and different developmental significance, at different stages of development.

Continuity of disorder or component

Not only does the degree of continuity and discontinuity need to be established, it is also necessary to determine the extent to which the continuity is that of the whole complex of hyperactivity or the individual components separately. In the first case, one would expect that all the components of hyperactivity would predict all the others since each component predicts later disturbance to the extent that it is correlated with the major risk factor of hyperactivity. In the second case each component predicts itself but not the other aspects. Inattentiveness leads to inattentiveness; impulsiveness leads to impulsiveness; but there is no necessary crossover between the two. If this is the pattern of development, then we will clearly need to think in terms of different behavioural tracks rather than a single disorder. The developmental evidence does not yet allow us to make clear conclusions.

Continuity of dimension or category

The longitudinal studies of population groups referred to earlier have for the most part been based on continuously distributed measurements of dimensions on which the whole population of children can be ranked. The implication from these is that subclinical levels of hyperactive behaviour are asociated with lesser degrees of adverse outcome: that there is in effect a continuum of risk. However, the point is not yet established beyond doubt. Some studies based on clinical diagnosis have suggested that no seriously adverse outcome is encountered in children with raised but subclinical levels of hyperactive behaviour (Gittelman *et al.* 1985). There is still much work to do before these apparent contradictions can be resolved.

Risks and prognostic factors

The outcome studies have shown that there is heterogeneity in psychological sequelae, ranging from severe impairment to very good social function. It is not yet possible to say what predicts outcome, and new generations of longitudinal studies will be needed to explore and differentiate the risks involved.

Genetic influences on hyperactive behaviour are known to be strong (Taylor 1994). It is also quite possible that genetic factors influence the course over time that the disorder takes. Longitudinal studies of twins should be informative for disentangling these influences from the effects of disorder itself and of the environment. The severity of initial hyperactivity is likely to be one of the factors determining risk; but severity is often associated with other types of comorbidity and it is not possible to distinguish completely which is responsible. Within groups of children who show ADHD, the presence of conduct disorder predicts a worse social adjustment in later development (August *et al.* 1983, Barkley *et al.* 1990). There are also several indications that hyperactivity predicts a particularly adverse outcome in children with conduct disorder. Schoolchildren with reliably identified conduct disorder have been followed into their adolescence by Schachar *et al.* (1981), Farrington *et al.* (1990), and Magnusson and Bergman (1990) with the finding that those who showed high levels of hyperactivity when first studied had more antisocial outcomes than those who had not been hyperactive.

Present knowledge admits of several possible developmental formulations about the interplay of childhood hyperactivity and conduct disorder.There might be a unitary disorder that can manifest with either or both of the problems, and whose outcome is a function of overall severity rather than of which type of disorder is predominant. Conduct disorder might constitute the developmental risk. According to this hypothesis, hyperactivity in the absence of conduct disorder would not be a risk for later adjustment and the degree of hyperactivity would not predict outcome once the degree of conduct disorder had been allowed for. Conversely, hyperactivity might be the major developmental risk factor and conduct disorder an epiphenomenon. As another possibility, hyperactivity and conduct disorder might be differentiated risk factors, each with a characteristic type of outcome. They would then have separate implications for developmental course that would not necessarily interact. Children with hyperactivity would be predicted to be at risk for hyperactivity but not for conduct disorder later (once initial comorbidity with conduct disorder was allowed for); children with conduct disorder would be at risk for conduct disorder later but not for hyperactivity. Finally, the developmental risk might be present only for a subgroup, e.g. for those children who show both problems.

These differential predictions call for more studies in which all the four groups, defined by the presence or absence of hyperactivity or conduct disorder, are represented. The prognostic impact of other types of comorbid disorder, such as emotional problems and neurodevelopmental delays, need to be worked out in similar ways. Such studies will need to take account of the range of possible outcomes. Educational underachievement, unsatisfactory peer relationships, and substance misuse may all have different predictors so will need separate examination.

Continuity may also depend upon the psychological environment in which the children live. At present the most promising line of evidence focuses on the development of hostile and critical expressed emotion by parents. This measure, taken at age 7, is a reliable quantified rating of the affective tone with which parents talk about their children. In the London study cited (Taylor *et al.* 1996), hostile expressed emotion at the age of 7 predicted whether children with hyperactivity would have conduct disorder at the age of 17. Of course, as in the previous example, the hostile expressed emotion may very well have been brought about by the deviant behaviour of the children. Hyperactive behaviour is aversive to parents; when hyperactivity is reduced by medication for the child, then hostile expressed emotion by parents tends to fall. Nevertheless, the independently predictive significance of critical expressed emotion implies that it is not acting merely as a marker to the presence of behavioural disturbance in the child. Rather, once it has appeared, it may be responsible for determining the outcome.

Conclusions

This review of outcome in the hyperkinetic disorders of childhood has raised more questions than it has been able to answer from empirical evidence. A few conclusions are possible. They are subject to many qualifications, but they carry strong implications for the organization of clinical services. Disorders of attention and activity are risk factors for development. Some of this risk comes from the hyperactivity itself, rather than from associated comorbidity. Therefore, the reduction of hyperactive behaviour should be one of the targets of a successful mental health service. There is a range of effective treatments, whose value in controlled trials is beyond doubt. In spite of this, the outcome is still dismal. Some of the problematic outcome may arise simply because the treatments are not given well enough. Psychosocial treatments may not be given with enough intensity and attention to detail; medication may not be given for long enough. Even so, it seems likely that the available treatments do not alter all the components of the disorder and that there are risk factors such as the interpersonal relationships made by affected children that will need more attention by the treatment services. At present it is not possible to say with confidence that the long-term outcome is affected by the treatment given. The research that is needed has been outlined. It calls for a more sustained application of the concepts and techniques of developmental psychopathology.

References

Anderson, J.C., Williams, S., McGee, R., and Silva, P.A. (1987). DSM-III disorders in preadolescent children: prevalence in a large sample from the general population. *Archives of General Psychiatry*, **44**, 69–76.

APA (1994). *Diagnostic and statistical manual of mental disorders*, 4th edn. American Psychiatric Association, Washington, D.C.

August, G.J., Stewart, M.A., and Holmes, C.S. (1983). A four-year follow-up of hyperactive boys with and without conduct disorder. *British Journal of Psychiatry*, **143**, 192–198.

Barkley, R.A. (1990). *Attention deficit hyperactivity disorder: a handbook for diagnosis and treatment*. Guilford, New York.

Barkley, R.A., Fischer, M., Edelbrock, C.S., and Smallish, L. (1990). The adolescent outcome of hyperactive children diagnosed by research criteria: I. An 8-year prospective follow-up study. *Journal of the American Academy of Child and Adolescent Psychiatry*, **29**, 546–557.

Bird, H.R., Canino, G., Rubio-Stipec, M. *et al*. (1988). Estimates of the prevalence of childhood maladjustment in a community survey in Puerto Rico. The use of combined measures. *Archives of General Psychiatry*, **45**, 1120–1126.

Brown, R.T., Borden, K.A., Wynne, M.E., Schleser, R., and Clingerman, S.R. (1986). Methylphenidate and cognitive therapy with hyperactive children: A methodological reconsideration. *Journal of Abnormal Child Psychology*, **14**, 481–497.

Carter, C.M., Urbanowicz, M., Hemsley, R., Mantilla, L., Strobel, S., Graham, P.J., and Taylor, E. (1993). Effects of a few food diet in attention deficit disorder. *Archives of Disease in Childhood*, **69**, 564–568.

Charles, L. and Schain, R. (1981). A four-year follow-up study of the effects of methylphenidate on the behavior and academic achievements of hyperactive children. *Journal of Abnormal Child Psychology*, **9**, 495–505.

Dienske, H., de Jonge, G., and Sanders-Woudstra, J.A.R. (1985). Quantitative criteria for attention and activity in child psychiatric patients. *Journal of Child Psychology and Psychiatry*, **26**, 895–916.

Esser, G., Schmidt, M.H., and Woerner, W. (1990). Epidemiology and course of psychiatric disorders in school-age children—results of a longitudinal study. *Journal of Child Psychology and Psychiatry*, **31**, 243–263.

Farrington, D.P., Loeber, R., and van Kammen W.B. (1990). Long-term criminal outcomes of hyperactivity-impulsivity-attention deficit and conduct problems in childhood. In *Straight and devious pathways from childhood to adulthood*, ed. L.N. Robins and M. Rutter, pp 62–81. Cambridge University Press, Cambridge.

Fergusson, D.M., Horwood, L.J., and Lynskey, M.T. (1994a). The childhoods of multiple problem adolescents: A 15-year longitudinal study. *Journal of Child Psychology and Psychiatry*, **35**, 1077–1092

Fergusson, D.M., Horwood, L.J., and Lynskey, M.T. (1994b). Structure of DSM-III-R criteria for disruptive childhood behaviors: confirmatory factor models. *Journal of the American Academy of Child and Adolescent Psychiatry*, **33**, 1145–1155.

Fischer, M., Barkley, R.A., Fletcher, K.E., and Smallish, L. (1993). The stability of dimensions of behaviour in ADHD and normal children over an 8-year follow-up. *Journal of Abnormal Child Psychology*, **21**, 315–337.

Gillberg, C., Carlstrom, G., and Rasmussen, P. (1983). Hyperkinetic disorders in children with perceptual, motor and attentional deficits. *Journal of Child Psychology and Psychiatry*, **24**, 233–246.

Gillberg, C. and Gillberg, C.H. (1988). Generalized hyperkinesis: a follow-up study from age 7 to 13 years. *Journal of the American Academy of Child and Adolescent Psychiatry*, **27**, 55–59.

Gittelman, R., Mannuzza, S., Shenker, R., and Bonagura, N. (1985). Hyperactive boys almost grown up. 1. Psychiatric status. *Archives of General Psychiatry*, **42**, 937–947.

Hechtman, L., Weiss, G., and Perlman, T. (1984). Young adult outcome of hyperactive children who received long-term stimulant treatment. *Journal of the American Academy of Child Psychiatry*, **23**, 261–269

Hill, J.C. and Schoener, E.P. (1996). Age- dependent decline of attention deficit hyperactivity disorder. *American Journal of Psychiatry*, **153**, 1143–1146.

Hoy, E., Weiss, G., Minde, K., and Cohen, N. (1978). The hyperactive child at adolescence: cognitive, emotional, and social functioning. *Journal of Abnormal Child Psychology*, **6**, 311–324

Loney, J., Whaley-Klahn, M.A., Kosier, T., and Conboy, J. (1983). Hyperactive boys and their brothers at 21: Predictors of aggressive and antisocial outcomes. In *Prospective studies of crime and delinquency*, ed. K.T. van Dusen and S.A. Mednick, pp 181–206. Kluwer-Nijhoff, Boston.

McCall, R.B. and Carriger, M.S. (1993). A meta-analysis of infant habituation and recognition memory performance as predictors of later IQ. *Child Development*, **64**, 57–79.

McGee, R., Williams, S., and Silva, P.A. (1984). Background characteristics of aggressive, hyperactive and aggressive-hyperactive boys. *Journal of the American Academy of Child and Adolescent Psychiatry*, **23**, 280–284.

Magnusson, D. and Bergman L.R. (1990). A pattern approach to the study of pathways from childhood to adulthood. In *Straight and devious pathways from childhood to adulthood*, ed. L., Robins and M. Rutter, pp 101–115. Cambridge University Press, Cambridge.

Mannuzza, S., Klein, R.G., and Addalli K.A. (1991). Young adult mental status of hyperactive boys and their brothers: A prospective follow-up study. *Journal of the American Academy of Child and Adolescent Psychiatry*, **30**, 743–751.

Mannuzza, S., Klein, R.G., Bessler, A., Malloy, P., and LaPadula, M. (1993). Adult outcome of hyperactive boys. *Archives of General Psychiatry*, **50**, 565–576.

Milich, R., Loney, J., and Landau, S. (1982). The independent dimensions of hyperactivity and aggression: a validation with playroom observation data. *Journal of Abnormal Psychology*, **91**, 183–198.

Moffitt, T.E. (1990). Juvenile delinquency and attention deficit disorder: Boys' developmental trajectories from age 3 to 15. *Child Development.* **61**, 893–910.

Offord, D.R., Boyle, M.H., Szatmari, P., Rae-Grant, N.I., Links, P.S., Cadman, D.T., Byles, J.A., Crawford, J.W., Blum, H.M., Byrne, C., Thomas, H., and Woodward, C.A. (1987). Ontario Child Health Study. II. Six month prevalence of disorder and rates of service utilization. *Archives of General Psychiatry*, **44**, 832–836.

Porrino, L.J., Rapoport, J.L., Behar, D., Sceery, W., Ismond, D., and Bunney, W.E. (1983). A naturalistic assessment of the motor activity of hyperactive boys: I. Comparison with normal controls. *Archives of General Psychiatry*, **40**, 681–687.

Reichenbach, L., Sharma, V., and Newcorn, J.H. (1992). Childrens motor activity, reliability and relationship to attention and behaviour. *Developmental Neuropsychology*, **8**, 87–97.

Satterfield, J., Hoppe, C.M., and Schell, A.M. (1982). A prospective study of delinquency in 100 adolescent boys with attention deficit disorder and 88 normal adolescent boys. *American Journal of Psychiatry*, **139**, 795–798.

Schachar, R.J., Rutter, M., and Smith, A. (1981). The characteristics of situationally and pervasively hyperactive children: implications for syndrome definition. *Journal of Child*

Psychology and Psychiatry, **22**, 375–392.

Schachar, R., Tannock, R., and Cunningham, C. (1996). Treatment. In *Hyperactivity disorders of childhood*, ed. S. Sandberg, pp. 433–476. Cambridge University Press, Cambridge.

Shekim, W.O., Kashari, J., Beck, N. *et al.* (1985). The prevalence of attention deficit disorders in a rural midwestern community sample of nine-year-old children. *Journal of the American Academy of Child Psychiatry*, **24**, 765–770.

Sleator, E., Neumann, H., and Sprague, R. (1974). Hyperactive children: A continuous long-term placebo-controlled follow-up. *Journal of the American Medical Association*, **229**, 316–317.

Swanson, J.M., McBurnett, K., Wigal, T., Pfiffner, L.J., Lerner, M.A., Williams, L., Christian, D.L., Tamm, L., Willcutt, E., Crowley, K., Clevenger, W., Khouzam, N., Woo, C., Crinella, F.M., and Fisher, T.D. (1993). Effect of stimulant medication on children with attention deficit disorder: A review of reviews. *Exceptional Children*, **60**, 154–162.

Taylor, E. (1986). Attention deficit. In *The overactive child*, ed. E. Taylor. Clinics in Developmental Medicine No. 97, MacKeith Press; London/Blackwell Scientific/Oxford:

Taylor, E. (1994). Syndromes of attention deficit and overactivity. In *Child and adolescent psychiatry: modern approaches*, 3rd edn, ed. M. Rutter, E. Taylor, and L. Hersov, pp. 285–307. Blackwell Scientific, Oxford.

Taylor, E. (1995). Dysfunctions of attention. In *Developmental psychopathology, vol. 2: risk, disorder, and adaptation*, ed. D. Cicchetti and D.J. Cohen, pp. 243–273. Wiley, New York,

Taylor, E., Schachar, R., Thorley, G., Wieselberg, M., Everitt, B., and Rutter, M. (1987). Which boys respond to stimulant medication? A controlled trial of methylphenidate in boys with disruptive behaviour. *Psychological Medicine*, **17**, 121–143.

Taylor, E., Sandberg, S., Thorley, G., and Giles, S. (1991). *The epidemiology of childhood hyperactivity*. Maudsley Monographs No. 33, Oxford University Press, Oxford.

Taylor, E., Chadwick, O., Heptinstall, E., and Danckaerts, M. (1996). Hyperactivity and conduct problems as risk factors for adolescent development. *Journal of the American Academy of Child and Adolescent Psychiatry*, **35**, 1213–1226.

Velez, C.N., Johnson, J., and Cohen, P. (1989). A longitudinal analysis of selected risk factors for childhood psychopathology. *Journal of the American Academy of Child and Adolescent Psychiatry*, **28**, 861–864.

Wallander, J.L. (1988). The relationship between attention problems in childhood and antisocial behaviour eight years later. *Journal of Child Psychology and Psychiatry*, **29**, 53–61.

WHO (1990). *International classification of diseases*, 10th revision. World Health Organization, Geneva.

Woodward, L., Dowdney, L., and Taylor, E. (1997). Child, parent and family factors associated with the clinical referral of hyperactive children. *Journal of Child Psychology and Psychiatry*, **38**, 479–485.

Yule, W. (1986) Psychological treatments. In *The overactive child*, ed. E. Taylor. Clinics in Developmental Medicine No. 97, MacKeith Press, London/Blackwell Scientific, Oxford.

11 Conduct disorder and delinquency

David P. Farrington

Within the scope of a single chapter, it is obviously impossible to provide an exhaustive review of the topics of conduct disorder (CD) and delinquency. I will be very selective in focusing on results obtained in the more important studies, namely large-scale community surveys such as the Ontario Child Health Study (Offord *et al.* 1987), prospective longitudinal surveys such as the Cambridge Study in Delinquent Development (Farrington 1995), and randomized experiments such as the Montreal longitudinal-experimental study (Tremblay *et al.* 1995). Although the chapter has a developmental perspective, the main focus is on antisocial behaviour between ages 7–17 inclusive. CD is defined according to the DSM system (APA 1994), and the main thrust is on research carried out in North America, the UK, and other developed countries. Research specifically on aggression and violence will not be reviewed (Coie and Dodge 1998, Farrington 1998, Loeber and Farrington 1998). Most research concerns males, but studies of females are included where applicable. More extensive book length reviews of CD and delinquency are available elsewhere (Kazdin 1995, Rutter *et al.* 1998).

CLINICAL PICTURE

Definitions

Robins (1998) has traced the development of CD definitions over time. According to DSM-IV (APA 1994, p.85), the essential feature of CD is a repetitive and persistent pattern of behaviour in which the basic rights of others or major age-appropriate societal norms are violated. Also, the disturbance of behaviour must cause clinically significant impairment in social, academic or occupational functioning. According to the DSM-IV diagnostic criteria, 3 or more out of 15 specified behaviours must be present, including aggression to people or animals, property destruction, stealing or lying, and violating rules (e.g. truanting, running away). Frequent, serious, persistent behaviours shown in several different settings are most likely to be defined as symptoms of a disorder.

Two criticisms might be levied against the symptoms included in DSM-IV. The first is that they predominantly describe the kinds of aggressive acts committed by males (overt aggression) as opposed to females (indirect or relationship aggression; Bjorkqvist *et al.* 1992). The second is that they focus on behaviour rather than personality. Just as psychopathy includes both an antisocial life style and a callous, unemotional personality (Harpur *et al.* 1989), so, arguably, should CD (Christian *et al.* 1997).

Delinquency is defined according to acts prohibited by the criminal law, such as theft, burglary, robbery, violence, vandalism, and drug use. Other acts included in CD (e.g. truancy, running away from home) are defined as 'status offences' in the US. The main difference between CD and delinquency is that CD involves impairment in functioning. Interestingly, DSM-IV states that the CD diagnosis should be applied only when the behaviour is symptomatic of an underlying dysfunction within the individual and not simply a reaction to the immediate social context (e.g. a high crime area: APA 1994, p.88).

Comorbidity

Not surprisingly, in light of the similar definitions of CD and delinquency, these two constructs are highly correlated (Loeber *et al.* 1998, p. 168). In the Christchurch Study in New Zealand, Fergusson and Horwood (1995) reported that 90% of children with 3 or more CD symptoms at age 15 were self-reported frequent offenders at age 16 (compared with only 17% of children with no CD symptoms). Similarly, Foley *et al.* (1996) concluded that 90% of juvenile offenders met the criteria for CD.

CD is highly comorbid with oppositional defiant disorder (ODD) (Lahey *et al.* 1997) and attention deficit hyperactivity disorder (ADHD) (Biederman *et al.* 1991). It has been suggested that subgroups of children should be studied, such as those with both CD and ADHD, those with only CD, and those with only ADHD (McArdle *et al.* 1995). The comorbid children are generally more seriously impaired cases (Lewinsohn *et al.* 1995). There are some indications that CD girls have more comorbid conditions than CD boys (Loeber and Keenan 1994). CD is also comorbid with substance use (Boyle and Offord 1991) and with depression (Petersen *et al.* 1993). Its comorbidity with anxiety disorder is less clear; according to Russo and Beidel (1994), CD and anxiety are negatively associated in children but positively associated in adolescents.

Generally, delinquents are versatile rather than specialized in their offending. In the Cambridge Study, 86% of violent offenders also had convictions for non-violent offences (Farrington 1991b). Violent and non-violent but equally frequent offenders are very similar in their childhood and adolescent features (Capaldi and Patterson 1996). Studies of transition matrices summarizing the probability of one type of offence following another show that there is a small degree of specificity superimposed on a great deal of generality in juvenile delinquency (Farrington *et al.* 1988). Sex offenders tend to be the most specialized, and specialization tends to increase with age.

Epidemiology

Nottelman and Jensen (1995) have usefully summarized findings obtained in epidemiological studies of CD. One problem in interpreting prevalence results concerns the time period to which they refer, which may be 6 months, 12 months, or a period of years. Prevalence rates are different for males and females and different at different ages. Also, prevalence rates change as the DSM definitions change (Lahey *et al.* 1990).

Summarizing results obtained in some of the major community surveys, the 6 month prevalence of CD for boys was 6.5% at age 4–11 and 10.4% at age 12–16 in the Ontario Child Health Study (Offord *et al.* 1987). For girls, it was 1.8% at age 4–11 and 4.1% at age 12–16. In the New York State longitudinal study, the 12 month prevalence of CD for boys was 16.0% at age 10–13 and 15.8% at age 14–16 (Cohen *et al.* 1993a). For girls, it was 3.8% at age 10–13 and 9.2% at age 14–16. In the Dunedin longitudinal survey in New Zealand, the 12 month prevalence at age 15 of aggressive CD was 1.6% and of non-aggressive CD was 5.7%, for boys and girls combined (McGee *et al.* 1990).

Even when measured by convictions, the prevalence of delinquency is surprisingly high. In the Cambridge Study, the 12 month prevalence of convictions increased to a peak at age 17 and then declined (Farrington 1992a). It was 1.5 per 100 males at age 10, 5.4 at age 13, 11.2 at age 17, 6.4 at age 22, and 3.2 at age 30. The median age for most types of offences (burglary, robbery, theft of and from vehicles, shoplifting) was 17; for violence it was 20 and for fraud 21. The prevalence of delinquency according to self-reports is even higher, of course. In the large-scale Denver, Rochester, and Pittsburgh longitudinal studies, the 12 month prevalence rate for 'street crimes' (burglary, serious theft, robbery, aggravated assault, etc.) increased for males from less than 15% at age 11 to almost 50% at age 17 (Huizinga *et al.* 1993).

The cumulative prevalence of convictions in the Cambridge study was very high: 40% up to age 40 (Farrington *et al.* 1998). Nevertheless, it was true that only 6% of the sample—the chronic offenders—accounted for nearly half of all the convictions (Farrington and West 1993). Similarly, chronic offenders were disproportionally likely to commit other types of antisocial behaviour. In numerous other projects such as the Philadelphia cohort study of Wolfgang *et al.* (1987) and the Jyvaskyla (Finland) longitudinal study of Pulkkinen (1988), there was a similar concentration of offending in a small proportion of the sample.

Intervention studies and their effects

The focus here is especially on randomized experiments with reasonably large samples and with outcome measures of CD or delinquency, since the effect of any intervention on antisocial behaviour can be demonstrated most convincingly in such experiments (Farrington 1983, Farrington *et al.* 1986b). Excellent reviews of intervention studies have been provided by Tremblay and Craig (1995) and Wasserman and Miller (1998).

Early prevention

CD and delinquency can be prevented by intensive home visiting programmes. For example, in New York State, Olds *et al.* (1986a,b) randomly allocated 400 mothers either to receive home visits from nurses during pregnancy, or to receive visits both during pregnancy and during the first 2 years of life, or to a control group who received no visits. The home visitors gave advice about pre- and postnatal care of the child, about infant development, and about the importance of proper nutrition and avoiding smoking and drinking during pregnancy.

The results of this experiment showed that the postnatal home visits caused a decrease in recorded child physical abuse and neglect during the first 2 years of life, especially by poor unmarried teenage mothers; 4% of visited versus 19% of non-visited mothers of this type were guilty of child abuse or neglect. Olds *et al.* (1997) reported a 15 year follow-up showing that experimental mothers committed half as much child abuse and had half as many arrests as control mothers. Similar results were obtained by Larson (1980) and Kitzman *et al.* (1997) with similar interventions.

One of the most successful early prevention programmes has been the Perry preschool project carried out in Michigan by Schweinhart and Weikart (1980). This was essentially a 'Head Start' programme targeted on disadvantaged African-American children. The experimental children attended a daily preschool programme, backed up by weekly home visits, usually lasting 2 years (covering ages 3–4). The aim of the 'plan-do-review' programme was to provide intellectual stimulation, to increase thinking and reasoning abilities, and to increase later school achievement.

As demonstrated in several other Head Start projects, the experimental group showed gains in intelligence that were rather short-lived. However, they were significantly better in elementary school motivation, school achievement at age 14, teacher ratings of classroom behaviour at 6–9, self-reports of classroom behaviour at 15, and self-reports of offending at 15. Other projects (Consortium for Longitudinal Studies 1983, Horacek *et al.* 1987) also show that preschool intellectual enrichment programmes have long-term beneficial effects on school success.

A later follow-up of the Perry sample (Berrueta-Clement *et al.* 1984) showed that, at age 19, the experimental group was more likely to be employed, more likely to have graduated from high school, more likely to have received college or vocational training, and less likely to have been arrested. By age 27, the experimental group had accumulated only half as many arrests on average as the controls (Schweinhart *et al.* 1993). Also, they had significantly higher earnings and were more likely to be home-owners. More of the experimental women were married, and fewer of their children had been born out of wedlock. Hence, this preschool intellectual enrichment programme led to decreases in school failure, to decreases in offending, and to decreases in other undesirable outcomes. For every $1 spent on the programme, $7 were saved in the long run.

Parent training

Parent training is also an effective method of preventing CD and offending. Many different types of parent training have been used (Barlow 1997, Kazdin 1997), but the behavioural parent management training developed by Patterson (1982) in Oregon is one of the most hopeful approaches. His careful observations of parent–child interaction showed that parents of antisocial children were deficient in their methods of child rearing. These parents failed to tell their children how they were expected to behave, failed to monitor their behaviour to ensure that it was desirable, and failed to enforce rules promptly and unambiguously with appropriate rewards and penalties. The parents of antisocial children used more punishment (such as scolding, shouting, or threatening), but failed to make it contingent on the child's behaviour.

Patterson attempted to train these parents in effective child rearing methods, namely noticing what a child is doing, monitoring behaviour over long periods, clearly stating house rules, making rewards and punishments contingent on behaviour, and negotiating disagreements so that conflicts and crises did not escalate. His treatment was shown to be effective in reducing child stealing and antisocial behaviour over short periods in small-scale studies (Dishion *et al.* 1992, Patterson *et al.* 1982, 1992).

Skills training

The set of techniques variously termed cognitive-behavioural interpersonal social skills training have proved to be quite successful (Lipsey and Wilson 1998). For example, the 'Reasoning and Rehabilitation' programme developed by Ross and Ross (1995) in Canada aimed to modify the impulsive, egocentric thinking of delinquents, to teach them to stop and think before acting, to consider the consequences of their behaviour, to conceptualize alternative ways of solving interpersonal problems, and to consider the impact of their behaviour on other people, especially their victims. It included social skills training, lateral thinking (to teach creative problem solving), critical thinking (to teach logical reasoning), values education (to teach values and concern for others), assertiveness training (to teach non-aggressive, socially appropriate ways to obtain desired outcomes), negotiation skills training, interpersonal cognitive problem-solving (to teach thinking skills for solving interpersonal problems), social perspective training (to teach how to recognize and understand other people's feelings), role-playing, and modelling (demonstration and practice of effective and acceptable interpersonal behaviour). This programme led to a large decrease in reoffending by a small sample of delinquents.

Jones and Offord (1989) implemented a skills training programme in an experimental public housing complex in Ottawa and compared it with a control complex. The programme centred on non-school skills, both athletic (e.g. swimming and hockey) and non-athletic (e.g. guitar and ballet). The aim of developing skills was to increase self-esteem, to encourage children to use time constructively and to provide desirable role models. Participation rates were high; about three-quarters of age-eligible children in the experimental complex took at least one course in the first year. The programme was successful; delinquency rates decreased significantly in the experimental complex compared to the control complex.

School programmes

An important school-based prevention experiment was carried out in Seattle by Hawkins *et al.* (1991, 1992). This combined parent training, teacher training, and skills training. About 500 first grade children (aged 6) were randomly assigned to be in experimental or control classes. The children in the experimental classes received special treatment at home and school which was designed to increase their attachment to their parents and their bonding to the school, on the assumption that delinquency was inhibited by the strength of social bonds. Their parents were trained to notice and reinforce socially desirable behaviour in a programme called 'Catch them being good'. Their teachers were trained in classroom management, for example to provide clear instructions and expectations to children, to reward children for participation in desired behaviour, and to teach children prosocial (socially desirable) methods of solving problems (Hawkins *et al.* 1988).

In an evaluation of this programme 18 months later, when the children were in different classes, Hawkins *et al.* (1991) found that the boys who received the experimental programme were significantly less aggressive than the control boys, according to teacher ratings. This difference was particularly marked for white boys rather than African-American boys. The experimental girls were not significantly less aggressive, but they were less self-destructive, anxious, and depressed. By the fifth grade (age 10), the experimental children were less likely to have initiated delinquency and alcohol use. Among low income children, experimental boys were less likely to have initiated delinquency, and experimental girls were less likely to have initiated drug use (O'Donnell *et al.* 1995).

Several school-based programmes have been designed to decrease bullying. The most famous of these was implemented by Olweus (1993, 1994) in Norway. It aimed to increase awareness and knowledge of teachers, parents, and children about bullying and to dispel myths about it. A 30 page booklet was distributed to all schools in Norway describing what was known about bullying and recommending what steps schools and teachers could take to reduce it. Also, a 25 minute video about bullying was made available to schools. Simultaneously, the schools distributed to all parents a 4 page folder containing information and advice about bullying. In addition, anonymous self-report questionnaires about bullying were completed by all children.

The programme was evaluated in Bergen. Each of the 42 participating schools received feedback information from the questionnaire, about the prevalence of bullies and victims, in a specially arranged school conference day. Also, teachers were encouraged to develop explicit rules about bullying (e.g. do not bully, tell someone when bullying happens, bullying will not be tolerated, try to help victims, try to include children who are being left out) and to discuss bullying in class, using the video and role-playing exercises. Also, teachers were encouraged to improve monitoring and supervision of children, especially in the playground. The programme was successful in reducing the prevalence of bullying by half.

A similar programme was implemented in England in 23 Sheffield schools by Smith and Sharp (1994). The core program involved establishing a 'whole-school' anti-bullying policy, raising awareness of bullying and clearly defining roles and responsibilities of teachers and students, so that everyone knew what bullying was and what they should do about it. In addition, there were optional interventions tailored to particular schools: curriculum work (e.g. reading books, watching videos), direct work with students (e.g. assertiveness training for those who were bullied) and playground work (e.g. training lunchtime supervisors). This programme was successful in reducing bullying in primary schools, but had relatively small effects in secondary schools.

Multi-modal programmes

Multi-modal programmes including both skills training and parent training are likely to be more effective than either alone (Kazdin *et al.* 1992, Webster-Stratton and Hammond 1997). An important multi-modal programme was implemented by Tremblay *et al.* (1995) in Montreal. They identified about 250 disruptive (aggressive/hyperactive) boys at age 6 for a prevention experiment. Between ages 7 and 9, the experimental group received training to foster social skills and self-control. Coaching, peer modelling, role playing, and reinforcement contingencies were used in small group sessions on such topics as 'how to help', 'what to do when you are angry', and 'how to react to teasing'. Also, their parents were trained using the parent management training techniques developed by Patterson (1982). This prevention programme was quite successful. By age 12, the experimental boys committed less burglary and theft, were less likely to get drunk, and were less likely to be involved in fights than the controls. Also, the experimental boys had higher school achievement. At every age from 10 to

15, the experimental boys had higher self-reported delinquency scores than the control boys. Interestingly, the differences in antisocial behaviour between experimental and control boys increased as the follow-up progressed. However, there is the problem of identifying what is the active ingredient in this kind of multi-modal programme.

Intervention programmes that tackle several of the major risk factors for CD and delinquency are likely to be particularly effective. Henggeler *et al.* (1992, 1993) evaluated multi-systemic therapy (MST) for juvenile offenders, tackling family, peer, and school risk factors simultaneously in individualized treatment plans tailored to the needs of each family. MST was compared with the usual Department of Youth Services treatment, involving out-of-home placement in the majority of cases. In a randomized experiment with 84 offenders, MST was followed by fewer arrests, lower self-reported delinquency, and less peer-oriented aggression. Borduin *et al.* (1995) also showed that MST was more effective in decreasing arrests and antisocial behaviour than was individual therapy.

The results were somewhat less favourable in a real world implementation of MST using therapists recruited and trained in each site. Previous experiments had been implemented and closely monitored by MST experts. Henggeler *et al.* (1997) randomly allocated 155 chronic and violent juvenile offenders either to MST or to the usual services (which in this case mainly involved probation and restitution). MST led to a decrease in arrests, self-reported delinquency, and antisocial behaviour, but only when treatment fidelity was high. They concluded that, in real world applications, therapist adherence to MST principles was a crucial factor.

Short-term and long-term outcomes

Outcomes of CD

CD in childhood and adolescence is disproportionally followed by antisocial personality disorder (APD) in adulthood (Rutter 1995). In a longitudinal survey of African-American males in St. Louis, Robins and Ratcliff (1978) related 9 types of childhood antisocial behaviour (under age 15) to 10 types of adult antisocial behaviour (age 25–35). Childhood drug use, sexual intercourse, and delinquency were the best predictors of the number of adult behaviours. Conversely, the number of childhood behaviours best predicted adult criminality, welfare dependency, and a deviant lifestyle (e.g. hanging about on the street or in bars). The number of childhood behaviours predicted the number of adult behaviours; 41% of males showing three or more childhood behaviours also showed four or more adult behaviours (compared to only 14% of males showing no childhood antisocial behaviour).

These results were replicated and applied more explicitly to CD and APD diagnoses in the ECA project by Robins *et al.* (1991). Again, the number of adult antisocial symptoms increased linearly with the number of childhood conduct problems (under age 15). Looking forwards, 26% of children who fulfilled the criteria for CD (three or more symptoms) also fulfilled the criteria for APD, although 46% of children with six or more CD symptoms fulfilled the criteria for APD. The total prevalence of APD in the ECA was only 2.6%. The best childhood predictors of APD were running away and delinquency. Looking backwards, 95% of APD adult males had at least one CD symptom, and 76% fulfilled the criteria for childhood CD. CD girls were less likely to develop adult externalizing disorders (APD, drug and alcohol problems) than were CD boys, but CD girls were more likely to develop adult internalizing disorders than CD boys (Robins 1986). For both males and females, CD predicted adverse adult life events such as moving home, losing a job, and breaking up with lovers or spouses.

There have been a number of follow-ups of CD children into adulthood. Storm-Mathisen and Vaglum (1994) conducted a 20 year follow-up in Oslo and reported that one-third of CD children became APD adults. Also, a quarter of CD children developed an anxiety disorder, and a quarter had a substance abuse disorder. In Sydney, Australia, Rey *et al.* (1995) followed up 14 year old adolescents to age 20, and found that 36% of CD children became APD adults, but half of those with cooccurring CD and ADHD became APD adults.

Numerous studies show that childhood conduct problems predict adult offending (Loeber and LeBlanc 1990, Hodgins 1994). In the Cambridge study, conduct problems at age 8–10 predicted juvenile convictions, juvenile self-reported delinquency, adult convictions, and chronic offending independently of HIA (hyperactivity–impulsivity–attention deficit; Farrington *et al.* 1990). After reviewing existing studies, Lynam (1996) concluded that children with co-occurring CD and HIA were at greatest risk of becoming chronic offenders.

Also in the Cambridge Study, antisocial personality scales were developed at ages 10, 14, 18, and 32 (Farrington 1991a). The scales at ages 10 and 14 included many CD symptoms. The scales at ages 18 and 32 measured teenage and adult deviance, including delinquency, drug use, heavy drinking, conflict with spouses and parents, unemployment, and anti-establishment attitudes. All the scales were significantly intercorrelated. Adult deviance at age 32 was predicted by conduct problems at ages 10 ($r = 0.30$), 14 ($r = 0.42$), and 18 ($r = 0.55$). Of the most antisocial boys at age 18, 60% were still among the most antisocial at age 32 (compared to only 14% of the remainder).

Zoccolillo *et al.* (1992) also documented how far childhood CD up to age 15 was followed by adult social dysfunction at age 26, reflecting problems of crime, work, sex/love, and social relationships. Of the CD males, 13% had problems in all four adult areas, and a further 30% had problems in three (most commonly, crime, sex/love, and work). Of the CD females, 7% had problems in all four adult areas, and a further 30% had problems in three (most commonly, sex/love, work, and social relationships). CD also predicts teenage childbearing (Kessler *et al.* 1997), which in turn predicts delinquency of the ensuing children (Nagin *et al.* 1997).

Outcomes of delinquency

The Cambridge Study shows that delinquency is associated with many short-term and long-term antisocial outcomes. The boys who were convicted before age 18 (most commonly for offences of dishonesty, such as burglary and theft) were significantly more deviant than the non-delinquents on almost every factor that was investigated at that age (West and Farrington 1977). The convicted delinquents drank more beer, they got drunk more often, and they were more likely to say that drink made them violent. They smoked more cigarettes, they had started smoking at an earlier age, and they were more likely to be heavy gamblers. They were more likely to have been convicted for minor motoring offences, to have driven after drinking at least 10 units of alcohol (e.g. 5 pints of beer), and to have been injured in road accidents. The delinquents were more likely to have taken prohibited drugs such as marijuana or LSD, although few of them had convictions for drug offences. Also, they were more likely to have had sexual intercourse, especially with a variety of different girls, and especially beginning at an early age, but they were less likely to use contraceptives.

The convicted delinquents at age 18 tended to hold relatively well paid but low status (unskilled manual) jobs, and they were more likely to have erratic work histories including periods of unemployment. They were more likely to be living away from home, and they tended not to get on well with their parents. They were more likely to be tattooed, possibly reflecting their 'macho' orientation. The delinquents were more likely to go out in the evenings, and were especially likely to spend time hanging about on the street. They tended to go around in groups of four or more, and were more likely to be involved in group violence or vandalism. They were much more likely to have been involved in fights, to have started fights, to have carried weapons, and to have used weapons in fights. They were also more likely to express aggressive and anti-establishment attitudes on a questionnaire (negative to police, school, rich people, and civil servants). Also, the delinquents tended to show adult social dysfunction at age 32 (Farrington 1989a).

Continuity versus discontinuity

Conduct disorder

There is considerable continuity or absolute stability in CD, at least over a few years and in the 7–17 age range. In the Ontario Child Health Study, 45% of children aged 4–12 who displayed CD in 1983 still displayed CD 4 years later, compared with only 5% of those who had no disorder in 1983 (Offord *et al.* 1992). CD was more stable than ADHD or emotional disorder. Also, stability was greater for children aged 8–12 (60% persisting) than for children aged 4–7 (25% persisting). However, the interpretation of results was complicated by comorbidity; 35% of those with CD in 1983 had ADHD 4 years later, and conversely 34% of those with ADHD in 1983 had CD 4 years later.

Similar results have been reported by other researchers. In their New York State study, Cohen *et al.* (1993b) found that 43% of CD children aged 9–18 still displayed CD 2.5 years later (compared with 10% of non-CD children). There were no significant age or gender differences in stability, but stability increased with the severity of CD. In the Developmental Trends Study, Lahey *et al.* (1995) reported that half of CD boys aged 7–12 still displayed CD 3 years later. Persistence was predicted by parental APD and by the boy's low verbal IQ, but not by age, socioeconomic status, or ethnicity. It is also important to study factors that predict discontinuity in CD over time (Fergusson *et al.* 1996).

Turning to studies of relative stability, Achenbach *et al.* (1995a) reported stability correlations over 3 years on the CBCL, TRF, and YSR for an American national sample of children initially aged 4–18. The mean correlation for delinquency scales was 0.45. Correlations were higher on the CBCL (0.53 for boys, 0.57 for girls) than on the TRF (0.41, 0.38) or YSR (0.34, 0.47). In a separate analysis focusing on youth aged 16–19, stability correlations were 0.59 (boys) and 0.47 (girls) on the CBCL and 0.51 (boys) and 0.38 (girls) on the YSR (Achenbach *et al.* 1995b).

Verhulst and his colleagues have provided the most extensive data on relative stability, using the CBCL, TRF, and YSR in their longitudinal study of Dutch children initially aged 4–12. Beginning with the CBCL, the average 4 year stability correlation over all ages and both genders for delinquency scales was 0.31 (Verhulst *et al.* 1990). It was lowest for children aged 4–5 (e.g. only 0.13 for girls aged 4–5), possibly reflecting low scores and a highly skewed distribution of scores. In the whole sample, the stability correlation for delinquency was 0.40 over 4 years and 0.36 over 6 years (Verhulst and van der Ende 1992b). When scores were dichotomized at the 90th percentile, the odds ratio for delinquency over 6 years was 4.2. Verhulst and van der Ende (1992a) also traced developmental pathways over the 6 years. For example, 13% of children who were above the 90th percentile on delinquency initially were also above the 90th percentile at the 2 year, 4 year and 6 year follow-ups. Stability correlations over 8 years were 0.43 (boys) and 0.32 (girls) for those initially aged 7–10 and 0.33 (boys) and 0.20 (girls) for those initially aged 4–6 (Verhulst and van der Ende 1995). Absolute scores tended to decrease over time.

Stability correlations were not reported for the delinquency scale on the TRF. On the Externalizing scale, the average 4 year correlation over all ages and both genders was 0.34 for boys and 0.55 for girls (Verhulst and van der Ende 1991). Problem scores tended to increase over time. On the YSR for youth aged 15–18 initially, the 4 year correlation for delinquency was 0.43 for boys and 0.39 for girls (Ferdinand *et al.* 1995). Since the mean scores were the same at all ages, there was absolute as well as relative stability in CD during this time period.

Delinquency

Generally, there is significant continuity between delinquency in one age range and delinquency in another. In the Cambridge study, nearly three-quarters (73%) of those convicted as juveniles at age 10–16 were reconvicted at age 17–24, in comparison with only 16% of those not convicted as juveniles (Farrington 1992a). Nearly half (45%) of those convicted as juveniles were reconvicted at age 25–32, in comparison with only 8% of those not convicted as juveniles. Furthermore, this continuity over time did not merely reflect continuity in police reaction to delinquency. For 10 specified offences, the significant continuity between delinquency in one age range and offending in a later age range held for self-reports as well as official convictions (Farrington 1989b).

Other studies (e.g. Hamparian *et al.* 1985, McCord 1991, Tracy and Kempf-Leonard 1996) show similar continuity in delinquency. For example, in Sweden, Stattin and Magnusson (1991) reported that nearly 70% of males registered for crime before age 15 were registered again between ages 15 and 20, and nearly 60% were registered between ages 21 and 29. Also, the number of juvenile offences is an effective predictor of the number of adult offences (Wolfgang *et al.* 1987). There was considerable continuity in offending between ages 10 and 25 in both London and Stockholm (Farrington and Wikström 1994).

As already indicated, relative continuity is quite compatible with absolute change. In other words, the relative ordering of people on some underlying construct such as delinquency potential can remain significantly stable over time, even though the absolute level of delinquency potential declines on average for everyone. For example, in the Cambridge study, the prevalence of self-reported offending declined significantly between ages 18 and 32, but there was a significant tendency for the worst offenders at 18 also to be the worst offenders at 32 (Farrington 1990a).

Risk and prognostic factors

Because of the difficulty of establishing causal effects of factors that vary only between individuals (e.g. gender and ethnicity), and because such factors have no practical implications for prevention (e.g. it is not practicable to change males into females), unchanging variables are not reviewed here. In any case, their effects on offending are usually explained by reference to other, modifiable, factors (Farrington 1987). For example, gender differences in offending have been explained on the basis of different socialization methods used by parents with boys and girls, or different opportunities for offending of men and women. Similarly, risk factors that are or might be measuring the same underlying construct as CD or delinquency (e.g. physical aggression or peer delinquency) or that are comorbid conditions (e.g. ADHD or ODD) are not reviewed; the focus is on risk factors that might have causal effects. Risk factors are discussed one by one; additive, interactive, independent, or sequential effects are not exhaustively reviewed, although these are important issues. Because of limitations of space, biological and community factors are not reviewed (see Farrington *et al.* 1993, Raine *et al.* 1997), nor are protective factors, and neither are theories of the mechanisms by which risk factors have their effects.

Low IQ and attainment

Low IQ and low school attainment are important predictors of CD and delinquency. In an epidemiological study of 13 year old twins, low IQ of the child predicted conduct problems independently of social class and of the IQ of parents (Goodman *et al.* 1995). Low achievement was a strong correlate of CD in the Pittsburgh Youth Study (Loeber *et al.* 1998). In both the Ontario Child Health Study (Offord *et al.* 1989) and the New York State longitudinal study (Velez *et al.* 1989), failing a grade predicted CD. Underachievement, defined according to a discrepancy between achievement and IQ, is also characteristic of CD children, as Frick *et al.* (1991) reported in the Developmental Trends Study.

Low IQ measured in the first few years of life predicts later delinquency. In a prospective longitudinal survey of about 120 Stockholm males, low IQ measured at age 3 significantly predicted officially recorded offending up to age 30 (Stattin and Klackenberg-Larsson 1993). Frequent offenders (with 4 or more offences) had an average IQ of 88 at age 3, whereas non-offenders had an average IQ of 101. All of these results held up after controlling for social class. Similarly, low IQ at age 4 predicted arrests up to age 27 in the Perry preschool project and court delinquency up to age 17 in the Collaborative Perinatal Project (Lipsitt *et al.* 1990, Schweinhart *et al.* 1993).

In the Cambridge study, twice as many of the boys scoring 90 or less on a non-verbal IQ test (Raven's Progressive Matrices) at age 8–10 were convicted as juveniles as of the remainder (West and Farrington 1973). However, it was difficult to disentangle low IQ from low school attainment, because they were highly intercorrelated and both predicted delinquency. Low non-verbal IQ predicted juvenile self-reported delinquency to almost exactly the same degree as juvenile convictions (Farrington 1992c), suggesting that the link between low IQ and delinquency was not caused by the less intelligent boys having a greater probability of being caught. Also, measures of low IQ and attainment predicted measures of offending independently of other variables such as low family income and large family size (Farrington 1990b).

Low IQ may lead to delinquency through the intervening factor of school failure, as Hirschi and Hindelang (1977) suggested. The association between school failure and delinquency has been demonstrated consistently in longitudinal surveys (Wolfgang *et al.* 1972, Polk *et al.* 1981). In the Pittsburgh Youth Study, Lynam *et al.* (1993) concluded that low verbal IQ led to school failure and subsequently to self-reported delinquency, but only for African-American boys. Another plausible explanatory factor underlying the link between low IQ and delinquency is the ability to manipulate abstract concepts. Children who are poor at this tend to do badly in IQ tests and in school attainment, and they also tend to commit offences, mainly because of their poor ability to foresee the consequences of their offending and to appreciate the feelings of victims (i.e. their low empathy; see Cohen and Strayer 1996). Delinquents often do better on non-verbal performance IQ tests, such as object assembly and block design, than on verbal IQ tests (Walsh *et al.* 1987), suggesting that they find it easier to deal with concrete objects than with abstract concepts. Similarly, Rogeness (1994) concluded that CD children had deficits in verbal IQ but not in performance IQ.

Temperament and personality

Personality traits such as sociability or impulsiveness describe broad predispositions to respond in certain ways, and temperament is basically the childhood equivalent of personality. The modern study of child temperament began with the New York longitudinal study of Chess and Thomas (1984). Children in their first 5 years of life were rated on temperamental dimensions by their parents, and these dimensions were combined into three broad categories of easy, difficult, and 'slow to warm up' temperament. Having a difficult temperament at age 3–4 (frequent irritability, low amenability and adaptability, irregular habits) predicted poor psychiatric adjustment at age 17–24. Guerin *et al.* (1997) found that a difficult temperament at age 1.5 years predicted CD up to age 12, and similar results were reported by Sanson *et al.* (1993) in the Australian Temperament Project.

Studies using classic personality inventories such as the MMPI and CPI (Wilson and Herrnstein 1985, pp. 186–98) often seem to produce essentially tautological results, such as that delinquents are low on socialization. The Eysenck personality questionnaire has yielded more promising results (Eysenck 1996). In the Cambridge Study, those high on both Extraversion and Neuroticism tended to be juvenile self-reported delinquents, adult official offenders, and adult self-reported offenders, but not juvenile official delinquents (Farrington *et al.* 1982). Furthermore, these relationships held independently of other variables such as low family income, low intelligence, and poor parental child rearing behaviour. However, when individual items of the personality questionnaire were studied, it was clear that the significant relationships were caused by the items measuring impulsivity (e.g. doing things quickly without stopping to think). Impulsivity has often been identified as an important predictor of

CD and delinquency (Farrington 1992c; Tremblay *et al.* 1994), but it is not reviewed in detail here because of its conceptual link with ADHD.

Child rearing behaviour

In the Pittsburgh Youth Study, poor parental supervision was an important risk factor for CD (Loeber *et al.* 1998). Poor maternal supervision and low persistence in discipline predicted CD in the Developmental Trends Study (Frick *et al.* 1992), but not independently of parental APD. Rothbaum and Weisz (1994) carried out a meta-analysis and concluded that parental reinforcement, parental reasoning, parental punishments, and parental responsiveness to the child were all related to Externalizing child behaviour.

The classic longitudinal studies by McCord (1979) in Boston and Robins (1979) in St. Louis show that poor parental supervision, harsh discipline, and a rejecting attitude all predict delinquency. Similar results were obtained in the Cambridge study. Harsh or erratic parental discipline, cruel, passive, or neglecting parental attitudes, and poor parental supervision, all measured at age 8, all predicted later juvenile convictions and self-reported delinquency (West and Farrington 1973). Generally, the presence of any of these adverse family background features doubled the risk of a later juvenile conviction.

There seems to be significant intergenerational transmission of aggressive and violent behaviour from parents to children, as Widom (1989) found in a retrospective study of over 900 abused children in Indianapolis. Children who were physically abused up to age 11 were significantly likely to become violent offenders in the next 15 years (Maxfield and Widom 1996). Similarly, in the Cambridge study, harsh parental discipline and attitude predicted both violent and persistent offending up to age 32 (Farrington 1991b). The extensive review by Malinosky-Rummell and Hansen (1993) confirms that being physically abused as a child predicts later violent and non-violent offending.

Parental conflict and separation

Parental conflict is related to childhood Externalizing behaviour, irrespective of whether the information about both comes from parents or children (Jenkins and Smith 1991). In the Pittsburgh Youth Study, CD boys tended to have parents who had unhappy relationships (Loeber *et al.* 1998), and the meta-analysis by Buehler *et al.* (1997) confirms the link between parental conflict and child problem behaviours. Parental conflict also predicts delinquency (West and Farrington 1973).

Parental separation and single parent families predict CD children. In the Christchurch Study in New Zealand, separations from parents in the first 5 years of a child's life (especially) predicted CD and ODD at age 15 (Fergusson *et al.* 1994). In the New York State longitudinal study, CD was predicted by parental divorce, but far more strongly by having a never-married lone mother (Velez *et al.* 1989). In the Ontario Child Health Study, coming from a single parent family predicted CD, but this was highly related to poverty and dependence on welfare benefits (Blum *et al.* 1988). The analyses of Morash and Rucker (1989) suggest that women who have children as teenagers and then become lone mothers are particularly likely to have delinquent children.

Many studies show that broken homes or disrupted families predict delinquency. In the Newcastle Thousand-Family Study, Kolvin et al. (1988) reported that marital disruption (divorce or separation) in a boy's first 5 years predicted his later convictions up to age 32. Similarly, in the Dunedin study in New Zealand, Henry et al. (1993) found that children who were exposed to parental discord and many changes of the primary care-giver tended to become antisocial and delinquent.

The cause of the broken home is emphasized in the English National Survey of Health and Development (Wadsworth 1979). Boys from homes broken by divorce or separation had an increased likelihood of being convicted or officially cautioned up to age 21, in comparison with those from homes broken by death or from unbroken homes. Homes broken while the boy was under age 5 especially predicted delinquency, whereas homes broken while the boy was between ages 11 and 15 were not particularly criminogenic. Remarriage (which happened more often after divorce or separation than after death) was also associated with an increased risk of delinquency, suggesting a possible negative effect of step-parents. The meta-analysis by Wells and Rankin (1991) also shows that broken homes are more strongly related to delinquency when they are caused by parental separation or divorce rather than by death.

In the Cambridge study, both permanent and temporary separations from a biological parent before age 10 (usually from the father) predicted convictions and self-reported delinquency, providing that they were not caused by death or hospitalization (Farrington 1992c). However, homes broken at an early age (under age 5) were not unusually criminogenic (West and Farrington 1973). Separation before age 10 predicted both juvenile and adult convictions (Farrington 1992b) and predicted convictions up to age 32 independently of all other factors such as low family income or poor school attainment (Farrington 1990b 1993).

Antisocial parents and large families

It is clear that CD children disproportionally have antisocial parents. In the Developmental Trends Study, parental APD was the best predictor of childhood CD (Frick et al. 1992) and parental substance use was an important predictor of the onset of CD (Loeber et al. 1995). Similarly, in the New York State longitudinal study, parental APD was a strong predictor of Externalizing child behaviour (Cohen et al. 1990). In the Pittsburgh Youth Study, parents with behaviour problems and substance use problems tended to have CD boys (Loeber et al. 1998).

In their classic longitudinal studies, McCord (1977) and Robins et al. (1975) showed that criminal parents tended to have delinquent sons. In the Cambridge Study, the concentration of offending in a small number of families was remarkable. Less than 6% of the families were responsible for half of the criminal convictions of all members (fathers, mothers, sons, and daughters) of all 400 families (Farrington et al. 1996). Having a convicted mother, father, brother, or sister significantly predicted a boy's own convictions. Furthermore, convicted parents and delinquent siblings were related to a boy's self-reported as well as official offending (Farrington 1979). CD symptoms also tend to be concentrated in families (Szatmari et al. 1993).

Many studies show that large families predict delinquency (Fischer 1984). For example, in the English National Survey, Wadsworth (1979) found that the percentage of boys who were officially delinquent increased from 9% for families containing one child to 24% for families containing four or more children. The Newsons in their Nottingham study also concluded that large family size was one of the most important predictors of delinquency (Newson *et al.* 1993).

In the Cambridge Study, if a boy had four or more siblings by his tenth birthday, this doubled his risk of being convicted as a juvenile (West and Farrington 1973). Large family size predicted self-reported delinquency as well as convictions (Farrington 1979), and adult as well as juvenile convictions (Farrington 1992b). Also, large family size was the most important independent predictor of convictions up to age 32 in a logistic regression analysis (Farrington 1993).

Socioeconomic status

It is clear that CD children disproportionally come from familiesof low socioeconomic status. In the Ontario Child Health Study, CD children tended to come from low income families, with unemployed parents, living in subsidized housing and dependent on welfare benefits (Offord *et al.* 1986). In the New York State longitudinal study, low socioeconomic status, low family income, and low parental education predicted CD children (Velez *et al.* 1989). In the Developmental Trends Study, low socioeconomic status predicted the onset of CD (Loeber *et al.* 1995); and, in the Pittsburgh Youth Study, family dependence on welfare benefits was characteristic of CD boys (Loeber *et al.* 1998).

Low socioeconomic status is a less consistent predictor of delinquency (Hindelang *et al.* 1981). However, a lot depends on whether it is measured by income and housing or by occupational prestige. In the Cambridge Study, low family income and poor housing predicted official and self-reported, juvenile and adult delinquency, but low parental occupational prestige predicted only self-reported delinquency (Farrington 1992b,c). Unemployment is related to delinquency. Between ages 15 and 18, the Cambridge study boys were convicted at a higher rate when they were unemployed than when they were employed (Farrington *et al.* 1986a), suggesting that unemployment in some way causes crime, and conversely that employment may lead to desistence from offending. Since crimes involving material gain (e.g. theft, burglary, robbery) especially increased during periods of unemployment, it seems likely that financial need is an important link in the causal chain between unemployment and crime.

School influences

It is clear that the prevalence of delinquency varies dramatically between different secondary schools, as Power *et al.* (1967) showed many years ago in London. Characteristics of schools with high delinquency rates are well known (Graham 1988). For example, such schools have high levels of distrust between teachers and students, low commitment to school by students, and unclear and inconsistently enforced rules. However, what is far less clear is how much of the variation between schools should be attributed to differences in school organization, climate, and practices, and how much to differences in the composition of the student body.

In the Cambridge study, the effects of secondary schools on delinquency were investigated by following boys from their primary schools to their secondary schools (Farrington 1972). The best primary school predictor of juvenile delinquency was the rating of the boy's troublesomeness at age 8–10 by peers and teachers, showing the continuity in antisocial behaviour. The secondary schools differed dramatically in their official delinquency rates, from one school with 21 court appearances per 100 boys per year to another where the corresponding figure was only 0.3. Moreover, going to a secondary school with a high delinquency rate was a significant predictor of later convictions (Farrington 1993). It was, however, very noticeable that the most troublesome boys tended to go to the schools with high delinquency rates, whereas the least troublesome boys tended to go to the schools with low delinquency rates. Furthermore, it was clear that most of the variation between schools' delinquency rates could be explained by differences in their intakes of troublesome boys. The secondary schools themselves had only a very small effect on the boys' offending.

The most famous study of school effects on delinquency was also carried out in London, by Rutter *et al.* (1979). They studied 12 comprehensive schools, and again found big differences in official delinquency rates between them. Schools with high delinquency rates tended to have high truancy rates, low ability pupils, and low social class parents. However, the differences between the schools in delinquency rates could not be entirely explained by differences in the social class and verbal reasoning scores of the pupils at intake (age 11). Therefore, they must have been caused by some aspect of the schools themselves or by other, unmeasured factors. Rutter *et al.* (1979) found that the main school factors associated with delinquency were a high amount of punishment and a low amount of praise given by teachers in class. Unfortunately, it is difficult to know whether much punishment and little praise are causes or consequences of antisocial school behaviour, which in turn may be linked to offending outside school.

Conclusions

Although the definition of CD emphasizes impairment of functioning, the diagnostic criteria focus on delinquent and antisocial behaviour. Consideration should be given to including personality measures in the diagnostic criteria, such as low empathy, low guilt, callous/ unemotional, and manipulative. Also, the definition focuses on overt, typically male behaviour. Consideration should be given to including types of antisocial behaviour committed more often by females, such as spreading rumours, saying things calculated to upset others, ostracizing and rejecting certain children, and other types of indirect or relational aggression.

Comorbidity poses major challenges to the understanding of CD. It is hard to know how far any results are characteristic of CD children as opposed to children with multiple problems. Similarly, it is hard to know how far conclusions about delinquency are driven by the minority of chronic offenders. The relationship betwen levels of CD and levels of delinquency needs to be studied. More research is needed on types of people. The Moffitt (1993) typology is a useful beginning, but far more detailed typologies are needed, focusing on a wide variety of possibly causal factors as well as on patterns of antisocial behaviour. More research is needed focusing on individuals rather than variables (Bergman and Magnusson 1997).

Research on the epidemiology of CD is limited. Studies are needed on a wider range of features of antisocial careers; not just prevalence and onset but also frequency, seriousness, duration, escalation, de-escalation, desistance, remission, motivation, and situational influences (Farrington 1997). More studies are needed with multiple informants and frequent measurements. A great deal is known about risk factors for CD and delinquency, but little is known about risk factors for persistence or escalation after onset, for example. How far risk factors are the same for males and females, different ethnic groups, or at different ages is less clear. More cross-cultural comparisons of risk factors are needed (Farrington and Loeber 1999).

Often, multiple risk factors lead to multiple outcomes. How far any given risk factor predicts a variety of different outcomes generally (as opposed to predicting specifically one or two outcomes) and how far each outcome is predicted by a variety of different risk factors generally (as opposed to being predicted by only one or two risk factors specifically) is unclear. An increasing number of risk factors seems to lead to an increasing probability of negative outcomes, almost irrespective of the particular risk factors included in the prediction measure, but more research is needed on this. There is insufficient space in this chapter to review theories explaining the links between risk factors and CD and delinquency, but these have to be based on knowledge about the additive, independent, interactive, and sequential effects of risk factors.

More research is needed to identify protective factors. Although there is marked continuity in CD and delinquency over time, it is important to investigate discontinuities, and especially why people who are antisocial at one time improve (absolutely or relatively) at a later time. Such research could help in designing intervention programmes. Research is specifically needed on the linkage between anxiety and associated factors (e.g. social isolation, being shy or withdrawn) and CD and delinquency. It is unclear how far anxiety is comorbid with CD and how far it might be a protective factor.

There are many examples of successful intervention programmes for CD and delinquency, although many experiments are based on small samples and short follow-up periods. Often, the most successful programmes are multi-modal, making it difficult to identify the active ingredient. Successful multi-modal programmes should be followed by more specific experiments targeting single risk factors. These could be very helpful in establishing which risk factors have causal effects. More efforts are needed to tailor types of interventions to types of people. Ideally, an intervention should be preceded by a screening or needs assessment to determine which problems need to be rectified and which children are most likely to be amenable to treatment. It is important to establish how far interventions are successful with the most extreme cases (e.g. chronic offenders), in order to identify where the benefits will be greatest in practice. Cost–benefit analyses should be carried out, as in the Perry project.

A great deal has been learned about CD and delinquency in the last 20 years, especially from longitudinal and experimental studies. More investment in these kinds of studies is needed in the next 20 years in order to advance knowledge about and decrease these troubling social problems.

Acknowledgement

I am very grateful to Rolf Loeber for sharing some of his encyclopaedic knowledge about CD with me, for helpful comments on an earlier version of this chapter, and for numerous stimulating and insightful discussions over the years.

References

Achenbach, T.M., Howell, C.T., McConaughty, S.H., and Stanger, C. (1995a). Six-year predictors of problems in a national sample of children and youth. I. Cross-informant syndromes. *Journal of the American Academy of Child and Adolescent Psychiatry*, **34**, 336–347.

Achenbach, T.M., Howell, C.T., McConaughty, S.H., and Stanger, C. (1995b). Six-year predictors of problems in a national sample of children and youth. III. Transitions to young adult syndromes. *Journal of the American Academy of Child and Adolescent Psychiatry*, **34**, 658–669.

APA (1994). *Diagnostic and statistical manual of mental disorders*, 4th edn. American Psychiatric Association, Washington, D.C.

Barlow, J. (1997). *Systematic review of the effectiveness of parent-training programmes in improving behaviour problems in children aged 3–10 years.* Health Services Research Unit, Oxford.

Bergman, L.R. and Magnusson, D. (1997). A person-oriented approach in research on developmental psychopathology. *Development and Psychopathology*, **9**, 291–319.

Berrueta-Clement, J.R., Schweinhart, L.J., Barnett, W.S., Epstein, A.S., and Weikart, D.P. (1984). *Changed lives*. High/Scope, Ypsilanti, M.I.

Biederman, J., Newcorn, J., and Sprich, S. (1991). Comorbidity of attention deficit hyperactivity disorder with conduct, depressive, anxiety and other disorders. *American Journal of Psychiatry*, **148**, 564–577.

Bjorkqvist, K., Lagerspetz, K.M.J., and Kaukiainen, A. (1992). Do girls manipulate and boys fight? Developmental trends in regard to direct and indirect aggression. *Aggressive Behaviour*, **18**, 117–127.

Blum, H.M., Boyle, M.H., and Offord, D.R. (1988). Single-parent families: Child psychiatric disorder and school performance. *Journal of the American Academy of Child and Adolescent Psychiatry*, **27**, 214–219.

Borduin, C.M., Mann, B.J., Cone, L.T., Henggeler, S.W., Fucci, B.R., Blaske, D.M., and Williams, R.A. (1995). Multisystemic treatment of serious juvenile offenders: Long-term prevention of criminality and violence. *Journal of Consulting and Clinical Psychology*, **63**, 569–578.

Boyle, M.H. and Offord, D.R. (1991). Psychiatric disorder and substance use in adolescence. *Canadian Journal of Psychiatry*, **36**, 699–705.

Buehler, C., Anthony, C., Krishnakumar, A., Stone, G., Gerard, J., and Pemberton, S. (1997). Interparental conflict and youth problem behaviours: A meta-analysis. *Journal of Child and Family Studies*, **6**, 233–247.

Capaldi, D.M. and Patterson, G.R. (1996). Can violent offenders be distinguished from frequent offenders? Prediction from childhood to adolescence. *Journal of Research in Crime and Delinquency*, **33**, 206–231.

Chess, S. and Thomas, A. (1984). *Origins and evolution of behaviour disorders: From infancy to early adult life*. Brunner/Mazel, New York.

Christian, R.E., Frick, P.J., Hill, N.L., Tyler, L., and Frazer, D.R. (1997). Psychopathy and conduct problems in children. II. Implications for subtyping children with conduct problems. *Journal of the American Academy of Child and Adolescent Psychiatry*, **36**, 233–241.

Cohen, D. and Strayer, J. (1996). Empathy in conduct-disordered and comparison youth. *Developmental Psychology*, **32**, 988–998.

Cohen, P., Brook, J.S., Cohen, J., Velez, C.N., and Garcia, M. (1990). Common and uncommon pathways to adolescent psychopathology and problem behaviour. In *Straight and devious pathways from childhood to adulthood*, ed. L.N. Robins and M. Rutter, pp. 242–258. Cambridge University Press, Cambridge.

Cohen, P., Cohen, J., Kasen, S., Velez, C.N., Hartmark, C., Johnson, J., Rojas, M., Brook, J.S., and Struening, E.L. (1993a) An epidemiological study of disorders in late childhood and adolescence. I. Age and gender-specific prevalence. *Journal of Child Psychology and Psychiatry*, **34**, 851–867.

Cohen, P., Cohen, J., and Brook, J. (1993b) An epidemiological study of disorders in late childhood and adolescence. II. Persistence of disorders. *Journal of Child Psychology and Psychiatry*, **34**, 869–877.

Coie, J.D. and Dodge, K.A. (1998). Aggression and antisocial behaviour. In *Handbook of child psychology*, 5th edn, vol. 3: *Social, emotional and personality development*, ed. W.Damon and N.Eisenberg, pp. 779–862. Wiley, New York.

Consortium for Longitudinal Studies (1983). *As the twig is bent..Lasting effects of pre-school programmes*. Erlbaum, Hillsdale, N.J.

Dishion, T.J., Patterson, G.R., and Kavanagh, K.A. (1992). An experimental test of the coercion model: Linking theory, measurement and intervention. In *Preventing antisocial behaviour*, ed. J.McCord and R.Tremblay, pp. 253–282. Guilford, New York.

Eysenck, H.J. (1996). Personality and crime: Where do we stand? *Psychology, Crime and Law*, **2**, 143–152.

Farrington, D.P. (1972). Delinquency begins at home. *New Society*, **21**, 495–497.

Farrington, D.P. (1979). Environmental stress, delinquent behaviour, and convictions. In *Stress and anxiety*, vol. 6, ed. I.G. Sarason and C.D. Spielberger, pp. 93–107. Hemisphere, Washington, D.C.

Farrington, D.P. (1983). Randomized experiments on crime and justice. In *Crime and justice*, vol. 4, ed. M. Tonry and N.Morris, pp. 257–308. University of Chicago Press, Chicago.

Farrington, D.P. (1987). Epidemiology. In *Handbook of juvenile delinquency*, ed. H.C. Quay, pp. 33–61. Wiley, New York.

Farrington, D.P. (1989a). Later adult life outcomes of offenders and non-offenders. In *Children at risk: Assessment, longitudinal research, and intervention*, ed. M.Brambring, F. Losel, and H.Skowronek, pp. 220–244. De Gruyter, Berlin.

Farrington, D.P. (1989b). Self-reported and official offending from adolescence to adulthood. In *Cross-national research in self-reported crime and delinquency*, ed. M.W. Klein, pp. 399–423. Kluwer, Dordrecht.

Farrington, D.P. (1990a). Age, period, cohort, and offending. In *Policy and theory in criminal justice: Contributions in honour of Leslie T. Wilkins*, ed. D.M. Gottfredson and R.V. Clarke, pp. 51–75. Avebury, Aldershot.

Farrington, D.P. (1990b). Implications of criminal career research for the prevention of offending. *Journal of Adolescence*, **13**, 93–113.

Farrington, D.P. (1991a). Antisocial personality from childhood to adulthood. *Psychologist*, **4**, 389–394.

Farrington, D.P. (1991b). Childhood aggression and adult violence: Early precursors and later life outcomes. In *The development and treatment of childhood aggression*, ed. D.J. Pepler and K.H. Rubin, pp. 5–29. Erlbaum, Hillsdale, N.J.

Farrington, D.P. (1992a). Criminal career research in the United Kingdom. *British Journal of Criminology*, **32**, 521–536.

Farrington, D.P. (1992b). Explaining the beginning, progress and ending of antisocial behaviour from birth to adulthood. In *Facts, frameworks and forecasts: Advances in criminological theory*, vol. 3, ed. J. McCord, pp. 253–286. Transaction, New Brunswick, N.J.

Farrington, D.P. (1992c). Juvenile delinquency. In *The school years*, 2nd edn, ed. J.C. Coleman, pp. 123–163. Routledge, London.

Farrington, D.P. (1993). Childhood origins of teenage antisocial behaviour and adult social dysfunction. *Journal of the Royal Society of Medicine*, **86**, 13–17.

Farrington, D.P. (1995). The development of offending and antisocial behaviour from childhood: Key findings from the Cambridge Study in Delinquent Development. *Journal of Child Psychology and Psychiatry*, **36**, 929–964.

Farrington, D.P. (1997). Human development and criminal careers. In *The Oxford handbook of criminology*, 2nd edn ed. M. Maguire, R. Morgan and R. Reiner, p. 361–408. Clarendon Press, Oxford.

Farrington, D.P. (1998). Predictors, causes and correlates of youth violence. In *Youth violence*, ed. M. Tonry and M.H. Moore, pp. 421–475. University of Chicago Press, Chicago.

Farrington, D.P. and Loeber, R. (1999). Transatlantic replicability of risk factors in the development of delinquency. In *Where and when: Historical and geographical influences on psychopathology*, ed. P.Cohen, C. Slomkowski and, L.N. Robins, pp. 299–329. Erlbaum, Mahwah, NJ.

Farrington, D.P. and West, D.J. (1993). Criminal, penal and life histories of chronic offenders: Risk and protective factors and early identification. *Criminal Behaviour and Mental Health*, **3**, 492–523.

Farrington, D.P. and Wikström, P-O.H. (1994). Criminal careers in London and Stockholm: A cross-national comparative study. In *Cross-national longitudinal research on human development and criminal behaviour*, ed. E.G.M. Weitekamp and H.J. Kerner, pp. 65–89. Kluwer, Dordrecht.

Farrington, D.P., Biron, L., and LeBlanc, M. (1982). Personality and delinquency in London and Montreal. In *Abnormal offenders, delinquency, and the criminal justice system*, ed. J.Gunn and, D.P. Farrington, pp. 153–201. Wiley, Chichester.

Farrington, D.P. Gallagher, B., Morley, L., St. Ledger, R.J., and West, D.J. (1986a). Unemployment, school leaving, and crime. *British Journal of Criminology*, **26**, 335–356.

Farrington, D.P., Ohlin, L.E., and Wilson, J.Q. (1986b) *Understanding and controlling crime: Toward a new research strategy*. Springer-Verlag, New York.

Farrington, D.P., Snyder, H.N., and Finnegan, T.A. (1988). Specialization in juvenile court careers. *Criminology*, **26**, 461–487.

Farrington, D.P., Loeber, R., and van Kammen, W.B. (1990). Long-term criminal outcomes of hyperactivity-impulsivity-attention deficit and conduct problems in childhood. In *Straight and devious pathways from childhood to adulthood*, ed. L.N. Robins and M. Rutter, pp. 62–81. Cambridge University Press, Cambridge.

Farrington, D.P., Sampson, R.J., and Wikström, P-O. (ed.) (1993). *Integrating individual and ecological aspects of crime.* National Council for Crime Prevention, Stockholm.

Farrington, D.P., Barnes, G., and Lambert, S. (1996). The concentration of offending in families. *Legal and Criminological Psychology*, **1**, 47–63.

Farrington, D.P., Lambert, S., and West, D.J. (1998). Criminal careers of two generations of family members in the Cambridge Study in Delinquent Development. *Studies on Crime and Crime Prevention*, **7**, 85–106.

Ferdinand, R.F., Verhulst, F.C., and Wiznitzer, M. (1995). Continuity and change of self-reported problem behaviours from adolescence into young adulthood. *Journal of the American Academy of Child and Adolescent Psychiatry*, **34**, 680–690.

Fergusson, D.M. and Horwood, L.J. (1995). Predictive validity of categorically and dimensionally scored measures of disruptive childhood behaviours. *Journal of the American Academy of Child and Adolescent Psychiatry*, **34**, 477–485.

Fergusson, D.M., Horwood, J., and Lynskey, M.T. (1994). Parental separation, adolescent psychopathology, and problem behaviours. *Journal of the American Academy of Child and Adolescent Psychiatry*, **33**, 1122–1131.

Fergusson, D.M., Lynskey, M.T., and Horwood, L.J. (1996). Factors associated with continuity and changes in disruptive behaviour patterns between childhood and adolescence. *Journal of Abnormal Child Psychology*, **24**, 533–553.

Fischer, D.G. (1984). Family size and delinquency. *Perceptual and Motor Skills*, **58**, 527–534.

Foley, H.A., Carlton, C.O., and Howell, R.J. (1996). The relationship of attention deficit hyperactivity disorder and conduct disorder to juvenile delinquency: Legal implications. *Bulletin of the American Academy of Psychiatry and Law*, **24**, 333–345.

Frick, P.J., Kamphaus, R.W., Lahey, B.B., Loeber, R., Christ, M.A.G., Hart, E.L., and Tannenbaum, L.E. (1991). Academic underachievement and the disruptive behaviour disorders. *Journal of Consulting and Clinical Psychology*, **59**, 289–294.

Frick, P.J., Lahey, B.B., Loeber, R., Stouthamer-Loeber, M., Christ, M.A.G., and Hanson, K. (1992). Familial risk factors to oppositional defiant disorder and conduct disorder: Parental psychopathology and maternal parenting. *Journal of Consulting and Clinical Psychology*, **60**, 49–55.

Goodman, R., Simonoff, E., and Stevenson, J. (1995). The impact of child IQ, parent IQ and sibling IQ on child behavioural deviance scores. *Journal of Child Psychology and Psychiatry*, **36**, 409–425.

Graham, J. (1988). *Schools, disruptive behaviour and delinquency.* HMSO, London.

Guerin, D.W., Gottfried, A.W., and Thomas, C.W. (1997). Difficult temperament and behaviour problems: A longitudinal study from 1.5 to 12 years. *International Journal of Behavioural Development*, **21**, 71–90.

Hamparian, D.M., Davis, J.M., Jacobson, J.M., and McGraw, R.E. (1985). *The young criminal years of the violent few.* Office of Juvenile Justice and Delinquency Prevention, Washington, D.C.

Harpur, T.J., Hare, R.D., and Hakstian, A.R. (1989). Two-factor conceptualization of psychopathy: Construct validity and assessment implications. *Psychological Assessment*, **1**, 6–17.

Hawkins, J.D., Doueck, H.J., and Lishner, D.M. (1988). Changing teaching practices in mainstream classrooms to improve bonding and behaviour of low achievers. *American Educational Research Journal*, **25**, 31–50.

Hawkins, J.D., von Cleve, E., and Catalano, R.F. (1991). Reducing early childhood aggression: Results of a primary prevention programme. *Journal of the American Academy of Child and Adolescent Psychiatry*, **30**, 208–217.

Hawkins, J.D., Catalano, R.F., Morrison, D.M., ODonnell, J., Abbott, R.D., and Day, L.E. (1992). The Seattle social development project: Effects of the first four years on protective factors and problem behaviours. In *Preventing antisocial behaviour*, ed. J. McCord and R. Tremblay, pp. 139–161. Guilford, New York.

Henggeler, S.W., Melton, G.B., and Smith, L.A. (1992). Family preservation using multi-systemic therapy: An effective alternative to incarcerating serious juvenile offenders. *Journal of Consulting and Clinical Psychology*, **60**, 953–961.

Henggeler, S.W., Melton, G.B., Smith, L.A., Schoenwald, S.K., and Hanley, J.H. (1993). Family preservation using multi-systemic treatment: Long-term follow-up to a clinical trial with serious juvenile offenders. *Journal of Child and Family Studies*, **2**, 283–293.

Henggeler, S.W., Melton, G.B., Brondino, M.J., Scherer, D.G., and Hanley, J.H. (1997). Multisystemic therapy with violent and chronic juvenile offenders and their families: The role of treatment fidelity in successful dissemination. *Journal of Consulting and Clinical Psychology*, **65**, 821–833.

Henry, B., Moffitt, T., Robins, L., Earls, F., and Silva, P. (1993). Early family predictors of child and adolescent antisocial behaviour: Who are the mothers of delinquents? *Criminal Behaviour and Mental Health*, **2**, 97–118.

Hindelang, M.J., Hirschi, T., and Weis, J.G. (1981). *Measuring delinquency*. Sage, Beverly Hills, CA.

Hirschi, T. and Hindelang, M.J. (1977). Intelligence and delinquency: A revisionist review. *American Sociological Review*, **42**, 571–587.

Hodgins, S. (1994). Status at age 30 of children with conduct problems. *Studies on Crime and Crime Prevention*, **3**, 41–62.

Horacek, H.J., Ramey, C.T., Campbell, F.A., Hoffmann, K.P., and Fletcher, R.H. (1987). Predicting school failure and assessing early intervention with high-risk children. *Journal of the American Academy of Child and Adolescent Psychiatry*, **26**, 758–763.

Huizinga, D., Loeber, R., and Thornberry, T.P. (1993). Longitudinal study of delinquency, drug use, sexual activity and pregnancy among children and youth in three cities. *Public Health Reports*, **108**, 90–96.

Jenkins, J.M. and Smith, M.A. (1991). Marital disharmony and children's behaviour problems: Aspects of a poor marriage that affect children adversely. *Journal of Child Psychology and Psychiatry*, **32**, 793–810.

Jones, M.B. and Offord, D.R. (1989). Reduction of antisocial behaviour in poor children by non-school skill-development. *Journal of Child Psychology and Psychiatry*, **30**, 737–750.

Kazdin, A.E. (1995). *Conduct disorders in childhood and adolescence*, 2nd edn. Sage, Thousand Oaks, CA.

Kazdin, A.E. (1997). Parent management training: Evidence, outcomes and issues. *Journal of the American Academy of Child and Adolescent Psychiatry*, **36**, 1349–1356.

Kazdin, A.E., Siegel, T.C., and Bass, D. (1992). Cognitive problem-solving skills training and parent management training in the treatment of antisocial behaviour in children. *Journal of Consulting and Clinical Psychology*, **60**, 733–747.

Kessler, R.C., Berglund, P.A., Foster, C.L., Saunders, W.B., Stang, P.E., and Walters, E.E. (1997). Social consequences of psychiatric disorders, II. Teenage parenthood. *American Journal of Psychiatry*, **154**, 1405–1411.

Kitzman, H., Olds, D.L., Henderson, C.R., Hanks, C., Cole, R., Tatelbaum, R., McConnochie, K.M., Sidora, K., Luckey, D.W., Shaver, D., Engelhardt, K., James, D., and Barnard, K. (1997). Effects of prenatal and infancy home visitation by nurses on pregnancy outcomes, childhood injuries, and repeated childbearing. *Journal of the American Medical Association*, **278**, 644–652.

Kolvin, I., Miller, F.J. W., Fleeting, M., and Kolvin, P.A. (1988). Social and parenting factors affecting criminal-offence rates: Findings from the Newcastle Thousand Family Study (1947–1980). *British Journal of Psychiatry*, **152**, 80–90.

Lahey, B.B., Loeber, R., Stouthamer-Loeber, M., Christ, M.A. G., Green, S., Russo, M.F., Frick, P.J., and Dulcan, M. (1990). Comparison of DSM-3 and DSM-3R diagnoses for prepubertal children: Changes in prevalence and validity. *Journal of the American Academy of Child and Adolescent Psychiatry*, **29**, 620–626.

Lahey, B.B., Loeber, R., Hart, E.L., Frick, P.J., Applegate, B., Zhang, Q., Green, S.M., and Russo, M.F. (1995). Four-year longitudinal study of conduct disorder in boys: Patterns and predictors of persistence. *Journal of Abnormal Psychology*, **104**, 83–93.

Lahey, B.B., Loeber, R., Quay, H.C., Frick, P.J., and Grimm, J. (1997). Oppositional defiant disorder and conduct disorder. In *DSM-4 sourcebook*, vol. 3, ed. T.A. Widiger, A.J. Frances, H.A. Pincus, R. Ross, M.B. First, and W. Davis, pp. 189–209. American Psychiatric Association, Washington, D.C.

Larson, C. (1980). Efficacy of prenatal and postpartum home visits on child health and development. *Pediatrics*, **66**, 191–197.

Lewinsohn, P.M., Rohde, P., and Seeley, J.R. (1995). Adolescent psychopathology. III. The clinical consequences of comorbidity. *Journal of the American Academy of Child and Adolescent Psychiatry*, **34**, 510–519.

Lipsey, M.W. and Wilson, D.B. (1998). Effective intervention for serious juvenile offenders: A synthesis of research. In *Serious and violent juvenile offenders: Risk factors and successful interventions*, ed. R. Loeber and D.P. Farrington, pp. 313–345. Sage, Thousand Oaks, CA.

Lipsitt, P.D., Buka, S.L., and Lipsitt, L.P. (1990). Early intelligence scores and subsequent delinquency: A prospective study. *American Journal of Family Therapy*, **18**, 197–208.

Loeber, R. and Farrington, D.P. (ed.) (1998). *Serious and violent juvenile offenders: Risk factors and successful interventions*. Sage, Thousand Oaks, CA.

Loeber, R. and Keenan, K. (1994). Interaction between conduct disorder and its comorbid conditions: Effects of age and gender. *Clinical Psychology Review*, **14**, 497–523.

Loeber, R. and LeBlanc, M. (1990). Toward a developmental criminology. In *Crime and justice* vol.12, ed. M. Tonry and N. Morris, pp 375–473. University of Chicago Press, Chicago.

Loeber, R., Green, S.M., Keenan, K., and Lahey, B.B. (1995). Which boys will fare worse? Early predictors of the onset of conduct disorder in a six-year longitudinal study. *Journal of the American Academy of Child and Adolescent Psychiatry*, **34**, 499–509.

Loeber, R., Farrington, D.P., Stouthamer-Loeber, M., and van Kammen, W.B. (1998). *Antisocial behaviour and mental health problems: Explanatory factors in childhood and adolescence*. Erlbaum, Mahwah, N.J.

Lynam, D. (1996). Early identification of chronic offenders: Who is the fledgling psychopath? *Psychological Bulletin*, 120, 209–234.

Lynam, D., Moffitt, T.E., and Stouthamer-Loeber, M. (1993). Explaining the relation between IQ and delinquency: Class, race, test motivation, school failure or self-control? *Journal of Abnormal Psychology*, **102**, 187–196.

Malinosky-Rummell, R. and Hansen, D.J. (1993). Long-term consequences of childhood physical abuse. *Psychological Bulletin*, **114**, 68–79.

Maxfield, M.G. and Widom, C.S. (1996). The cycle of violence revisited 6 years later. *Archives of Pediatrics and Adolescent Medicine*, **150**, 390–395.

McArdle, P., OBrien, G., and Kolvin, I. (1995). Hyperactivity: Prevalence and relationship with conduct disorder. *Journal of Child Psychology and Psychiatry*, **36**, 279–303.

McCord, J. (1977). A comparative study of two generations of native Americans. In *Theory in criminology*, ed. R.F. Meier, pp. 83–92. Sage, Beverly Hills, CA.

McCord, J. (1979). Some child-rearing antecedents of criminal behaviour in adult men. *Journal of Personality and Social Psychology*, **37**, 1477–1486.

McCord, J. (1991). Family relationships, juvenile delinquency, and adult criminality. *Criminology*, **29**, 397–417.

McGee, R., Feehan, M., Williams, S., Partridge, F., Silva, P.A., and Kelly, J. (1990). DSM-3 disorders in a large sample of adolescents. *Journal of the American Academy of Child and Adolescent Psychiatry*, **29**, 611–619.

Moffitt, T.E. (1993). Adolescence-limited and life-course-persistent antisocial behaviour: A developmental taxonomy. *Psychological Review*, **100**, 674–701.

Morash, M. and Rucker, L. (1989). An exploratory study of the connection of mother's age at childbearing to her children's delinquency in four data sets. *Crime and Delinquency*, **35**, 45–93.

Nagin, D.S., Pogarsky, G., and Farrington, D.P. (1997). Adolescent mothers and the criminal behaviour of their children. *Law and Society Review*, **31**, 137–162.

Newson, J., Newson, E., and Adams, M. (1993). The social origins of delinquency. *Criminal Behaviour and Mental Health*, **3**, 19–29.

Nottelman, E.D. and Jensen, P.S. (1995). Comorbidity of disorders in children and adolescents: Developmental perspectives. In *Advances in Clinical Child Psychology*, vol. 17, ed. T.H. Ollendick and R.J. Prinz, pp. 109–155. Plenum, New York.

O'Donnell, J., Hawkins, J.D., Catalano, R.F., Abbott, R.D., and Day, L.E. (1995). Preventing school failure, drug use, and delinquency among low-income children: Long-term intervention in elementary schools. *American Journal of Orthopsychiatry*, **65**, 87–100.

Offord, D.R., Alder, R.J., and Boyle, M.H. (1986). Prevalence and sociodemographic correlates of conduct disorder. *American Journal of Social Psychiatry*, **6**, 272–278.

Offord, D.R., Boyle, M.H., Szatmari, P., Rae-Grant, N.I., Links, P.S., Cadman, D.T., Byles, J.A., Crawford, J.W., Blum, H.M., Byrne, C., Thomas, H., and Woodward, C.A. (1987). Ontario Child Health Study. II. Six-month prevalence of disorder and rates of service utilization. *Archives of General Psychiatry*, **44**, 832–836.

Offord, D.R., Boyle, M.H., and Racine, Y. (1989). Ontario Child Health Study: Correlates of disorder. *Journal of the American Academy of Child and Adolescent Psychiatry*, **28**, 856–860.

Offord, D.R., Boyle, M.H., Racine, Y.A., Fleming, J.E., Cadman, D.T., Blum, H.M., Byrne, C., Links, P.S., Lipman, E.L. Macmillan, H.L., Rae-Grant, N.I., Sanford, M.N., Szatmari, P., Thomas, H., and Woodward, C.A. (1992). Outcome, prognosis and risk in a longitudinal follow-up study. *Journal of the American Academy of Child and Adolescent Psychiatry*, **31**, 916–923.

Olds, D.L., Henderson, C.R., Chamberlain, R., and Tatelbaum, R. (1986a). Preventing child abuse and neglect: A randomized trial of nurse home visitation. *Pediatrics*, **78**, 65–78.

Olds, D.L., Henderson, C.R., Tatelbaum, R., and Chamberlain, R. (1986b). Improving the delivery of prenatal care and outcomes of pregnancy: A randomized trial of nurse home visitation. *Pediatrics*, **77**, 16–28.

Olds, D.L., Eckenrode, J., Henderson, C.R., Kitzman, H., Powers, J., Cole, R., Sidora, K., Morris, P., Pettitt, L.M., and Luckey, D.W. (1997). Long-term effects of home visitation on maternal life course and child abuse and neglect. *Journal of the American Medical Association*, **278**, 637–643.

Olweus, D. (1993). *Bullying at school*. Blackwell, Oxford.

Olweus, D. (1994). Bullying at school: Basic facts and effects of a school based intervention programme. *Journal of Child Psychology and Psychiatry*, **35**, 1171–1190.

Patterson, G.R. (1982). *Coercive family process*. Castalia, Eugene, OR.

Patterson, G.R., Chamberlain, P., and Reid, J.B. (1982). A comparative evaluation of a parent training programme. *Behaviour Therapy*, **13**, 638–650.

Patterson, G.R., Reid, J.B., and Dishion, T.J. (1992). *Antisocial boys*. Castalia, Eugene, OR.

Petersen, A.C., Compas, B.E., Brooks-Gunn, J., Stemmler, M., Ey, S., and Grant, K.E. (1993). Depression in adolescence. *American Psychologist*, **48**, 155–168.

Polk, K., Alder, C., Bazemore, G., Blake, G., Cordray, S., Coventry, G., Galvin, J., and Temple, M. (1981). *Becoming adult*. Final Report to the National Institute of Mental Health, Washington, D.C.

Power, M.J., Alderson, M.R., Phillipson, C.M., Shoenberg, E., and Morris, J.N. (1967). Delinquent schools? *New Society*, **10**, 542–543.

Pulkkinen, L. (1988). Delinquent development: Theoretical and empirical considerations. In *Studies of psychosocial risk*, ed. M. Rutter, pp. 184–199. Cambridge University Press. Cambridge:

Raine, A., Brennan, P.A., Farrington, D.P., and Mednick, S.A. (ed.) (1997). *Biosocial bases of violence*. Plenum, New York.

Rey, J.M., Morris-Yates, A., Singh, M., Andrews, G., and Stewart, G.W. (1995). Continuities between psychiatric disorders in adolescents and personality disorders in young adults. *American Journal of Psychiatry*, **152**, 895–900.

Robins, L.N. (1979). Sturdy childhood predictors of adult outcomes: Replications from longitudinal studies In *Stress and mental disorder*, ed. J.E. Barrett, R.M. Rose, and G.L. Klerman, pp. 219–235. Raven Press, New York.

Robins, L.N. (1986). The consequences of conduct disorder in girls. In *Development of antisocial and prosocial behaviour*, ed. D.Olweus, J. Block, and M.R. Yarrow, pp. 385–414. Academic Press, Orlando, FL.

Robins, L.N. (1999). A 70-year history of conduct disorder: Variations in definition, prevalence and correlates. In *Where and when: Historical and geographical influences on psychopathology*, ed. P.Cohen, C. Slomkowski, and L.N. Robins. Erlbaum, Mahwah, NJ.

Robins, L.N. and Ratcliff, K.S. (1978). Risk factors in the continuation of childhood antisocial behaviour into adulthood. *International Journal of Mental Health*, **7**, 96–116.

Robins, L.N., West, P.J., and Herjanic, B.L. (1975). Arrests and delinquency in two generations: A study of black urban families and their children. *Journal of Child Psychology and Psychiatry*, **16**, 125–140.

Robins, L.N., Tipp, J., and Przybeck, T. (1991). Antisocial personality. In *Psychiatric disorders in America*, ed. L.N. Robins and, D.A. Regier, pp. 259–290. Macmillan/Free Press, New York.

Rogeness, G.A. (1994). Biologic findings in conduct disorder. *Child and Adolescent Psychiatric Clinics of North America*, **3**, 271–284.

Ross, R.R. and Ross, R.D. (1995). (ed.) *Thinking straight: The reasoning and rehabilitation programme for delinquency prevention and offender rehabilitation.* Air Training and Publications, Ottawa, Canada.

Rothbaum, F. and Weisz, J.R. (1994). Parental caregiving and child externalizing behaviour in nonclinical samples: A meta-analysis. *Psychological Bulletin*, **116**, 55–74.

Russo, M.F. and Beidel, D.C. (1994). Comorbidity of childhood anxiety and externalizing disorders: Prevalence, associated characteristics, and validation issues. *Clinical Psychology Review*, **3**, 199–221.

Rutter, M. (1995). Relationships between mental disorders in childhood and adulthood. *Acta Psychiatrica Scandinavica*, **91**, 73–85.

Rutter, M., Maughan, B., Mortimore, P., and Ouston, J. (1979). *Fifteen thousand hours*. Open Books, London.

Rutter, M., Giller, H., and Hagell, A. (1998). *Antisocial behaviour by young people*. Cambridge University Press, Cambridge.

Sanson, A., Smart, D., Prior, M., and Oberklaid, F. (1993). Precursors of hyperactivity and aggression. *Journal of the American Academy of Child and Adolescent Psychiatry*, **32**, 1207–1216.

Schweinhart, L.J. and Weikart, D.P. (1980). *Young children grow up*. High/Scope, Ypsilanti, M.I.

Schweinhart, L.J., Barnes, H.V., and Weikart, D.P. (1993). *Significant benefits*. High/Scope, Ypsilanti, M.I.

Smith, P.K. and Sharp, S. (1994). *School bullying*. Routledge, London.

Stattin, H. and Klackenberg-Larsson, I. (1993). Early language and intelligence development and their relationship to future criminal behaviour. *Journal of Abnormal Psychology*, **102**, 369–378.

Stattin, H. and Magnusson, D. (1991). Stability and change in criminal behaviour up to age 30. *British Journal of Criminology*, **31**, 327–346.

Storm-Mathisen, A. and Vaglum, P. (1994). Conduct disorder patients 20 years later: A personal follow-up study. *Acta Psychiatrica Scandinavica*, **89**, 416–420.

Szatmari, P., Boyle, M.H., and Offord, D.R. (1993). Familial aggregation of emotional and behavioural problems of childhood in the general population. *American Journal of Psychiatry*, **150**, 1398–1403.

Tracy, P.E. and Kempf-Leonard, K. (1996). *Continuity and discontinuity in criminal careers*. Plenum, New York.

Tremblay, R.E. and Craig, W.M. (1995). Developmental crime prevention. In *Building a safer society: Strategic approaches to crime prevention*, ed. M. Tonry and D.P. Farrington, pp. 151–236. University of Chicago Press, Chicago.

Tremblay, R.E., Pihl, R.O., Vitaro, F., and Dobkin, P.L. (1994). Predicting early onset of male antisocial behaviour from pre-school behaviour. *Archives of General Psychiatry*, **51**, 732–739.

Tremblay, R.E., Pagani-Kurtz, L., Vitaro, F., Masse, L.C., and Pihl, R.D. (1995). A bimodal preventive intervention for disruptive kindergarten boys: Its impact through mid-adolescence. *Journey of Consulting and Clinical Psychology*, **63**, 560–568.

Velez, C.N., Johnson, J., and Cohen, P. (1989). A longitudinal analysis of selected risk factors for childhood psychopathology. *Journal of the American Academy of Child and Adolescent Psychiatry*, **28**, 861–864.

Verhulst, F.C. and van der Ende, J. (1991). Four-year follow-up of teacher-reported problem behaviours. *Psychological Medicine*, **21**, 965–977.

Verhulst, F.C. and van der Ende, J. (1992a). Six-year developmental course of internalizing and externalizing problem behaviours. *Journal of the American Academy of Child and Adolescent Psychiatry*, **31**, 924–931.

Verhulst, F.C. and van der Ende, J. (1992b). Six-year stability of parent-reported problem behaviour in an epidemiological sample. *Journal of Abnormal Child Psychology*, **20**, 595–610.

Verhulst, F.C. and van der Ende, J. (1995). The eight-year stability of problem behaviour in an epidemiologic sample. *Pediatric Research*, **38**, 612–617.

Verhulst, F.C., Koot, H.M. and Berden, G.F. M.G. (1990). Four-year follow-up of an epidemiological sample. *Journal of the American Academy of Child and Adolescent Psychiatry*, **29**, 440–448.

Wadsworth, M. (1979). *Roots of delinquency*. Martin Robertson, London.

Walsh, A., Petee, T.A., and Beyer, J.A. (1987). Intellectual imbalance and delinquency: Comparing high verbal and high performance IQ delinquents. *Criminal Justice and Behaviour*, **14**, 370–379.

Wasserman, G.A. and Miller, L.S. (1998). The prevention of serious and violent juvenile offending. In *Serious and violent juvenile offenders: Risk factors and successful interventions*, ed. R. Loeber and D.P. Farrington, pp. 197–247. Sage, Thousand Oaks, CA.

Webster-Stratton, C. and Hammond, M. (1997). Treating children with early-onset conduct problems: A comparison of child and parent training interventions. *Journal of Consulting and Clinical Psychology*, **65**, 93–109.

Wells, L.E. and Rankin, J.H. (1991). Families and delinquency: A meta-analysis of the impact of broken homes. *Social Problems*, **38**, 71–93.

West, D.J. and Farrington, D.P. (1973). *Who becomes delinquent?* Heinemann, London.

West, D.J. and Farrington, D.P. (1977). *The delinquent way of life*. Heinemann, London.

Widom, C.S. (1989). The cycle of violence. *Science*, **244**, 160–166.

Wilson, J.Q. and Herrnstein, R.J. (1985). *Crime and human nature*. Simon and Schuster, New York.

Wolfgang, M.E., Figlio, R.M., and Sellin, T. (1972). *Delinquency in a birth cohort*. University of Chicago Press, Chicago.

Wolfgang, M.E., Thornberry, T.P., and Figlio, R.M. (1987). *From boy to man, from delinquency to crime*. University of Chicago Press, Chicago.

Zoccolillo, M., Pickles, A., Quinton, D., and Rutter, M. (1992). The outcome of childhood conduct disorder: Implications for defining adult personality disorder and conduct disorder. *Psychological Medicine*, **22**, 971–986.

12 Substance use disorders

Yifrah Kaminer and and Ralph E. Tarter

There is mounting concern regarding the physical and mental health outcomes among adolescents who use psychoactive drugs for non-medical reasons. This concern among professionals and policymakers is based on epidemiological data demonstrating a continued increase in the incidence of substance use among youth (Johnston *et al.* 1996), a decrease in the age of first diagnosis of substance use disorder (SUD) (Reich *et al.* 1988), the lifetime prevalence of substance abuse and dependence in the adolescent population (Lewinsohn *et al.* 1996), and the observation that alcohol and other drugs are leading causes of adolescent morbidity and mortality consequent to motor vehicle accidents, suicidal behavior, violence, drowning, and unprotected sexual behavior (US Department of Vital Statistics 1993, Kaminer 1994).

This chapter begins with a review of the literature pertaining to the clinical picture of adolescent substance use. Next, natural history is reviewed, particularly with respect to stability or continuity of substance use and diagnosis over time. An examination of intervention studies and their effects is then presented. The chapter concludes with a succinct presentation of the factors which augment risk for substance abuse in adolescents.

Clinical picture

Contemporary taxonomic systems do not distinguish SUD in youth from the adult condition. Although it is dubious whether the same criteria that are applied to adults are appropriate for youth (Martin *et al.* 1995), clinicians and researchers alike have nonetheless accepted adult criteria in formulating SUD diagnoses in adolescents. For example, neuroadaptation (chronic tolerance), and adverse psychosocial consequences typically occur after prolonged drug exposure. Inasmuch as young people have not typically had sufficient time to manifest the chronic consequences comprising the criteria for diagnosis, it is to be expected that adolescence is primarily the period prodromal to syndromal SUD. Those individuals that do, however, satisfy the criteria for SUD, are thus especially disturbed in view of the fact that the disorder occurred during a relatively compressed period of time following initial exposure. Not surprisingly, there are manifold behavioral, psychiatric, and social consequences resulting from this rapid momentum and escalation of alcohol and drug consumption and problems in adolescents who qualify for SUD diagnosis. These disturbances, manifest in multiple domains of everyday functioning, are highly intercorrelated and include precocious and risky sexual behavior, non-normative attitudes and antisocial behavior, and injury-prone behavior (Newcomb and Bentler 1988, Kaplan 1995, Mezzich *et al.* 1997). Suicide attempts and completion are also more common among adolescents who abuse alcohol and other drugs (Brent *et al.* 1987).

Historical factors, particularly post-traumatic stress disorder, family violence, physical/sexual abuse during childhood, and deficient social integration are found more commonly in substance-abusing youth compared to the general population (Clark and Kirisci 1996),. Homeless and runaway youth, as well as those coming in contact with the criminal justice system, commonly, if not typically, have a history of substance abuse (Bailey *et al.* in press). Adolescents with SUD score on average lower on tests of intelligence and academic achievement compared to those who do not quality for diagnosis (Moss *et al.* 1994). Neuropsychological tests suggest that the deficits are primarily circumscribed to language-based processes (Tarter *et al.* 1995). In contrast to these varied disturbances, physical health and nutrition are generally intact. Indeed, it is uncommon to detect signs of liver injury or disease (Arria *et al.* 1995).

It is significant to note that the pattern and natural history of drug use differs markedly between adolescent and adult onset SUD. Diagnosis of marijuana and hallucinogen abuse and dependence are more often observed in adolescents (Clark *et al.* 1998). Despite their younger age, adolescents with SUD are more likely than adults to have multiple SUD diagnoses, pointing to secular trends towards polydrug abuse as the typical pattern in contrast to the older population. In one recent study, Martin *et al.* (1994) found that 96% of adolescents who qualified for a diagnosis of alcohol abuse or dependence also used other drugs.

Adolescents qualifying for SUD typically come into treatment via three main routes. First, behavioral and emotional problems reach a point of unmanageability or conflict with others such that a referral is made to a social service or psychiatric facility. The referral may be precipitated by suspicion of substance use (e.g. finding drug paraphernalia or the drug itself, abrupt changes in the youngster's home behavior) or on the basis of the adolescent's emotional and behavioral disposition (e.g. irritability, depression, loss of motivation). In this latter instance, involvement with drugs or SUD is discovered during the course of an intake psychiatric interview or using a self-administered screening instrument such as the Drug Use Screening Inventory (Kirisci *et al.* 1995, Tarter 1995).

Second, in response to increasing recognition of the prevalence of substance use among youth, school personnel have become increasingly attuned to identifying students in need of treatment. Outreach programs by university health centers to schools under the aegis of health promotion provide another avenue for guiding adolescents into treatment. Although prevention of SUD has not traditionally been a school-based activity, recent trends indicate that treatment services are also increasingly offered.

Third, treatment is frequently initiated following contact with the criminal justice system. Although systematic research has not been conducted, driving an automobile while intoxicated is probably the most common situation for problem detection. Discovery of an alcohol or drug problem is often made following arrest for minor offenses, and occasionally major offenses, including drug possession, drug dealing, and sexual violence.

It is important to point out that it is not possible to characterize the typical adolescent with SUD or, for that matter, the typical adolescent who consumes alcohol or drugs but does not qualify for a disorder. For example, ethnic and gender characteristics have been reported frequently (Chavez *et al.* 1989, Groerer 1996). Also, demographic factors, changing circumstances pertaining to cost and availability, and secular trends in society affect consumption patterns (Altschuler and Brounstein 1991). As a case in point, cocaine use appears to be declining whereas marijuana use is increasing among US youth (Johnston *et al.* 1996).

Unlike certain other types of psychiatric disorder, substance consumption and its consequences comprise a continuum of severity. Beyond a somewhat arbitrary diagnostic threshold the person is deemed to qualify for a disorder of abuse, and in the more severe variant, dependence. Clinical phenomenology, even within the suprathreshold range, is very heterogeneous in the population with respect to substance use topography, psychiatric comorbidity, risk factors, and natural history. This heterogeneity is further magnified by the fact that there is a high degree of variation in the population with respect to environmental risk factors (family, school, culture, etc.), genetic predisposition, and socialization experience. Before addressing these latter topics, it is useful to review the nosology of SUD in adolescents.

Nosology

Consumption of drugs having abuse or dependence liability can be conceptualized along a dimension of severity. Surpassing a threshold based on the number of consequences of drug use qualifies the person as affected, i.e. manifesting a disorder of abuse or dependence.

Abuse liability is determined for the most part by the reinforcing pharmacological properties of the drug. Positive reinforcement occurs when the drug induces a euphoric effect or otherwise enhances cognitive, affective, or behavioral processes. Negative reinforcement occurs when the drug relieves or alleviates the person from a negative state. The likelihood of developing addiction or physical dependence is also affected to large degree by the speed the drug reaches the brain. Compounds that are inhaled (e.g. crack, nicotine, ethers, etc.) generally produce a dependence syndrome faster than drugs that require injection, which in turn produce addiction faster than drugs that are ingested. Because compounds having the pharmacological properties of positive and negative reinforcers are ubiquitous in society and hence are readily obtainable, it is not surprising that most youth experiment, and within this subpopulation, some become habitual consumers.

By age 18, 79.2% of youth in the US have been exposed to alcohol and 3.7% are daily users (Johnston *et al.* 1996). Cigarettes have been used by 63.5%, and 13% smoke half a pack a day. These data, reflecting the results of a 1996 survey, underscore the fact that, from a statistical perspective, consumption is normative, or at least not egregiously deviant.

The majority of adolescents who engage in substance use do not escalate to SUD as defined by DSM-IV criteria (APA 1994). However, approximately 8% of the population during their lifetime will qualify for a diagnosis of SUD. Although the threshold for assigning a diagnosis of abuse/dependence is somewhat arbitrary, particularly in adolescents (Rhode *et al.* 1996), clinical psychiatry has traditionally adopted this categorical orientation (e.g. normal vs. abnormal) despite its limitations with respect to understanding pathogenesis and treatment (Bukstein and Kaminer 1994).

In the DSM-IV (American Psychiatric Association 1994), SUD consists of two diagnostic categories: dependence and abuse (the residual disorder). Abuse is considered to be prodromal to dependence, and a less maladaptive disorder. Its residual category status, however, could jeopardize the availability of treatment for adolescents with this diagnosis since it implies that the disorder is not severe enough to warrant professional treatment. Significantly, only 63% of adolescents in one study who qualified for a diagnosis of dependence previously satisfied criteria for a diagnosis of abuse (Pollock and Martin 1996), indicating that abuse and dependence may not reflect an SUD continuum defined by severity. Part of the difficulty lies with the criteria utilized for the diagnosis of abuse. For example, it is possible to document impaired social role functioning due to problems at home or school as a symptom of abuse even if the consumption level is very low. In effect, the level of consumption is discordant with severity of consequence.

The diagnosis of abuse is applied if one or more symptoms are present during the prior 12 month period. The diagnosis of dependence is applied if the person demonstrates three or more symptoms during the prior 12 month period. Although the DSM-IV is an improvement over previous taxonomic systems, its applicability to adolescents remains unproven. For example, the symptoms have markedly different salience. In particular, legal problems and hazardous use have higher severity than the other symptoms in the abuse category (Martin *et al.* 1996a). Also, males are more likely to qualify for symptoms due merely to the higher presence of conduct disorder. Moreover, about 25% of habitual adolescent disorders are 'diagnostic orphans'; that is, they exhibit symptoms of dependence but do not satisfy the criteria for a diagnosis (Pollock and Martin 1996). Notably, a recent study of the timing of symptom appearance employing survival analysis procedures did not support the validity of the DSM-IV taxonomic system (Martin *et al.* 1996b). Clearly, additional research is needed to either adapt the adult criteria to adolescents or to devise a nosological system specific to this developmental stage.

Diagnostic subtypes

Research on alcoholics has revealed two main variants, known as type 1 and type 2 (Cloninger 1987, Sigvardsson *et al.* 1996). This dichotomy was renamed type A–type B based on psychosocial and treatment history factors (Babor *et al.* 1992). Specifically, the type 2 or type B variant is first diagnosed during adolescence. It is characterized by an early age onset of alcohol-seeking behavior, a rapid acceleration of alcohol (and other drug) involvement, severe alcohol-related symptoms, antisocial behavior, and poor prognosis. Three personality characteristics, high novelty seeking, low harm avoidance, and low reward dependence have been implicated to characterize this variant (Cloninger 1987) although empirical evidence in support of this profile is inconsistent. Tarter and colleagues (1994) used the difficult temperament index to classify adolescent alcoholics. The clusters obtained were similar to the adult subtypes reported by Cloninger (1987) and Babor *et al.* (1992). The smaller subset of adolescents manifesting behavioral dyscontrol and hypophoria were included in cluster 2 while those with primarily negative affect were classified in cluster 1. Cluster 2 patients had an earlier age of onset of first substance use, younger age of first substance abuse diagnosis, and younger age of first psychiatric diagnosis than subjects in cluster 1. Moreover, adolescents with a difficult temperament displayed a high probability of developing psychiatric disorders such as conduct disorder, attention deficit hyperactivity disorder (ADHD), anxiety disorders, and mood disorders (Tarter *et al.* 1994). Recently, Tarter *et al.* (1997) reported that cluster 1 and cluster 2 were identified within each sex.

Psychiatric comorbidity

A number of psychiatric disorders are commonly associated with SUD in youth (Bukstein *et al.* 1989). Conduct disorder commonly accompanies adolescent SUD (Loeber 1988, Milin *et al.* 1991). Clinical populations of adolescents with SUD show rates of conduct disorder ranging from 50% to 80%. ADHD is also frequently observed in youth using and abusing substances; however, this association is probably due to the high level of comorbidity between conduct disorder and ADHD (Alterman and Tarter 1986, Wilens *et al.* 1994).

In addition, mood disorders, especially depression, are frequently concurrent with substance use and SUD in adolescents (Bukstein *et al.* 1992, Deykin *et al.* 1992). The prevalence of depressive disorders ranges from 24% to 50%. The empirical literature also supports an association between SUDs and suicidal behavior in adolescents (Kaminer 1996). Adolescent suicide victims are frequently under the influence of alcohol or other drugs at the time of suicide (Brent *et al.* 1987, Mezzich *et al.* 1997). Possible mechanisms underlying this relationship include acute pharmacological effects of psychoactive substances. Acute intoxication may be experienced as a transient but intense dysphoric state with accompanying behavioral disinhibition and impaired judgment. In addition, substance use may exacerbate pre-existing depression to produce a suicide attempt. Although not extensively researched, episodic behaviors, such as violence or suicide, most likely reflect the combined influences of predisposing vulnerability, direct pharmacological effects, and contextual factors at the time of intoxication.

Studies of clinical samples have observed a high rate of anxiety disorder among youth with SUD (Clark and Sayette 1993, Clark *et al.* 1995). Prevalence estimates range from 7% to 40% (Stowell 1991, Clark *et al.* 1995). The order of appearance of anxiety and SUD is variable, depending on the specific anxiety disorder. Social phobia usually precedes substance abuse, whereas panic and generalized anxiety disorder more often follow the onset of SUD (Kushner *et al.* 1990). Adolescents with SUD often have a history of post traumatic stress disorder (PTSD) consequent to a history of physical or sexual abuse (Van Hasselt *et al.* 1993, Clark *et al.* 1995). Bulimia nervosa (Bulik 1987) and gambling behavior (Griffiths 1995) are also commonly found in adolescents who have SUD.

In summary, psychiatric comorbidity is common, indeed typical of adolescents with SUD. As pointed out earlier, this is not surprising considering that drug abuse and dependence developing at a young age are expected to be associated with behavioral and emotional problems. Overtly, this is manifest as multiple comorbid disorders, the specific configuration and progression of severity being highly variable in the adolescent SUD population (Mezzich *et al.* 1994, Martin *et al.* 1996a). Externalizing disorder is more common in males, whereas internalizing disorder is more common in females (Mezzich *et al.* 1993); however, it is not uncommon to observe a mixed profile of comorbidity consisting of SUD with both internalizing and externalizing psychiatric disorder in males and females.

Studies of natural course

Kandel (1982), the initial proponent of the 'gateway' theory, argued that there are at least four distinct developmental stages in drug use involvement. The stages are:

- use of beer or wine
- use of cigarettes or hard liquor
- use of marijuana
- use of other illicit drugs.

Many adolescents who use illicit drugs (approximately 26%) progress to the next stage, compared to only 4% who have never used marijuana. Thus, once exposure to marijuana occurs, the person is at much higher risk of using drugs such as opiates and cocaine. A study by Golub and Johnson (1994) indicates that alcohol is losing its importance as a precursor to marijuana. On the other hand, marijuana's role as a gateway drug appears to have increased. This finding concurs with epidemiological trends pointing to increased use of marijuana as normative behavior.

Little is known about the natural history of adolescents who qualify for SUD. In one study, Doyle *et al.* (1994) conducted a 4 year follow-up of inpatients who were under age 21 (not necessarily adolescent) at the time of treatment. It was found that 61% had persisting alcohol problems. Poor school performance, aggression, and self-injurious behavior were also associated with poor prognosis.

In a 10 year outcome study of 15–16 year old adolescent substance users, Kandel *et al.* (1986) found that the strongest predictor of drug use is prior drug use. Bates and Labouvie (1997) followed a large sample of 12–18 year old adolescents for 15 years. Drug use levels in late adolescence mediated the effects of risk factors first assessed during adolescence. A retrospective analysis of the Epidemiological Catchment Area data also indicated that drug use portends future drug use (Anthony and Petronis 1995). Nevertheless, the association is not necessarily fixed. Moreover, drug use in early adolescence does not invariably bring problems. For example, in a long-term follow-up study, Jessor *et al.* (1991) found that problem drinking in junior high school students did not always present as problem drinking at ages 25–27: only about 25% of females and 50% of males continued to be problem drinkers. However, problem drinking in junior high school was not without its long-term adverse consequences; these individuals as young adults were more likely to smoke cigarettes, have an arrest record, get divorced, and not complete college. Other studies have found little association, or only a weak one, between alcohol and drug use in adolescence and a variety of outcome measures (Newcomb and Bentler 1988). These results are consistent with the observation that adolescents who experimented with psychoactive substances had healthier psychological outcomes than either frequent users or abstainers (Shedler and Block 1990). Although it is not in accordance with current social policy, it appears that modest exposure may be a component of normative socialization (Newcomb 1995) and does not necessarily reflect a current problem or portend a poor prognosis.

Intervention studies

A review of 47 studies on the treatment outcome of adolescents with SUD concluded that treatment is better than no treatment. However, the effects of treatment are not uniform. Substantial variability is observed with respect to outcome status post-treatment (Catalano *et al.* 1990–91, Kaminer 1994).

The majority of studies aimed at predicting outcome have focused on patient characteristics measured at the time treatment is initiated. Factors such as age, race, socioeconomic status, severity of drug use, and mental health status have been postulated to be associated with prognosis. Although some studies provide evidence of a relationship between pre-treatment patient characteristics and outcome across studies, the findings are not consistent. Variables such as severity of alcohol problems, severity of other drug use, severity of internalizing symptoms, and level of self-esteem are prognostic of treatment completion in American, Canadian, and Irish adolescents (Kaminer *et al.* 1992, Blood and Cornwall 1994, Doyle *et al.* 1994). Psychopathology, particularly conduct disorder, is negatively correlated with treatment completion and post-treatment abstinence (Myers *et al.* 1995).

Most studies on treatment outcome of adolescents with SUD have focused on completion of treatment rather than follow-up status. There are no published studies comparing short-term to long-term outcomes, although several studies concerning this issue are presently under way. Reports of results from short-term follow-up studies indicate that relapse rates are high, 35–85% (Brown *et al.* 1989, Catalano *et al.* 1990–91, Doyle *et al.* 1994). The high relapse rate is associated with social pressures. It is notable, however, that abstinent teens experience decreased interpersonal conflict, improve their academic performance, and demonstrate increased involvement in normative social and occupational activities (Vik *et al.* 1992, Brown *et al.*1994).

Time in treatment

Time in treatment has been shown to be a less informative predictor of treatment outcome than staff characteristics, program environment, and treatment services. Research has, however, shown that the longer the adolescent remains in treatment, the better the prognosis (Catalano *et al.* 1990–91, Kaminer 1994). Because time covaries with amount of treatment exposure, more treatment produces more opportunities for improvement. How patient characteristics and the various components of treatment interact to affect treatment retention has not yet been studied.

Staff characteristics

Staff characteristics which foster treatment success include length of professional experience, competence in applying a problem-solving approach, and availability of volunteers who interact with patients (Friedman *et al.* 1989). Staff who are themselves recurring addicts do not enhance treatment outcome (Catalano *et al.* 1990–91).

Program environment and treatment services

Recent data suggest that the treatment setting (e.g. inpatient, residential treatment, out-patient) is less important for outcome than the modality of treatment (Kaminer 1994). Two interventions, family therapy and cognitive-behavioral therapy (CBT), have demonstrated enhanced clinical utility in the treatment of adolescents with SUD. The involvement of the family increases the likelihood that the client will complete treatment and reduces problem behavior during treatment (Barrett *et al.* 1988). Several investigators have demonstrated the benefits of family-based approaches in treating adolescent SUD (Szapocznik *et al.* 1988, Liddle and Dakof 1995). The multi-systemic therapy (MST) model is a highly successful family-ecological systems approach in which interventions simultaneously target family functioning and communication, school and peer functioning, and adjustment in the community (Henggeler *et al.* 1992, 1996).

Behavioral treatment has been reported to be superior to supportive counseling (Azrin *et al.* 1994). A number of CBT approaches, including many previously used with adults (e.g. relapse prevention), have also shown promise for adolescents (Kaminer 1994). Manual guided therapy has been shown to be helpful for improving drug refusal skills, problem-solving, and social skills (Kaminer 1994). Comparison of the effectiveness of two 12 week psychosocial interventions revealed that adolescents enrolled in a CBT program fared better than those who participated in interactional therapy (IT). According to the outcome variables measured by the Teen-Addiction Severity Index (T-ASI; Kaminer *et al.* 1991,1993) and controlled by the Teen-Treatment Services Review (Kaminer *et al.* 1998a), those assigned to CBT demonstrated a statistically significant reduction in severity of substance use compared to those assigned to IT (Kaminer *et al.* 1998b). Improvements were also observed in the areas of family function, school adjustment, peer/social relationship, legal problems, and psychiatric disturbance in patients receiving CBT, although the difference was not statistically significant (Kaminer *et al.* 1998b).

Friedman *et al.* (1989) reported that prognosis is enhanced by the provision of special services. The types of services include relaxation techniques and counseling in the areas of school, work, recreation, and contraception. Finally, pharmacotherapy of adolescent SUD is a neglected therapeutic modality that has recently shown promise mostly in the form of single case studies and small open-label studies (Kaminer 1995).

Treatment outcome studies have yielded an array of inconclusive and conflicting results. This is not surprising in view of the heterogeneity of the SUD population and lack of standardization of treatment procedures. Generally, the results indicate that relapse 1 year post-treatment is comparable between adolescents and adults with SUD. A relapse rate of the order of 50% is generally observed (Brown 1993). Among adolescents with SUD, in contrast to youth who use drugs but do not qualify for diagnosis, it is common for the disorder to persist into adulthood (Benson 1985, Bry and Krinsky 1992). In a reanalysis of Brown *et al.*'s (1993) data, Vik (1994) found that the 4 year outcome status was predicted more by the social risk factors for SUD than by the severity of substance involvement at the onset of treatment. Notably, in several treatment outcome studies, it was found that moderate drug use post-treatment was not associated with significant negative consequences even though the aim of treatment was abstinence (Alford *et al.* 1991, Brown *et al.* 1994, Doyle *et al.* 1994). Currently, abstinence is the goal of treatment in virtually all programs for adolescents (Ross 1994); however, there is meager empirical information documenting the factors that could prevent relapse. Available data suggest that coping skills enhancement and reduction of family conflict (Brown *et al.* 1994) potentiate long-term prognosis; nevertheless, there is little information regarding the modes of treatment which are most effective for particular individuals.

Patient–treatment matching

An emphasis in psychotherapy is to determine the intervention modality which best produces specific changes by particular therapists in specified settings in particular individuals (Waltz *et al.* 1993). One promising treatment strategy for adult substance abusers involves matching the patient to the treatment modality according to the needs and characteristics of the client (Kadden *et al.* 1989, Litt *et al.* 1992). Research on patient–treatment matching does not focus on whether one intervention is more effective than another, but rather on the interaction between intervention modality and client variables. Kadden *et al.* (1989), for example, reported that adult alcoholics scoring high on measures of sociopathy or global psychopathology have a better prognosis using a coping skills approach, whereas patients low on either of these two dimensions have a better outcome employing interpersonal group treatment. A review of more than 30 studies indicates that patient–treatment matching may maximize treatment prognosis in adults (Mattson *et al.* 1994). As yet, however, no studies have been published on patient–treatment matching in adolescent substance abusers.

A comorbid psychiatric disorder may be the primary reason adolescents with psychoactive SUD seek treatment. Indeed, Friedman and Glickman (1986) reported that 28% of adolescents applied for treatment because of an emotional or psychiatric problem. The impact of psychiatric comorbidity on treatment outcome in comorbidly diagnosed adolescents has been reported in two studies. Friedman and Glickman (1987) studied court-referred male drug abusers in a day treatment program. The findings indicated that the number of psychiatric symptoms correlated with treatment outcome. Kaminer and colleagues (1992) investigated patient variables that may distinguish treatment completers from non-completers in hospitalized dually diagnosed adolescents. Significant differences between groups were not found on any of the following variables: age, parent/care-giver education, socioeconomic status, sex, race, domicile, legal status at admission, and history of psychiatric and/or substance abuse treatment. The two groups also did not differ with respect to the prevalence of psychiatric disorders in their parents. The two groups were, however, distinguishable according to psychiatric diagnosis. Mood and adjustment disorders were significantly more frequent among treatment completers, whereas non-completers were more likely to have a conduct disorder diagnosis.

Because existing treatments are generally associated with only modest prognosis, there is the need to develop and test innovative psychosocial treatment approaches (Crits-Christoph and Siqueland 1996). The development of manual-guided therapies will ensures fidelity in the application of treatment procedures. Another area of interest pertains to the dissemination of research findings that is needed to augment clinical practice (Clark 1995).

Risk and prognostic factors

Temperament deviations have been shown to be associated with psychopathology and substance abuse. Children with a 'difficult temperament' commonly manifest externalizing and internalizing behavior problems by middle childhood (Earls and Jung 1987) and in adolescence (Maziade *et al.* 1990). Difficult temperament in childhood is also predictive of later alcohol and drug use (Lerner and Vicary 1984). This temperament configuration, first delineated by Thomas and Chess (1977), is characterized by poor capacity to regulate behavior, affect, and biological rhythms (e.g. sleep–waking cycle). Significantly, because temperament is strongly rooted in genetics (Plomin *et al.* 1990), it can be inferred that risk for SUD in adolescents accordingly has a strong genetic basis. This conclusion is reinforced by the observation that the early onset variant of alcoholism has a stronger genetic contribution than later (adult) onset alcoholism (Cloninger *et al.* 1988). Inasmuch as temperament traits are measurable in infancy and tend to be relatively stable, although modifiable, investigating their contribution to SUD etiology is a heuristic avenue of research.

High behavioral activity level has been noted in youth at high risk for substance abuse as well as those manifesting SUD. High activity level is also correlated with the severity of the disorder (Tarter *et al.* 1990a; b). In the most extreme form, this is manifest as ADHD. Other deviations found in youth at high risk include low attention span–persistence (Schaffer *et al.* 1984), high impulsivity (Noll *et al.* 1992), negative affect (Chassin *et al.* 1991), irritability (Brook *et al.* 1990), and emotional reactivity (Blackson 1994).

As the child matures, the psychological repertoire expands via socialization, learning, and environmental exposures. Acquired dispositional characteristics that are associated with an increased risk for SUD include impulsive aggression, high sensation seeking, low harm avoidance, inability to delay gratification, and low achievement motivation. A personality profile or 'type' has not been discovered, although as noted above, several traits are associated with increased risk.

Cognitive factors, particularly the executive cognitive functions, have also been observed to be integral to risk for SUD (Giancola *et al.* 1996). In aggregate, these processes encompass the mental capacities involved in strategic goal planning, attentional control, working memory, abstraction, self-monitoring, and thinking flexibility. Internal language ('thinking') is an important component of executive cognitive functions insofar as it comprises the mechanism regulating the relationship between thought and action. Significantly, high risk youth are deficient in language competence compared to youth at average risk (Najam and Tarter 1997). Finally, it is noteworthy that the latency and amplitude of the P3 wave component of the event-related potential is diminished in high risk youth (Polich *et al.* 1994); this neurophysiological process underlies attention and working memory.

Family contextual factors that are most common include stressful life events, lack of parental support or supervision, and poor discipline practices by parents. Contextual social factors include affiliation with deviant or delinquent peers, perception of high drug availability, social norms facilitating drug use, and relaxed laws and regulatory policies (Kaplan 1995, Institute of Medicine 1996, Clark *et al.* in press). No particular risk or environmental factor is, however, responsible for initiation and maintenance of drug use. Rather, manifold risk factors, each having different salience, interactively determine the severity of the person's risk status (Tarter and Vanyukov 1994).

Throughout development, individual liability factors (cognitive, affective, behavioral) interact with numerous and changing environments (family, peers, school, neighborhood, job, etc.). The resulting interactions determine risk for use initiation. Following initiation or first exposure, the momentum of the trajectory to diagnoses of abuse and dependence is determined by social selection and contagion effects operating in conjunction with the adolescent's vulnerabilities and environmental contexts (Tarter and Mezzich 1992). This in turn, influences ontogeny such that the social niche occupied by the adolescent assumes increasing importance regarding availability of other drugs, and predisposes the youngster to ever-increasing problems. However, it is important to emphasize although adolescence is a time of heightened risk, heavy use is often 'adolescence-limited'. That is, the progression does not invariably continue to increasing severity culminating in dependence. Indeed, moderation of even cessation may occur during or following adolescence (Labouvie 1996).

Conclusion

It is essential to recognize the importance of individual differences in the etiological pathway to drug abuse. Drug use in most adolescents subsides or stops by adulthood. However, adolescents with behavioral or affective dysregulation, poor social skills, a limited social network, and substance use during late adolescence, are at increased risk for developing substance dependence in adulthood. Research is needed, however, to clarify the developmental emergence and interaction between individual and contextual risk factors. Understanding person–environment processes within a developmental perspective will not only yield a better understanding of etiology but also inform us about taxonomy, prevention, and treatment. From such a knowledge base, it will be possible to determine the type of treatment which maximizes prognosis in both prevention and treatment based on a profile of the client's psychiatric, behavioral, and social history and presentation.

References

Alterman, A.I. and Tarter, R.E. (1986). An examination of selected topologies: Hyperactivity, familial and antisocial alcoholism. In *Recent Developments in Alcoholism*, Vol. 4. Plenum Press, New York.

Alford, G., Koehler, R., and Leonard, J. (1991). Alcoholics Anonymous–Narcotics Anonymous model inpatient treatment of chemically dependent adolescents. A 2-year outcome study. *Journal of Studies on Alcohol*, *52*, 118–126.

Altschuler, D. and Brounstein, P. (1991). Patterns of drug use, drug trafficking and other delinquency among inner-city adolescent males in Washington, D.C. *Criminology*, **29**, 589–622.

Anthony, J.C. and Petronis, K.R. (1995). Early-onset drug use and risk of later drug problems. *Drug and Alcohol Dependence*, **40**, 9–15.

APA (1994). *Diagnostic and statistical manual of mental disorders*, 4th edn. American Psychiatric Association, Washington, DC.

Arria, A., Dohey, M., Mezzich, A., Bukstein, O., and Van Thiel, D. (1995). Self-reported health problems and physical symptomatology in adolescent alcohol abusers. *Journal of Adolescent Health*, **16**, 226–231.

Azrin, N.H., Donohue, B., and Besalel, V.A. (1994). Youth drug abuse treatment: A controlled outcome study. *Journal of Child and Adolescent Substance Abuse*, **3**, 1–16.

Babor, T.F., Hoffman, M., Del Boca, F., Hesselbrock, V., and Kaplan, R.F. (1992). Types of alcoholics I: Evidence for an empirically-derived typology based on indicators of vulnerability and severity. *Archives of General Psychiatry*, **49**, 599–608.

Bailey, S., Camlin, S., and Ennett, S. (in press). Substance use and risky sexual behavior among homeless and runaway youth. *Journal of Adolescent Health*.

Barrett, M.E., Simpson, D.D., and Lehman, W.E. (1988). Behavioral changes of adolescents in drug abuse intervention programs. *Journal of Clinical Psychology*, **44**, 461–473.

Bates, M.E. and Labouvie, E.W. (1997). Adolescent risk factors and the prediction of persistent alcohol and drug use into adulthood. *Alcoholism: Clinical and Experimental Research,* **211**, 944–950.

Benson, G. (1985). Course and outcome of drug abuse and medical and social conditions in selected young drug abusers. *Acta Psychiatrica Scandinavia*, **71**, 48–86.

Blackson, T.C. (1994). Temperament: A salient correlate of risk factors for alcohol and drug abuse. *Drug and Alcohol Dependence*, **36**, 205–214.

Blood, L. and Cornwall, A. (1994). Pretreatment variables that predict completion of an adolescent substance abuse treatment program. *Journal of Nervous and Mental Disease,* **182**, 14–19.

Brent, D.A., Perper, J.A., and Allman, C. (1987). Alcohol, firearms and suicide among youth: Temporal trends in Allegheny County, Pennsylvania, 1960 to 1983. *Journal of the American Medical Association,* **257**, 3369–3372.

Brook, J.S., Whiteman, M., Gordon, A.S., and Brook, D.W. (1990). The psychosocial etiology of adolescent drug use: A family interactional approach. *Genetic, Social, and General Psychology Monographs,* **116**, 113–267.

Brown, S. (1993). Recovery patterns in adolescent substance abuse. In *Addictive behaviors acropss the life span,* ed. J. Baer, G. Marlatt, and R.McMahon. Sage, London.

Brown, S.A., Vik, P.N., and Creamer, V. (1989). Characteristics of relapse following adolescent substance abuse treatment. *Addictive Behaviors,* **14**, 291–300.

Brown, S.A., Myers, M.G., Mott, M.A., and Vik, P.W. (1994). Correlates of success following treatment for adolescent substance abuse. *Applied And Preventive Psychology,* **3**, 61–73.

Bry, H. and Krinskey, K. (1992). Booster sessions and long-term effects of behavioral family therapy on adolescent substance use and school performance. *Journal of Behavior Therapy and Experimental Psychiatry,* **23**, 183–189.

Bukstein, O.G., Brent, D.A., and Kaminer, Y. (1989). Comorbidity of substance abuse and other psychiatric disorders in adolescents. *American Journal of Psychiatry,* **146**, 1131–1141.

Bukstein, O., Glancy, L.J., and Kaminer, Y. (1992). Patterns of affective comorbidity in a clinical population of dually-diagnosed substance abusers. *Journal of the American Academy of Child and Adolescent Psychiatry,* **31**, 1041–1045.

Bukstein, O.G. and Kaminer, Y. (1994). The nosology of adolescent substance abuse. *American Journal of Addictions,* **3**, 1–13.

Bulik, C.M. (1987). Drug and alcohol abuse by bulimic women and their families. *American Journal of Psychiatry,* **144**, 1604–1606.

Catalano, R.F., Hawkins, J.D., Wells, E.A., Miller, J., and Brewer, D. (1990–91). Evaluation of the effectiveness of adolescent drug abuse treatment, assessment of risks for relapse, and promising approaches for relapse prevention. *International Journal of Addiction,* **25**, 1085–1140.

Chassin, L., Rogosh, F., and Barrera, M. (1991). Substance use and symptomatology among adolescent children of alcoholics. *Journal of Abnormal Psychology,* **100**, 449–463.

Chavez, E., Edwards, R., and Oetting, R. (1989). Mexican American and White American school dropouts drug use, health status and involvement in violence. *Public Health Reports,* **104**, 594–604.

Clark, G.N. (1995). Improving the transition from basic efficacy research to effectiveness studies: Methodological issues and procedures. *Journal of Consulting and Clinical Psychology,* **63**, 718–725.

Clark, D.B., Bukstein, O.G., Smith, M.G., Kaczynski, N.A., Mezzich, A.C., and Donovan, J.E. (1995). Identifying anxiety disorders in adolescents hospitalized for alcohol abuse or dependence. *Psychiatric Services,* **46**, 618–620.

Clark, D. and Kirisci, L. (1996). Post traumatic stress disorder, depression, substance use disorder and quality of life in adolescents. *Anxiety,* **2**, 228–233.

Clark, D., Kirisci, L., and Tarter, R. (1998). Adolescent versus adult onset and the development of substance use disorders. *Drug and Alcohol Dependence*, **79**: 115–121.

Clark, D., Neighbors, B., Lesnick, L., Lynch, K., and Donovan, J. (1998). Family functioning and adolescent alcohol use disorders. *Journal of Family Psychology*, **121**, 81–92.

Clark, D.B. and Sayette, M.A. (1993). Anxiety and the development of alcoholism. *American Journal of Addiction*, **2**, 56–76.

Cloninger, C.R. (1987). Neurogenetic adaptive mechanisms in alcoholism. *Science*, **236**, 410–415.

Cloninger, C., Sigvardson, S., and Bohman, M. (1988). Childhood personality predicts alcohol abuse in young adults. *Alcoholism: Clinical and Experimental Research*, **12**, 494–505.

Crits-Christoph, P. and Siqueland, L. (1996). Psychosocial treatment for drug abuse: Selected review and recommendations for national health care. *Archives of General Psychiatry*, **53**, 749–756.

Deykin, E.Y., Buka, S.L., and Zeena, T.H. (1992). Depressive Illness among chemically dependent adolescents. *American Journal of Psychiatry*, **149**, 1341–1347.

Doyle, H., Delaney, W., and Trobin, J. (1994). Follow-up study of young attendees at an alcohol unit. *Addiction*, **89**, 183–189.

Earls, F. and Jung, K. (1987). Temperament and home environment characteristics in the early development of child psychopathology. *Journal of American Academy and Child Psychiatry*, **26**, 491–498.

Friedman, A.S. and Glickman, N.W (1986). Program characteristics for successful treatment of adolescent drug abuse. *Journal of Nervous and Mental Disease*, **174**, 669–679.

Friedman, A.S. and Glickman, N.W. (1987).Effects of psychiatric symptomatology on treatment outcome for adolesent male drug abusers. . *Journal of Nervous and Mental Disease*, **175**, 425–430

Friedman, A.S. and Utada, A. (1989). A method for diagnosing and planning the treatment of adolescent drug abusers (The Adolescent Drug Abuse Diagnosis [ADAD] Instrument). *Journal of Drug Education*, **19**, 285–312.

Friedman, A.S., Schwartz, R., and Utada, A. (1989). Outcome of a unique youth drug abuse program: A follow-up study of clients of Straight, Inc. *Journal of Substance Abuse Treatment*, **6**, 259–268.

Giancola, P., Martin, C., Tarter, R., Moss, H., and Pelham, W. (1996). Executive cognitive functioning and aggressive behavior in preadolescent boys at high risk for substance abuse. *Journal of Studies on Alcohol*, **57**, 352–359.

Golub, A. and Johnson, B.D. (1994). The shifting importance of alcoholand marijuana as gateway substances among serious drug abusers. *Journal of Studies on Alcohol*, **55**, 607–614.

Griffiths, M. (1995). *Adolescent gambling*. Routledge, London.

Groerer, J. (1996). Special populations, sensitive issues, and the use of computer assisted interviewing in surveys. In *Health survey research*, ed. R. Warnecke. DHHS Publication No. (PHS) 96–1013.

Henggeler, S.W., Melton, G.B., and Smith, L.A. (1992). Family preservation using multi-systemic therapy: An effective alternative to incarcerating serious juvenile offenders. *Journal of Consulting and Clinical Psychology*, **66**, 953–961.

Henggeler, S.W., Pickrel, S.G., Brondino, M.J., and Crouch, J.L. (1996). Eliminating treatment dropout of substance abusing or dependent delinquents through home-based multisystemic therapy. *American Journal of Psychiatry*, **153**, 427–428.

Institute of Medicine (1996). *Pathways of addiction*. National Academy Press, Washington, D.C.

Jessor, R.,. Donovan, J.E., and Costa, F.M. (1991*). Beyond adolescence: problem behavior and youth adult development*. Cambridge University Press, New York.

Johnson, L.D., OMalley, P., and Bachman, J. (1996). *National survey results on drug use from the monitoring the future study*, 1975–1995. NIH Publication No 96–4139. Superintendent of Documents, US Government Printing Office, Washington, D.C.

Kadden, R.M., Cooney, N.L., Getter, H., and Litt, M.B. (1989). Matching alcoholics to coping skills or interactional therapies: Post-treatment results. *Journal of Consulting and Clinical Psychology*, **57**, 698–704.

Kaminer, Y. (1994). *Adolescent Substance Abuse: A Comprehensive Guide to Theory and Practice*. Plenum Press, New York.

Kaminer, Y. (1995). Issues in pharmacological treatment of adolescent substance abuse. *Journal of Child and Adolescent Psychopharmacology*, **5**, 93–106.

Kaminer, Y. (1996). Adolescent substance abuse and suicidal behavior. In *Adolescent substance abuse and dual disorders*, ed. S.L. Jaffe, Child Adolescent Psychiatry Clinics in North America, W.B. Saunders, Philadelphia, P.A.

Kaminer, Y., Bukstein, O.G., and Tarter, R. (1991). The Teen-Addiction Severity Index: rationale and reliability. *International Journal of Addiction*, **26**, 219–226.

Kaminer, Y., Tarter, R., Bukstein, O.G., and Kabene, M. (1992). Comparison between treatment completers and noncompleters among dual-diagnosed substance-abusing adolescents. *Journal of the American Academy of Child and Adolescent Psychiatry*, **31**, 1046–1049.

Kaminer, Y., Wagner, E., Plummer, B., and Seifer, R. (1993). Validation of the Teen Addiction Severity Index (T-ASI). *American Journal of Addiction*, **2**, 250–254.

Kaminer, Y., Blitz, C., Burleson, J.A., and Sussman, J. (1998a). The Teen Treatment Services Review (T-TSR): rationale and reliability. *Journal of Substance Abuse and Treatment*, **15**, 291–300.

Kaminer, Y., Burleson, J.A., Blitz, C., Sussman, J., and Rounsaville, B.J. (1998b). Psychotherapies for adolescent substance abusers: Treatment outcomes. *Journal of Nervous and Mental Disease*, **186**1, 684–690.

Kandel, D.B. (1982). Epidemiological and psychosocial perspective on adolescent drug use. *Journal of the American Academy of Child Psychiatry*, **20**, 328–347.

Kandel, D.B. Davies, M., Karus, D., and Yamaguchi, K. (1986). The consequences in young adulthood of adolescent drug involvement. *Archives of General Psychiatry*, **43**, 746–754.

Kaplan, H. (ed.) (1995). *Drugs, crime and other deviant adaptations*. Plenum, New York.

Kirisci, L., Mezzich, A., and Tarter, R. (1995). Norms and sensitivity of the adolescent version of the Drug Use Screening Inventory. *Addictive Behaviors*, **20**, 149–157.

Kushner, M.G., Sher, K.J., and Beitman, B.D. (1990). The relation between alcohol problems and anxiety disorders. *American Journal of Psychiatry*, **147**, 685–695.

Labouvie, E. (1996). Maturing out of substance use: Selection and self-correction. *Journal of Drug Issues*, **26**, 455–474.

Lerner, J. and Vicary, J. (1984). Difficult temperament and drug use: Analyses from the New

York Longitudinal Study. *Journal of Drug Education*, **14**, 1–8.

Lewinsohn, P.M., Rohde, P., and Seeley, J. (1996). Alcohol consumption in high school adolescents: Frequency of use and dimensional structure of associated problems. *Addiction*, **91**, 375–390.

Liddle, H.A. and Dakof, G.A. (1995). Family-based treatment for adolescent drug use: State of the science. In *Adolescent drug abuse: clinical assessment*, ed. E. Rahdert and D. Czechowicz. NIDA Monograph 156, U.S. Department of Health and Human Services, Rockville, Maryland.

Litt, M.B., Babor, T.F., DelBoca, F., Kadden, R.M., and Cooney, N.L. (1992). Types of alcoholics, II: Application of empirically derived typology to treatment matching. *Archives of General Psychiatry*, **49**, 609–614.

Loeber, R. (1988). Natural histories of conduct problems, delinquency and associated substance use. In *Advances in Clinical Child Psychology*, ed. B.B. Lahey and A.E. Kazdin, pp. 73–124, Plenum, New York.

Martin, C., Earleywine, M., Blackson, T., Vanyukov, T., Moss, H., and Tarter, R. (1994). Aggressivity, inattention, hyperactivity, and impulsivity in boys at high and low risk for substance abuse. *Journal of Abnormal Child Psychology*, **22**, 177–203.

Martin, C.S., Kaczynski, N.A., Maisto, S.A., Bukstein, O.G., and Moss, H.B. (1995). Patterns of DSM-IV alcohol abuse and dependence symptoms in adolescent drinkers. *Journal of Studies on Alcohol*, **56**, 672–680.

Martin, C., Langenbucher, J., Kaczynski, N., and Chang, T. (1996a). Staging in the onset of DSM-IV alcohol abuse and dependence symptoms in adolescent drinkers. *Journal of Studies on Alcohol*, **57**, 549–558.

Martin, C.S., Kaczynski, N.A., Maisto, S.A., and Tarter, R. (1996b). Polydrug use in adolescent drinkers with and without DSM-IV alcohol abuse and dependence. *Alcoholism: Clinical and Experimental Research*, **20**, 1099–1108.

Mattson, M.E., Allen, J.P., Longabaugh, R., Nickless, C.J., Connors, G.J., and Kadden, R.M. (1994). A chronological review of empirical studies matching alcoholic clients to treatment. *Journal of Studies on Alcohol*, Suppl 12, 16–29.

Maziade, M., Caron, C., Cote, P., Boutin, P., and Thivierge, J. (1990). Extreme temperament and diagnosis. A study in a psychiatric sample of consecutive children. *Archives of General Psychiatry*, **47**, 477–484.

Mezzich, A., Tarter, R., Kirisci, L., Clark, D., Bukstein, O., and Martin, C. (1993). Subtypes of early age onset alcoholism. *Alcoholism: Clinical and Experimental Research*, **17**, 767–770.

Mezzich, A., Moss, H., Tarter, R., Wolfenstein, M., Hsieh, Y., and Mauss, R. (1994). Gender differences in conduct disordered adolescents. *American Journal of Addiction*, **3**, 289–295.

Mezzich, A., Tarter, R., Giancola, P., Lu, S., Kirisci, L., and Parks, S. (1997). Substance use and risky behavior in female adolescents. *Drug and Alcohol Dependence*, **44**, 157–166.

Mezzich, A., Giancola, P., Tarter, R., Lu, S., Parks, S., and Barrett, C. (1997). Violence, suicidality, and drug/alcohol use in female adolescent substance abusers. *Journal of Studies on Alcohol*, **21**, 1300–7.

Milin, R., Halikas, J.A., Meller, J.E., and Morse, C. (1991). Psychopathology among substance abusing juvenile offenders. *Journal of the American Academy of Child and Adolescent Psychiatry*, **30**, 569–574.

Moss, H., Kirisci, L., Gordon, H., and Tarter, R. (1994). The neuropsychologic profile of adolescent alcoholics. *Alcoholism: Clinical and Experimental Research*, **18**, 159–163.

Myers, M.G., Brown, S.A., and Mott, M.A. (1995). Preadolescent conduct disorder behaviors predict relapse and progression of addiction for adolescent alcohol and drug abusers. *Alcoholism: Clinical and Experimental Research*, **19**, 1528–1536.

Najam, N. and Tarter, R.E. (1997). Language deficits in children at high-risk for drug abuse. *Journal of Child and Adolescent Substance Abuse*, **6**, 69–80.

Newcomb, M.D. (1995). Identifying high-risk youth: Prevalence and patterns of adolescent drug abuse. In *Adolescent drug abuse: clinical assessment and therapeutic interventions*, eds E.Rahdert and D. Czechowicz, pp. 7–38. NIH Publication 95–3908, Rockville, M.D.

Newcomb, M.D. and Bentler, P. (1988). *Consequences of adolescent drug use.* Sage, Newbury Park, C.A.

Noll, R.B., Zucker, R.A., Fitzgerald, H.E., and Curtis, W.J. (1992). Cognitive and motoric functioning of sons of alcoholic fathers and controls: The early childhood years. *Developmental Psychology*, **28**, 665–675.

Plomin, R., DeFries, J., and McClearn, G. (1990). *Behavior genetics: a primer*, 2nd edn. Freeman , New York.

Polich, J., Pollock, V., and Bloom, F. (1994). Meta-analysis of P300 amplitude for males at risk for alcoholism. *Psychological Bulletin*, **15**, 55–73.

Pollock, N.K. and Martin, C. (1996). Alcohol use disorders in adolescents: how well do the DSM-II-R and DSM-IV work? Presented at the symposium Adolescents with alcohol and other substance abuse disorders, Annual Meeting of the American Academy of Child and Adolescent Psychiatry, Philadelphia, P.A.

Reich, T., Cloninger, P., Van-Eerdevegh, J.P., Rice, J.R., and Mullaney, J. (1988). Secular trends in the familial transmission of alcoholism. *Alcoholism: Clinical and Experimental Research*, **12**, 458–464.

Rhode, P., Lewinsohn, P.M., and Seeley, J.R. (1996). Psychiatric comorbidity with problematic alcohol use in high school students. *Journal of the American Academy of Child and Adolescent Psychiatry*, **35**, 101–109.

Ross, G. (1994). *Treating adolescent substance abuse.* Allyn and Bacon, Boston.

Schaeffer, K., Parson, O., and Yohman, J. (1984). Neuropsychological differences between male familial alcoholics and nonalcoholics. *Alcoholism: Clinical and Experimental Research*, **8**, 347–351.

Shedler, J. and Block, J. (1990). Adolescent drug use and psychological health. A longitudinal inquiry. *American Psychology*, **45**, 612–630.

Sigvardsson, S., Bohman, M., and Cloninger, C.R. (1996). Replication of the stockholm adoption study of alcoholism: Confirmatory cross-fostering analysis. *Archives of General Psychiatry*, **53**, 681–688.

Stowell, R.J. (1991). Dual diagnosis issues. *Psychiatry Annals*, **21**, 98–104.

Szapocznik, J., Perez-Vidal, A., Briskman, A.L., Foote, F.H., Santisteban, D., and Hervis, O. (1988). Engaging adolescent drug abusers and their families in treatment. *Journal of Consulting and Clinical Psychology*, **56**, 552–557.

Tarter, R. (1995). Rationale and method of client treatment matching. *The Counsellor* (July), 26–30.

Tarter, R. and Mezzich, A. (1992). Ontogeny of substance abuse: Perspective and findings.

In *Vulnerability to drug abuse*, ed. M. Glantz and R. Pickens. American Psychological Association Press, Washington, D.C.

Tarter, R. and Vanyukov, M. (1994). Alcoholism: A developmental disorder. *Journal of Consulting and Clinical Psychology*, **62**, 1096–1107.

Tarter, R., Laird, S.B., and Moss, H.B. (1990a). Neuropsychological and neurophysiological characteristics of children of alcoholics. In *Children of alcoholics: critical perspectives*, eds. M. Windel and J.S. Searles, pp 73–98. Guilford Press, New York.

Tarter, R., Laird, S.B., Kabene, M., Bukstein, O.G., and Kaminer, Y. (1990b). Drug abuse severity in adolescents is associated with magnitude of deviation in temperamental traits. *British Journal of Addiction*, **85**, 1501–1504.

Tarter, R., Kirisci, L., Hegedus, A., Mezich, A., and Yanyukov, M. (1994). Heterogeneity of adolescent alcoholism. In *Types of alcoholics: evidence from clinical, experimental and genetic research*, ed. T.F. Babor, V. Hesselbrock, R.E. Meyer, and W.Shoemaker), pp. 172- 180. Annals of the New York Academy of Science, New York.

Tarter, R., Mezzich, A., Hsieh, Y., and Parks, S. (1995). Cognitive capacities in female adolescent substance abusers: Association with severity of drug abuse. *Drug and Alcohol Dependence*, **39**, 15–21.

Tarter, R., Kirisci, L., and Mezzich, A. (1997). Multivariate typology of adolescents with alcohol use disorder. *American Journal on Addictions*, **6**, 150–158.

Thomas, A. and Chess, S. (1977). *Temperament and development*. Brunner/Mazel, New York.

US Department of Vital Statistics (1993). Bureau of Mortality Statistics.

Van Hasselt, V.B., Null, J.A., Kempton, T., and Bukstein, O.G. (1993). Social skills and depression in adolescent substance abusers. *Addictive Behaviors*, **18**, 9–18.

Vik, P. (1994). Adolescent substance abuse recovery: A path analysis. Paper presented at the annual meeting of the American Psychological Association, Los Angeles, CA.

Vik, P.W., Grisel, K., and Brown, S.A. (1992). Social resource characteristics and adolescent substance abuse relapse. *Journal of Adolescent Chemical Dependency*, **2**, 59–74.

Waltz, J., Addis, M.E., Koerner, K., and Jacobson, N.S. (1993). Testing the integrity of a psychotherapy protocol: Assessment of adherence and competence. *Journal of Consulting and Clinical Psychiatry*, **61**, 620–630.

Wilens, T.E., Biederman, J., Spencer, T.J., and Frances, R.J. (1994). Comorbidity of attention-deficit disorder and psychoactive substance use disorders. *Hospital and Community Psychiatry*, **45**, 421–435.

13 Eating disorders

Hans-Christoph Steinhausen

The eating disorders comprise the two syndromes of anorexia nervosa and bulimia nervosa. A substantial proportion of affected patients suffer from a chronic form of one of these disorders. There is a large body of literature on the clinical course and outcome of anorexia nervosa that has been accumulated over more than four decades. In contrast, studies that deal with the course and outcome of bulimia nervosa are still relatively limited because of the rather recent definition of the disorder in a seminal paper by Russell (1979). The present chapter is thus divided into two major but unequal parts.

Anorexia nervosa

Clinical picture

Anorexia nervosa occurs most commonly in adolescent girls and young women and rarely in girls before menarche, in older women, or in the male sex. The core symptoms include:

- a significant loss of body weight or a failure to make the expected weight gain during the period of growth in prepubertal patients
- various measures to lose weight, i.e. dieting, self-induced purging, excessive exercise, use of appetite suppressants and/or diuretics
- a disordered body image with a dread of fatness as an intrusive, overvalued idea
- various indicators of a widespread endocrine disorder involving the hypothalamic–pituitary–gonadal axis with amenorrhoea as a leading symptom in women and a loss of sexual interest and potency in men.

Studies of natural course

The number of studies addressing the natural history of eating behavior, attitudes, and disorders is relatively small, as shown by a recent review (Rathner 1992). The majority of these studies are based on questionnaires that deal with eating attitudes and behavior; only a minority have assessed eating disorders that fulfil clinical criteria of diagnoses and assessment. Among the latter, more information is provided on the natural course of bulimia nervosa (see below) than on anorexia nervosa. In conjunction with other studies on eating attitudes and behavior, they provide some limited evidence that a substantial proportion of subjects at risk and untreated cases remain stable with regard to their condition across a considerable time span (Rathner 1992).

Intervention studies and their effects

Despite the plethora of monographs and reviews on the treatment of anorexia nervosa, controlled intervention studies are rare. Recent reviews of pharmacotherapy indicate that no drug has yet been demonstrated to have clinically significant use (Heebink and Halmi 1995, Walsh 1995). Clinical features other than anorexia nervosa alone, e.g. depression, may dictate the use of medication. So far, no study has assessed the long-term effects of any medication.

A broad range of psychotherapeutic approaches is commonly advocated for the treatment of anorexia nervosa. However, surprisingly little research in terms of controlled studies has been performed so far. Among the few exceptions is the study by Crisp *et al.* (1991) which shows that outcome in a treatment group is better than in a waiting list control group. Furthermore, the authors of the Maudsley studies initially showed that adolescent anorectic patients with a relatively short history of their illness responded significantly better to family therapy than to individual supportive therapy (Russell *et al.* 1987). This is also the only study that has documented the stability of treatment effects over at least a 5 year period (Eisler *et al.* submitted for publication). For the older, more chronic anorectic and bulimic patients the benefits of the treatments were less clear cut. There was a trend for these patients to respond more favorably to individual supportive therapy. Subsequent research showed that conjoint family sessions and family counseling as two different forms of family therapy produced similar results in terms of symptomatic relief (Le Grange *et al.* 1992). One other group (Robin *et al.* 1994, Robin *et al.* 1995) compared behavioral systems therapy versus ego-oriented individual therapy and found that both treatments produced significant reductions in negative communication and parent–adolescent conflict, eating attitudes, and psychopathology. The improvements in eating-related conflict were maintained at a 1 year follow-up.

The application of cognitive-behavioral principles has gained extensive support through controlled trials only in bulimia nervosa; the efficacy of similar strategies in anorexia nervosa still has to be established (Bemis Vitousek 1995). There is sufficient evidence from the earlier generation of controlled studies based on behavioral interventions that operant conditioning is an effective short-term method of weight restoration in anorexia nervosa (Bemis 1987). However, the scarcity of long-term follow-up data after more than two decades of investigation of the effects of behavior therapy in anorexia nervosa is puzzling.

Short-term and long-term outcomes

Previous reviews of the outcome of anorexia nervosa have covered 45 studies in English and German published between 1953 and 1981 (Steinhausen and Glanville 1983), and a further 23 follow-up studies published in major English- and German-language journals between 1981 and 1989 (Steinhausen et al. 1991). Recently, Fichter and Quadflieg (1995) provided a similar analysis and review of 37 more recent studies including studies on the outcome of bulimia nervosa. In addition to these reviews, the author identified 15 outcome studies that were published between 1993 and 1996: those by Norring and Sohlberg (1993), Smith *et al.* (1993), Deter and Herzog (1994), van der Ham *et al.* (1994), Wonderlich *et al.* (1994), Gillberg *et al.* (1994, 1995), Råstam *et al.* (1995), Eckert *et al.* (1995), Herpertz-Dahlmann *et al.* (1996), Theander (1996), Bryant-Waugh *et al.* (1996), Steinhausen and Boyadjieva (1996), Kreipe and Piver Dukarm (1996), Casper and Jabine (1996), Sunday *et al.* (1996), and Fichter and

Quadflieg (1996). Thus, a total of 108 outcome studies on anorexia nervosa were suitable for the present analysis, although many are cited only in Table 13.5.

Outcome measures

Almost all studies contain data on crude mortality rates. However, only very few outcome studies assessed standardized mortality ratio. In these studies the ratio of observed to expected deaths represents the standard mortality ratio, which is calculated on the basis of census data for mortality.

The most common scheme of global outcome classification is the trichotomy between good, fair, or poor outcome. Although the studies vary, there is some general agreement that a 'good' outcome is marked by a recovery from all essential clinical symptoms of anorexia nervosa—i.e. disordered eating, weight loss, and amenorrhea—whereas a 'fair' outcome represents improvement with some residual symptoms, and a 'poor' outcome is synonymous with chronicity of the disorder. The core symptoms of weight, menstrual state, and eating behavior are less systematically reported in the literature.

Additional psychiatric diagnoses as well as the eating disorders are mentioned in a substantial number of studies. However, given the wide span of publications over more than four decades and the considerable changes in the classification of psychiatric disorders in recent years, it is uncertain to what extent similar criteria have been applied in the assessment of these other psychiatric disorders. In general, psychiatric status information is based on clinical interviews; research interviews for the assessment of psychopathology have been almost entirely neglected.

The following psychiatric diagnoses were extracted from the outcome studies:

- affective disorders in terms of a relatively broad category
- obsessive–compulsive disorders
- other neurotic disorders, including mainly anxiety disorders and phobias
- schizophrenia
- personality disorders, including borderline states
- substance use disorders.

A substantial number of studies also assessed psychosocial functioning at follow-up in terms of employment, marriage, relationships, and psychosexual development. However, the heterogeneity of data and information precludes any summarizing analysis.

Study characteristics

The 108 outcome series on anorexia nervosa comprised a total of 4990 patients ranging from a minimum of 6 to a maximum of 151 patients (mean = 46.2, SD = 31.0). There are considerable differences in study design, sample size, and methods. Few studies are prospectively organized, and even among the most recent outcome studies the vast majority are based on retrospective designs. In the recent past, diagnostic criteria have shifted to predominantly DSM categories, whereas more diverse criteria were used in the older studies. Male patients rarely present with anorexia nervosa, so almost no definite conclusions can be drawn from the literature as to whether or not their outcome is markedly different from female patients.

The age at onset ranges from relatively few studies containing a minority of prepubertal children as young as 7 years to a few studies that include individual patients beyond menopause and as old as 59 years. Because of the global descriptions of age that are given in the studies, precise parameters cannot be computed.

Similarly, no commonly accepted cut-offs could be extracted from the figures in the literature in order to test for the impact of age at onset on outcome. For the present review the studies were divided into two groups, one of studies containing only younger patients, i.e. no older than 17 years 11 months at onset, and one that also contained older patients. Admittedly, the age at onset partially overlaps in the two groups.

Unfortunately, the duration of follow-up is quite difficult to compute from the original studies. This problem is due not only to missing data but also to variations in the definition of the starting point—i.e. whether the length of follow-up is related to the onset of the disease or to either the onset or termination of treatment—or to the general trend of providing only ranges instead of precise sample parameters. Similarly, data on the follow-up period with a range from less than 1 year to a maximum of 29 years do not allow a more precise calculation of sample parameters. Almost all samples are characterized by a marked heterogeneity regarding the duration of follow-up. Thus, the present review is not in a position to differentiate between short-term and long-term outcomes.

Although a few studies were initially designed to evaluate certain treatment approaches, e.g. behavioral interventions or family therapy, the outcome literature on anorexia nervosa does not allow one to draw conclusions concerning the efficacy of treatment. There is a general lack of control conditions and a scarcity of precise information on treatment. The treatment approaches in internal medicine, pediatrics, adult psychiatry, and child and adolescent psychiatry are different, and various psychotherapeutic approaches were used. This diversity of interventions precludes any definite evaluation of treatment effects.

Finally, in a large number of studies, conclusions are jeopardized by a relatively high drop-out rate at follow-up. The mean drop-out rate for 108 studies with some relevant information is 13% (SD = 15, range = 0–77).

Follow-up findings

In the entire outcome literature, crude mortality rates based on a total of $N = 4786$ patients ranged from 0% to 21% with a mean of 5.49% (SD = 5.79). Five cohort studies found standard mortality ratios between 1.36 and 17.8, indicating an increase in deaths due to anorexia nervosa ranging from slight to almost 18-fold (Patton 1988, Crisp *et al*. 1992, Norring and Sohlberg 1993, Deter and Herzog 1994, Eckert *et al*. 1995). Because of the variations in the description of the follow-up periods, there is no way to determine how the length of the follow-up effects mortality rates.

For the surviving patients, the main findings based on all anorexia nervosa outcome studies are summarized in Table 13.1. Before turning to the findings, two important issues have to be considered. First, the sizes of the patient samples differ significantly for the various outcome measures, because not all variables were assessed in all studies. Second, for each measure there are rather wide standard deviations with extreme ranges across the studies, so that the means reflect a central trend only within very heterogeneous findings.

With this caveat in mind, there is a trend that only 45.1% of the patients make a full

Table 13.1 Outcome of anorexia nervosa based on 108 follow-up studies

Outcome	Sample size	Mean (%)	SD (%)	Range (%)
Recovery ('good')	4085	45.1	19.0	0—86
Improvement ('fair')	3951	33.0	17.5	0—69
Chronicity ('poor')	4395	19.8	12.3	0—63
Normalization of weight	2013	59.7	14.6	15—92
Normalization of menstruation	2420	57.2	16.8	25—96
Normalization of eating behavior	1824	45.9	18.9	0—97
Affective disorders	1778	22.0	15.2	2—67
Neurotic disorders	1203	26.2	15.4	7—61
Obsessive compulsive disorders	944	12.5	6.2	0—23
Schizophrenia	1054	4.6	5.8	1—28
Personality disorders	824	14.2	15.6	0—69
Substance use disorders	506	14.1	10.9	3—38

recovery, whereas 33.0% improve and 19.8% develop a chronic disorder. The outcome is slightly better for the core symptoms, with normalization of weight occurring in 59.7%, normalization of menstruation in 57.2%, and normalization of eating behavior in 45.9%. However, these slightly higher rates of normalization of the core symptoms, as compared to the global outcome rating, may be largely due to the smaller total sample sizes. Nevertheless, this gap remains, even after adapting for sample size when only those studies are considered that report both global outcome ratings and normalization of the core symptoms.

Furthermore, Table 13.1 shows that a large proportion of anorectic patients suffered from further psychiatric disorders. The term comorbidity has to be avoided in this context, because it is not clear from any outcome study that has so far been published to what extent these psychiatric disorders were actually coexistent or present as a single disorder in individuals with no further eating disorders. The most common diagnoses at follow-up were neurotic disorder, including anxiety disorders and phobias, followed by affective disorders, substance use disorders, obsessive–compulsive disorders, and personality disorders. Schizophrenia was only rarely observed at follow-up.

It was possible to control for three major factors that might influence outcome. Their influence was checked only for the global outcome of the eating disorder, in order to avoid conclusions that might be biased due to smaller sample size. The first factor was the drop-out rate. When comparing studies with a drop-out rate between 0–15% to studies with drop-out rates above 15%, as shown in Table 13.2, there was some indication that studies with high drop-out rates revealed slightly better findings based on the global outcome ratings. This leads to the conclusion that there may be a trend for patients with a less favorable outcome not to participate in outcome studies so that, in general, the above-mentioned outcome findings may be slightly too positive.

Age at onset of the disorder was checked as a second factor that might influence outcome. As will be shown in the next section, this is the factor that has been analyzed most frequently in the individual outcome studies. However, the total data from the 108 studies allowed a more

Table 13.2 Outcome of anorexia nervosa by drop-out rate

	Drop-out rate ⩽15%			Drop-out rate ⩾16%		
	N	Mean (%)	SD (%)	N	Mean (%)	SD (%)
Recovery ('good')	2400	44.2	21.2	1324	45.7	15.8
Improved ('fair')	2425	33.3	19.3	1180	31.6	14.5
Chronicity ('poor')	2799	20.6	12.6	1218	18.4	11.9

Table 13.3 Outcome of anorexia nervosa by age at onset

	Younger patients only			Younger and older patients		
	N	Mean (%)	SD (%)	N	Mean (%)	SD (%)
Recovery ('good')	798	51.1	19.5	3287	43.5	18.6
Improved ('fair')	690	28.8	14.5	3261	33.8	17.9
Chronicity ('poor')	892	18.9	10.5	3503	20.0	12.7

general though crude check across studies. When comparing the two age groups of patients (those with onset not later than 17;11 years and those with a much wider range), there was a trend for better global outcome among the younger patients, as indicated by the rates for recovery, improvement, and chronicity, as shown in Table 13.3.

The third effect tested was a potential time trend. Studies were allocated to four large date groups—the 1950s and 1960s, the 1970s, the 1980s, and the 1990s. As Table 13.4 shows, there was an increase of the proportion of fully recovered patients and a parallel linear decrease in the rates of improved patients. However, the trend for the rates of chronicity was not completely stable for the four respective periods. These global outcome measures indicate that the clinical course of anorectic patients has improved in the recent past. This may be due partly to an earlier identification of the patients with subsequent referral for treatment, and partly to refined and more effective modes of treatment. However, no ultimate test of these hypotheses is possible on the basis of our current knowledge.

Risks and prognostic factors

The distinction between risks and prognostic factors is that risks are associated variables at follow-up that increase the likelihood of a poor outcome, whereas prognostic factors are variables that predict the outcome by characteristics that are present at the onset of the disorder. Although prognostic factors have been examined repeatedly in the outcome literature on anorexia, there is very limited knowledge of risks, stemming mostly from more recent research.

Various recent studies point to a close link between comorbid depression and poor outcome of anorexia nervosa (Steiner et al. 1990, Eckert et al. 1995, Råstam et al. 1995, Herpertz-Dahlmann et al. 1996). A similar association has also been obtained for anxiety disorders and phobias (Eckert et al. 1995), personality disorders (Gillberg et al. 1995), and abnormal

Table 13. 4 Outcome of anorexia nervosa by time of study

Decade of publication	1950s/1960s			1970s			1980s			1990s		
	N	Mean (%)	SD (%)	N	Mean (%)	SD (%)	N	Mean (%)	SD (%)	N	Mean (%)	SD (%)
Recovery ('good')	257	40.3	20.6	653	44.4	19.5	1598	45.8	16.4	1137	51.7	19.2
Improved ('fair')	466	50.5	18.7	448	35.8	18.6	1483	30.2	14.9	1114	26.5	17.3
Chronicity ('poor')	670	19.6	10.8	787	16.7	8.4	1384	20.0	9.4	1114	16.3	11.6

personality features as obtained by questionnaires (Greenfeld et al. 1991, Schork et al. 1994).

A summary of the prognostic factors identified in anorexia nervosa is provided in Table 13.5. Findings are rather heterogeneous for the majority of factors. This may to a certain extent be due to the heterogeneity of sample composition, as outlined above. Most clearly, this interpretation applies to the ambiguous findings on age at onset. Owing to the wide variation of this variable, the trend of young age at onset as a favorable prognostic factor in the entire data set is largely obscured in a substantial number of individual studies. However, it should also be noted that prepubertal children obviously have a less favorable outcome owing to delay or arrest of puberty (Russell 1992).

More studies indicate that a short duration of symptoms prior to treatment is favorable for the outcome than otherwise. The impact of the duration of in-patient treatment is unclear because of ambiguous findings across the outcome studies. Similarly, no definite conclusions can be drawn as to whether or not a high weight loss at presentation has long-term effects on outcome. Although hyperactivity and dieting as weight reduction measures do not have any prognostic significance, it is quite clear from the literature that vomiting, bulimia, and purgative abuse imply an unfavorable prognosis. A few studies also show that premorbid developmental and clinical abnormalities, including eating disorders during childhood, carry the risk for a poor outcome. In contrast, a good parent–child relationship may protect the patient from poor outcome.

Furthermore, the data clearly show that chronicity leads to poor outcome, a finding that is partly tautological and partly implies that there are cases of anorexia nervosa in which treatment is refractory. A substantial number of studies provide evidence that histrionic personality features indicate a favorable outcome, whereas there are only two studies in young patients with depressive features at onset of the disorder who had a rather poor outcome (Bryant-Waugh et al. 1988, Herpertz-Dahlmann et al. 1996). Finally, no definite conclusions can be drawn from the outcome studies as to the relevance of socioeconomic status.

Continuity and discontinuity

The large body of follow-up studies of eating disorders has concentrated mainly on the outcome rather than on the course in terms of a process over time. Accordingly, very little is known about continuity and discontinuity of the eating disorders. Theoretically, three approaches could be followed.

The first assesses the individual eating disorder, i.e. either anorexia or bulimia nervosa. This

Table 13.5 Frequency of studies with identified prognostic factors in anorexia nervosa (study numbers in square brackets)

Prognostic factors	Favorable	References	Unfavorable	References	Not significant	References
Early age of onset	13	23, 30, 31, 32, 37, 45, 49, 53, 56, 57, 67, 69, 76	2	7, 74	11	6, 8A, 15, 24, 28, 33, 51, 60, 65, 66, 70, 75
Short duration of symptoms	12	8, 13, 15, 29, 37, 42, 48, 49, 53, 56, 59, 61	–		7	6, 7, 57, 60, 65, 66, 74
Short duration of in-patient treatment	7	7, 24, 31, 32, 61, 69, 77	–		7	6, 12, 49, 51, 57, 65, 66
High loss of weight	–		5	8, 8A, 12, 34, 37, 49, 66	6	7, 15, 28, 57, 60, 74
Hyperactivity and dieting	1	3	–		7	7, 31, 32, 53, 65, 66, 71
Vomiting	–		9	3, 11, 24, 30, 31, 37, 43, 51, 69	1	60
Bulimia and purgative abuse	–		10	3, 31, 37, 4, 43, 46, 63, 64, 69, 76	2	60, 66
Premorbid development/ clinical abnormalities	–		4	12, 48, 49, 65	1	66
Good parent-child relationship	8	7, 8, 11, 12, 37, 42, 48, 49, 53, 60	–		3	53, 60, 69
Chronicity	–		7	4, 8, 12, 27, 41, 42, 45	–	
Hysterical personality	8	5, 12, 27, 41, 42, 45, 58, 59	–		1	65
High socioeconomic status	6	24, 31, 32, 37, 41, 61	–		7	12, 15, 57, 60, 66, 69, 74

References: [1] Abraham *et al.* (1983), [2] Baell and Wertheim (1992), [3] Beumont *et al.* (1976), [4] Bhanji and Thompson (1974), [5] Blitzer *et al.* (1961), [6] Browning and Miller (1968), [7] Bryant-Waugh *et al.* (1988), [7A] Bryant-Waugh *et al.* (1996), [8] Burns and Crisp (1984), [8A] Casper and Jabine (1996), [9] Collings and King (1994), [10] Crisp *et al.* (1992), [11] Crisp *et al.* (1974), [1] Dally (1969), [13] Dally and Sargant (1966), [14] Deter and Herzog (1994), [15] Deter *et al.* (1992), [16] Eckert *et al.* (1995), [17] Fahy and Russell (1993), [18] Fairburn *et al.* (1987), [19] Fairburn *et al.* (1993), [20] Fairburn *et al.* (1995), [21] Fallon *et al.* (1991), [21A] Fichter and Quadflieg (1996), [22] Fichter *et al.* (1992), [23] Frazier (1965), [24] Garfinkel *et al.* (1977), [25] Gillberg *et al.* (1994), [26] Gillberg *et al.* (1995), [27] Goetz *et al.* (1977), [28] Greenfeld *et al.* (1991), [29] Hall *et al.* (1984), [30] Halmi (1991), [31] Halmi *et al.* (1973), [32] Halmi *et al.* (1976), [33] Hawley (1985), [34] Herpertz-Dahlmann *et al.* (1996), [35] Herzog *et al.* (1991), [36] Herzog *et al.* (1993), [37] Hsu and Holder (1986), [38] Hsu *et al.* (1979), [39] Johnson *et al.* (1990), [40] Johnson-Sabine *et al.* (1992), [41] Kalucy *et al.* (1976), [42] Kay and Shapira (1965), [42A] Kreipe and Piver Dukarm (1996), [43] Kreipe *et al.* (1989), [44] Lacey (1992), [45] Lesser *et al.* (1960), [46] Martin (1985), [47] Mitchell *et al.* (1989), [48] Morgan and Russell (1975), [49] Morgan *et al.* (1983), [50] Norring and Sohlberg (1993), [51] Nussbaum *et al.* (1985), [52] Patton (1988), [53] Pierloot *et al.* (1975), [54] Pope *et al.* (1985), [55] RŒstam *et al.* (1995), [56] Ratnasutiya *et al.* (1991), [57] Remschmidt *et al.* (1990), [58] Rollins and Blackwell (1968), [59] Rosenvinge and Mouland (1990), [60] Santonastaso *et al.* (1991), [61] Seidensticker and Tzagournis (1968), [62] Smith *et al.* (1993), [63] Sohlberg *et al.* (1989), [64] Steiner *et al.* (1990), [65] Steinhausen and Glanville (1983), [66] Steinhausen and Seidel (1993a), [66A] Steinhausen and Boyadjieva (1996), [67] Sturzenberger *et al.* (1977), [67A] Sunday *et al.* (1996), [68] Swift *et al.* (1987), [69] Theander (1970), [69A] Theander (1996)), [70] Tolstrup (1965), [71] Toner *et al.* (1986), [72] van der Ham *et al.* (1994), [73] Vandereycken and Pieters (1992), [74] Walford and McCune (1991), [75] Warren (1968), [76] Willi and Hagemann (1976), [77] Willi *et al.* (1989), [78] Wonderlich *et al.* (1994).

approach has been used in three German studies by Ziolko (1978), Steinhausen and Glanville (1984), and Remschmidt et al. (1990). In these studies anorectic patients were classified into four types:

- an acute course with complete remission of symptoms within a few months
- a simple chronic course with a duration of several years and a more or less marked remission of symptoms
- a chronic–relapsing or intermittent course
- a chronic–persistent course.

The three studies revealed markedly different proportions of these four types, with the two samples by Steinhausen and Glanville (1984) and Remschmidt et al. (1990) being more similar. The different sample composition in terms of age and other factors not yet identified may have been responsible for the discrepant findings. Deter and Herzog (1994) have graphically and quantitatively displayed the sequential course of anorexia nervosa in their sample by using the classical distinction of improvement, permanent recovery, and persistent illness. Clearly, both typological approaches warrant further study and analysis.

The second approach to studying the issue of continuity and discontinuity deals with the extent to which there is stability or change within the spectrum of eating disorders. Based on several studies, Hsu (1988) has concluded that

> ... (1) twice as many restrictive anorexics develop bulimia as do bulimic anorexics changing to restrictive anorexics; (2) most bulimic anorexics retain their bulimia; (3) restrictive anorexics who develop bulimia tend to gain weight (i.e. develop normal weight bulimia nervosa); (4) bulimia nervosa, normal weight or otherwise, is the commonest diagnosis after anorexia nervosa at follow-up. (p. 808)

Although some of these conclusions seem premature because of the very small database, there has recently been only very limited research on the course of anorexia nervosa. In two adolescent samples of anorectic patients at follow-up, Steinhausen and Seidel (1993a,b) and Herpertz-Dahlmann et al. (1996) observed partial syndromes of anorexia nervosa as the second most frequent diagnosis after recovery. This second approach of continuity and discontinuity within the spectrum of eating disorders also demands more detailed analysis based on larger samples.

A third approach would deal with the extent to which the eating disorders are followed by other psychiatric disorders. So far, this approach has not yet been addressed by empirical research. Although the above-mentioned findings on outcome have included psychiatric status at follow-up, neither the issue of comorbidity of other psychiatric disorders with eating disorders at follow-up nor the temporal succession of these disorders has been studied systematically.

Bulimia nervosa

Clinical picture

According to the ICD-10 (WHO 1992, p. 178), bulimia nervosa is characterized by 'repeated bouts of overeating and an excessive preoccupation with the control of the body, leading the patient to adapt extreme measures so as to mitigate the fattening effects of ingested food'. Bulimia nervosa shares the same psychopathology as anorexia nervosa, and it quite frequently follows an episode of anorexia nervosa.

In contrast to anorectics, the majority of bulimic patients are of normal weight for their height. They may suffer from many physical complications that are often serious in nature and that are frequently overlooked because the patients do not actively seek professional help. As with anorexia nervosa, the male sex is only rarely affected. The main symptoms are:

- a persistent preoccupation with eating, and an irresistible craving for food resulting in episodes of overeating in which large amounts of food are consumed in short periods of time

- various attempts to counteract the 'fattening' effects of food by self-induced vomiting, purgative abuse, alternating periods of starvation, and use of drugs such as appetite suppressants, thyroid preparations, or diuretics

- a morbid dread of fatness as the core psychopathological symptom.

Studies of natural course

There is a small series of longitudinal studies that have used either screening measures or a two-stage approach with a sequence of screening and interview that provide information on the natural history of bulimia nervosa. Several screening studies indicate that, in general, there is remarkable stability of symptoms and diagnoses across time (Yager *et al.* 1987, Drewnowski *et al.* 1988, Johnson *et al.* 1989, Striegel-Moore *et al.* 1989).

Studies using the two-stage approach consolidate the impression of stability in the natural course of bulimia nervosa. Based on a consecutive series of adults who were attending general practice, King (1989) found a high stability of diagnostic status at follow-up 12–18 months later. At the second follow-up 2–3 years after the first assessment (King 1991), three out of five of the original patients were still diagnosed as being bulimic, and there was little change in patients with the full syndrome of bulimia nervosa or in those with partial syndromes between the first and second follow-up.

In a large sample of female adolescents Patton *et al.* (1988) diagnosed bulimia nervosa or partial syndromes and calculated minimum point prevalence rates for these two categories that even increased from 2.8% to 8.1% at a 1 year follow-up. Finally, Keller *et al.* (1992) also reported very high rates of chronicity, relapse, recurrence, and psychosocial morbidity in 30 women with bulimia nervosa. Their findings show that almost one-third of the subjects remained in the index episode 3 years after entry into the study.

Intervention studies

In a thorough analysis of 15 drug studies and 19 controlled studies of psychotherapy, Mitchell *et al.* (1993) came to various critical conclusions. According to this review, the validity of findings is limited owing to the reliance on subject self-report measures of binge eating and purging episodes, the lack of adequate follow-up periods, the small numbers of subjects in most studies, and the problem of potential bias because the treatment assignment was not fully blind.

Among their tentative conclusions the authors state that treatment for bulimia nervosa can be successful in an outpatient setting and both individual and group approaches appear to be successful. Among the latter, cognitive-behavioral techniques (CBT) reduce target behavior and improve the accompanying psychopathology. However, the study of their efficacy requires further analysis of the impact of frequency of sessions and of specific elements of treatment. Recent studies using interpersonal therapy and psychodynamic approaches also appear promising but need further study to determine their relative efficacy. Among the effective drugs, no particular antidepressant is more effective than any other. The combination of antidepressant medication and CBT is not superior to CBT alone. Finally, two conclusions are of specific relevance for clinical practice: the limited knowledge about matching patients to treatments by defined predictor variables and the still insufficient effects of treatment. Although pharmacotherapy and psychotherapy result in substantial reductions of target eating behaviors, the majority of treated patients remains symptomatic at the end of treatment.

The lack of sufficient follow-up periods in these controlled intervention studies as a limiting factor for the derivation of conclusions pertaining to the long-term outcome does not apply to the most recent study by Fairburn *et al.* (1995). These authors compared three psychological treatments—CBT, behavior therapy, and focal interpersonal therapy—after a mean of close to 6 years. The three treatment approaches had different long-term effects. Both in terms of remission and abstinence from key behavioral features, those subjects who had received behavior therapy fared the worst. Although behavior therapy was comparable to CBT in short-term outcome, it obviously had a short-lived effect. So far, the study by Fairburn *et al.* (1995) is the only attempt to link evaluation of a controlled trial of treatment with the long-term outcome in bulimia nervosa.

Short-term and long-term outcomes

In their extensive review Fichter and Quadflieg (1995) summarized the findings of 22 follow-up studies of bulimia nervosa patients published between 1983 and 1994. With the exception of five retrospective studies, all studies employed a prospective design. In addition, two more recent publications (Fairburn *et al.* 1995, Fichter and Quadflieg 1996) were included in the present review. Similar outcome measures as described for anorexia nervosa were used in the bulimia nervosa follow-up studies, i.e. mortality rates, and the trichotomy of recovery, improvement, and chronicity. Furthermore, other psychiatric disorders were assessed and the issue of prognostic factors was ventilated.

Study characteristics

A total of 1383 patients are covered in these 24 studies. The smallest series contains 14 patients, and the maximum is 232 patients (mean = 57.6, SD = 46.1). Beacause of their recent origin—all studies were published between 1983 and 1994—almost all studies are based on patients who were diagnosed according to either DSM-III or DSM-III-R criteria. Two studies used Russell's (1979) criteria and one was even based on the recent DSM-IV criteria.

The mean age at onset of the disorder ranges from a minimum of 14.4 to a maximum of 22.2 years across the various samples. The majority of studies report on patients who received

Table 13. 6   Outcome of bulimia nervosa based on 24 follow-up studies

	Sample size	Mean (%)	SD (%)	Range (%)
Recovery ('good')	1303	47.5	14.4	22–66
Improvement ('fair')	1125	26.0	13.4	0–67
Chronification ('poor')	1164	26.0	14.0	0–43
Affective disorders	440	24.9	10.0	9–37
Neurotic disorders	329	12.9	5.0	2–18
Personality disorders	228	4.7	0.7	3–5
Substance use disorders	361	14.9	10.2	2–26

some sort of psychotherapy. Six studies used additional pharmacotherapy, and one study was based on additional medical treatment. Pharmacotherapy without further intervention was used in two studies. In contrast to anorexia nervosa, the majority of studies were based on outpatient treatment; inpatient treatment was used in only four of the studies.

The mean follow-up period was 30.7 months for 15 studies containing the respective information. Based on information provided by 10 studies, follow-up periods ranged from of 2 to 161 months,. Although no precise comparison is possible, an impression is given that the average follow-up period for bulimia nervosa patients is shorter than that for anorexia nervosa patients. Drop-out rates vary from between 0% and 37% with a mean of 12% (SD = 12.1).

Follow-up findings

Crude mortality rates amounted to a mean of 0.7% (SD = 1.5) and varied between 0% and 6%. These are considerably lower the corresponding figures for anorexia nervosa. Studies containing data on standard mortality ratios are not available.

The main outcome findings are summarized in Table 13.6. The ranges for the various outcome parameters are less extreme in comparison to the anorexia nervosa outcome studies, though they are still considerable. The mean proportion of full recovery (47.5%) is only slightly higher than in the anorexia nervosa patients (45%), whereas there are less improved cases (26% vs. 33%) and more chronic cases (26% vs. 20%) among the bulimic patients.

Among the various other psychiatric disorders, in bulimic patients at follow-up in contrast to anorectic patients there is a slightly higher rate of affective disorders (25% versus 22%) but a similar rate of substance abuse (15% versus 14%) and a lower rate of neurotic disorders (13% versus 26%). Personality disorders in former bulimic patients have only been mentioned, or perhaps even assessed, in one study (Fichter *et al.* 1992, Fichter and Quadflieg 1996), so no valid comparison with anorexia nervosa is possible.

Risks and prognostic factors

In the restricted series of outcome studies on bulimia nervosa there are only few reports on risk factors. According to Fallon *et al.* (1991), there is no association between outcome of bulimia nervosa and personality disorders according to DSM-III-R categories, whereas certain personality features have an impact, as is indicated in the study by Yager *et al.* (1995). These authors found that women with active bulimia were less likely to use active coping, planning, and seeking emotional support than recovered patients and controls and less likely to focus on and vent emotions than recovered patients. In addition, social problems were significantly associated with poor outcome in the study by Johnson-Sabine *et al.* (1992).

Because the outcome literature on bulimia nervosa is more scanty than for anorexia nervosa, less is also known about prognostic factors. The following factors have been identified.

- *Age at onset*: Two studies found younger age at onset to be favorably associated with outcome (Abraham *et al.* 1983, Johnson-Sabine *et al.* 1992), whereas four other studies found no significant effect for age at onset (Fairburn *et al.* 1987, Fallon *et al.* 1991, Fichter *et al.* 1992, Herzog *et al.* 1993).

- *Duration of illness*: A short duration of illness prior to treatment was found to be a positive predictor in four studies (Hsu and Holder 1986, Fallon *et al.* 1991, Fahy and Russell 1993, Herzog *et al.* 1993), whereas it was found to be insignificant in four other studies (Pope *et al.* 1985, Fairburn *et al.* 1987, Abraham *et al.* 1983, Baell and Wertheim 1992).

- *Clinical features*: The frequency of bulimic episodes or other scores of severity were not found to be a predictor of outcome in three studies (Hsu and Holder 1986, Swift *et al.* 1987, Mitchell *et al.* 1989), but was found to be a negative predictor in the two studies by Herzog *et al.* (1991) and Vandereycken and Pieters (1992). Weight was not significant as a predictor in two studies (Hsu and Holder 1986, Mitchell *et al.* 1989), but low weight was a negative predictor in the study by Herzog *et al.*(1993), as were vomiting and laxative abuse in the study by Vandereycken and Pieters (1992).

- *Premorbid clinical characteristics*: A history of anorexia nervosa preceding bulimia nervosa was not predictive of outcome in six studies (Abraham *et al.* 1983, Hsu and Holder 1986, Fairburn *et al.* 1987, Herzog *et al.* 1991, Johnson-Sabine *et al.* 1992, Fahy and Russell 1993). The same applies to premorbid substance or alcohol abuse, according to three studies (Fallon *et al.* 1991, Herzog *et al.* 1991, Fahy and Russell 1993) and to premorbid obesity (Hsu and Holder 1986).

- *Family variables*: A family history of alcohol abuse was detected as an unfavorable predictor in the study by Hsu and Holder (1986) but as a favorable sign for outcome in the study by Collings and King (1994), whereas a family history of depression turned out to be negative in the study by Hsu and Holder (1986) and was not found to be significant in the study by Fahy and Russell (1993).

- *Psychiatric features*: Various studies point to a concomitant personality disorder, including borderline symptoms, as being unfavorable for the outcome (Fairburn *et al.* 1987, Johnson *et al.* 1990, Herzog *et al.* 1991, Fichter *et al.* 1992, Fahy and Russell 1993). According to three studies (Fairburn *et al.* 1987, Herzog *et al.* 1991, 1993), depression was found to be insignificant. However, depression was significantly associated with poor outcome in the studies by Fichter *et al.* (1992), as was a comorbid anxiety disorder. Furthermore, suicide attempts (Abraham *et al.* 1983), low self-esteem (Baell and Wertheim 1992, Fairburn *et al.* 1993), and alcohol abuse (Lacey 1992) were found to be negative predictors of outcome, whereas impulsiveness was not found by Fahy and Russell (1993) to be significant.

- *Socioeconomic status*: Only one study found higher social class to be favorably associated with outcome (Johnson-Sabine *et al.* 1992), whereas it was not found to be significant in another study (Mitchell *et al.* 1989).

Continuity and discontinuity

In the corresponding section on anorexia nervosa, three approaches for the study of continuity and discontinuity were outlined. When using this distinction again for the study of developmental processes in bulimia nervosa, the first approach would require studies of the various types of remission, improvement, chronicity, and the like. These are entirely missing from the literature.

The very limited findings of the second approach, addressing the changes between anorexia and bulimia nervosa, were presented above. One additional study (Hsu and Sobkiewicz 1989) found that relapse into anorexia nervosa is very uncommon in bulimia nervosa.

Finally, the third approach for studying the temporal correlations between bulimia nervosa and other psychiatric disorders has, so far, also not been addressed by research.

Conclusions

In the past, definite statements on the outcome of the eating disorders have been limited by various methodological shortcomings pertaining to variations in patient selection, sample size, design of the studies, diagnostic criteria, assessment strategies, information on treatment, and follow-up periods. However, some progress has been made. In particular, recent outcome studies on bulimia nervosa have profited from methodological refinements in terms of prospective designs, adequate sample sizes, and reliable diagnostic criteria. Unfortunately the duration of follow-up in these studies is, in general, too short to allow definite conclusions. This, together with an unacceptably high drop-out rate in some of the studies, may obscure the impression that the outcome of bulimia nervosa patients is really slightly better than that of anorexia nervosa patients.

Future outcome studies would most definitely profit not only from more extended follow-up but also from a consistent follow-up period, which would reduce one potential source of outcome variation. The assessment procedures for the eating disorders have become more structured and detailed, but the diagnosis of further psychiatric disorders could benefit from the more precise, structured, and reliable interviews that are available. Furthermore, outcome studies should designate whether these psychiatric disorders are really coexistent with an additional persistent eating disorder, or whether they are *de novo* disorders without any further eating disorders. In the latter case, the term comorbidity is misleading.

There is still very little information on the natural course and developmental pattern of the various types of eating disorders, i.e. the continuity and discontinuity with each other of anorexia nervosa, bulimia nervosa, and further variants. In addition, the gap between treatment studies and outcome studies should be narrowed or closed. Inadequate follow-up periods are a shortcoming in most recent treatment studies, especially in bulimia nervosa, and the majority of outcome studies provide too little information on treatment. However, long-term outcome studies of the eating disorders must take into consideration that, besides professional intervention, other developmental factors that occur during the patient's life may have an effect. It is evident that only more complex and theory-driven research approaches will be able to analyze these issues.

References

Abraham S.F., Mira, M., and Llewellyn-Jones, D. (1983). Bulimia: a study of outcome. *International Journal of Eating Disorders*, **2**, 175–180.

Baell, W.K. and Wertheim, E.H. (1992). Predictors of outcome in the treatment of bulimia nervosa. *British Journal of Clinical Psychology*, **31**, 330–332.

Bemis, K.M. (1987). The present status of operant conditioning for the treatment of anorexia nervosa. *Behavior Modification*, **11**, 432–463.

Bemis Vitousek, K.B. (1995). Cognitive-behavioral therapy for anorexia nervosa. In *Eating disorders and obesity. A comprehensive handbook*, ed. K.D. Brownell and C.G. Fairburn, pp. 324–329. Guilford Press, New York.

Beumont, P.J.V., George, G.C.W., and Smart, D.E. (1976). Dieters and vomiters and purgers in anorexia nervosa. *Psychological Medicine*, **6**, 617–622.

Bhanji, S. and Thompson, J. (1974). Operant conditioning in the treatment of anorexia nervosa. *British Journal of Psychiatry*, **124**, 166–72.

Blitzer, J.R., Rollins, N., and Blackwell, A. (1961). Children who starve themselves: anorexia nervosa. *Psychosomatic Medicine*, **23**, 369–383.

Browning, C.H. and Miller, S.I. (1968). Anorexia nervosa: a study in prognosis and management. *American Journal of Psychiatry*, **124**, 1128–1132.

Bryant-Waugh, R., Knibbs, J., Fosson, A., Kaminski, Z., and Lask, B. (1988). Long term follow up of patients with early onset anorexia nervosa. *Archives of Disease in Childhood*, **63**, 5–9.

Bryant-Waugh, R., Hankins, M., Shafran, R., Lask, B., and Fosson, A. (1996). A prospective follow-up of children with anorexia nervosa. *Journal of Youth and Adolescence*, **25**, 431–437.

Burns, T. and Crisp, A.H. (1984). Outcome of anorexia nervosa in males. *British Journal of Psychiatry*, **145**, 319–325.

Casper, R.C. and Jabine, L.N. (1996). An eight-year follow-up: Outcome from adolescent compared to adult onset anorexia nervosa. *Journal of Youth and Adolescence*, **25**, 499–517.

Collings, S. and King, M. (1994). Ten-year follow-up of 50 patients with bulimia nervosa. *British Journal of Psychiatry*, **164**, 80–87.

Crisp, A.H., Harding, G., and McGuiness, B. (1974). Anorexia nervosa. Psychoneurotic characteristics of parents: relationship to prognosis. *Journal of Psychosomatic Research*, **18**, 167–173.

Crisp, A.H., Norton, K., Gowers, S., Halek, C., Bowyer, C., Yeldham, D., Levett, G., and Bhat, A. (1991). A controlled study of the effect of therapies aimed at adolescent and family psychopathology in anorexia nervosa. *British Journal of Psychiatry*, **159**, 325–323.

Crisp, A.H., Callendar, J.S., Halek, C., and Hsu, L.K. G. (1992). Long-term mortality in anorexia nervosa. *British Journal of Psychiatry*, **161**, 104–107.

Dally, P.J. (1969). *Anorexia nervosa*. Heinemann, London.

Dally, P.J. and Sargant, W. (1966). Treatment and outcome of anorexia nervosa. *British Medical Journal*, **ii**, 793–795.

Deter, H-C. and Herzog, W. (1994). Anorexia nervosa in a long-term perspective: Results of the Heidelberg–Mannheim study. *Psychosomatic Medicine*, **56**, 20–27.

Deter, H.C., Herzog, W., and Petzold, E. (1992). The Heidelberg–Mannheim study: Long-term follow-up of anorexia nervosa patients at the University Medical Center—background and preliminary results. In *The course of eating disorders. Long-term follow-up studies of anorexia and bulimia nervosa*, ed. W. Herzog, H.C. Deter, and W. Vanderdycken, pp. 71–84. Springer-Verlag, Berlin.

Drewnowski, A., Yee, D.K., and Krahn, D.D. (1988). Bulimia in college women—Incidence and recovery rates. *American Journal of Psychiatry*, **145**, 753–735.

Eckert, E.D., Halmi, K.A., Marchi, P., Grove, W., and Crosby, R. (1995). Ten-year follow-up of anorexia nervosa: Clinical course and outcome. *Psychological Medicine*, **25**, 143–56.

Eisler, I., Dare, F.C., Russell, G.F.M., Szmukler, G., Le Grange, D., and Dodge, E. (1997). Family and individual therapy in anorexia nervosa. *Archives of General Psychiatry*, **54**, 1025–1030.

Fahy, T. and Russell, G.F.M. (1993). Outcome and prognostic variables in bulimia nervosa. *International Journal of Eating Disorders*, **14**, 135–45.

Fairburn, C.G., Kirk, J., O'Connor, M., Anastasiades, P., and Cooper, P.J. (1987). Prognostic factors in bulimia nervosa. *British Journal of Clinical Psychology*, **26**, 223–224.

Fairburn, C.G., Peveler, R.C., Jones, R., Hope, R.A., and Doll, H.A. (1993). Predictors of 12-month outcome in bulimia nervosa and the influences of attitudes to shape and weight. *Journal of Consulting and Clinical Psychology*, **61**, 696–698.

Fairburn, C.G., Norman, P.A., Welch, S.L., OConnor, M.E., Doll, H.A., and Peveler, R.C. (1995). A prospective study of outcome in bulimia nervosa and the long-term effects of three psychological treatments. *Archives of General Psychiatry*, **52**, 304–312.

Fallon, B.A., Walsh, B.T., Sadik, C., Saoud, J.B., and Lukasik, V. (1991). Outcome and clinical course in inpatient bulimic women: A 2- to 9-year follow-up study. *Journal of Clinical Psychiatry*, **52**, 272–278.

Fichter, M.M. and Quadflieg, N. (1995). Comparative studies on the course of eating disorders in adolescents and adults. Is age at onset a predictor of outcome? In *Eating disorders in adolescence. Anorexia and bulimia nervosa*, ed. H-C. Steinhausen, pp. 301–37. de Gruyter, Berlin.

Fichter, M.M. and Quadflieg, N. (1996). Course and two-year outcome in anorexic and bulimic adolescents. *Journal of Youth and Adolescence*, **25**, 545–562.

Fichter, M.M., Quadflieg, N., and Rief, W. (1992). The German longitudinal bulimia nervosa study, I. In *The course of eating disorders: Long-term follow-up studies of anorexia and bulimia nervosa*, ed. W. Herzog, H-C. Deter, and W. Vandereycken, pp. 133–149. Springer-Verlag, Berlin.

Frazier, S.H. (1965). Anorexia nervosa. *Diseases of the Nervous System*, **26**, 155–159.

Garfinkel, P.E., Moldofsky, H., and Garner, D.M. (1977). The outcome of anorexia nervosa: Significance of clinical features. Body image and behavior modification. In *Anorexia nervosa*, ed. R.A. Vigersky, pp. 315–329. Raven Press, New York.

Gillberg, C., Råstam, M., and Gillberg, I.C. (1994). Anorexia nervosa: Physical health and neurodevelopment at 16 and 21 years. *Developmental Medicine and Child Neurology*, **36**, 567–575.

Gillberg, C., Råstam, M., and Gillberg, I.C. (1995). Anorexia nervosa 6 years after onset. 1. Personality disorders. *Comprehensive Psychiatry*, **36**, 61–69.

Goetz, P.L., Succop, R.A., Reinhart, J.B., and Miller, A. (1977). Anorexia nervosa in children: a follow-up study. *American Journal of Orthopsychiatry*, **47**, 597–603.

Greenfeld, D.G., Anyan, W.R., Hobart, M., Quinlan, D.M., and Plantes, M. (1991). Insight into illness and outcome in anorexia nervosa. *International Journal of Eating Disorders*, **10**, 101–9.

Hall, A., Slim, E., Hawker, F., and Salmond, C. (1984). Anorexia nervosa—long-term outcome in 50 female patients. *British Journal of Psychiatry*, **145**, 407–13.

Halmi, K.A. (1991). Course of anorexia nervosa: Ten year follow-up. In International Symposium of the International Society for Adolescent Psychiatry with the World Psychiatric Association (WPA)–Section on Eating Disorders Paris, 17–19 April.

Halmi, K.A., Brodland, G., and Loney, J. (1973). Prognosis in anorexia nervosa. *Annals of Internal Medicine*, **78**, 907–909.

Halmi, K.A., Brodland, G., and Rigs, C. (1976). A follow-up study of seventy-nine patients with anorexia patients with anorexia nervosa: An evaluation of prognostic factors and diagnostic criteria. In *Life history research in psychopathology* Vol. 4., ed. G. Writ, G. Winokur, and M. Roff, pp. 290–300. University of Minnesota Press, Minneapolis.

Hawley, R.M. (1985). The outcome of anorexia nervosa in younger subjects. *British Journal of Psychiatry*, **146**, 657–660.

Heebink, D., and Halmi, K.A. (1995). Psychopharmacology in adolescents with eating disorders. In *Eating disorders in adolescence. anorexia and bulimia nervosa*, ed. H-C. Steinhausen, pp. 271–285. de Gruyter, Berlin.

Herpertz-Dahlmann, B.M., Wewetzer, C., Schulz, E., and Remschmidt, H. (1996). Course and outcome in adolescent anorexia nervosa. *International Journal of Eating Disorders*, **19**, 335–345.

Herzog, T., Hartmann, A., Sandholz, A., and Stammer, H. (1991). Prognostic factors in outpatient psychotherapy of bulimia. *Psychotherapy and Psychosomatics*, **56**, 48–55.

Herzog, D.B., Sacks, N.R., Keller, M.B., Lavori, P.W., von Ranson, K.B., and Gray, H.M. (1993). Patterns and predictors of recovery in anorexia nervosa and bulimia nervosa. *Journal of the American Academy of Child and Adolescent Psychiatry*, **32**, 835–842.

Hsu, L.K.G. (1988). The outcome of anorexia nervosa: A reappraisal. *Psychological Medicine*, **18**, 807–812.

Hsu, L.K.G. and Holder, D. (1986). Bulimia nervosa: Treatment and short-term outcome. *Psychological Medicine*, **16**, 65–70.

Hsu, L.K.G. and Sobkiewicz, T.A. (1989). Bulimia nervosa: A four-to six-year follow-up study. *Psychological Medicine*, **19**, 1035–1038.

Hsu, L.K.G., Crisp, A.H., and Harding, B. (1979). Outcome of anorexia nervosa. *Lancet*, **1**, 61–65.

Johnson, C., Tobin, D.L., and Lipkin, J. (1989). Epidemiologic changes in bulimic behavior among female adolescents over a five-year period. *International Journal of Eating Disorders*, **8**, 647–55.

Johnson, C., Tobin, D.L., and Dennis, A. (1990). Differences in treatment outcome between borderline and nonborderline bulimics at one-year follow-up. *International Journal of Eating Disorders*, **9**, 617–627.

Johnson-Sabine, E., Reiss, D., and Dayson, D. (1992). Bulimia nervosa: A 5-year follow-up study. *Psychological Medicine*, **22**, 951–959.

Kalucy, R.S., Crisp, A.H., Harding, B., Chen, C.N., and Lacey, J.H. (1976). Nocturnal hormonal profiles in massive obesity, anorexia nervosa and normal females. *Journal of Psychosomatic Research*, **20**, 595–604.

Kay, D.W. and Shapira, K. (1965). The prognosis in anorexia nervosa. In *Anorexia nervosa*, ed. J.E. Meyer and H. Feldman, pp. 113–117. Thieme, Stuttgart.

Keller, M.B., Herzog, D.B., Lavori, P.W., Bradburn, I.S., and Mahoney, E.M. (1992). The naturalistic history of bulimia nervosa: Extraordinarily high rates of chronicity, elapse, recurrence, and psychosocial morbidity. *International Journal of Eating Disorders*, **12**, 1–9.

King, M.B. (1989). Eating disorders in a general practice population. Prevalence, characteristics and follow-up at 18 months. *Psychological Medicine (Monograph Suppl.)*, **14**, 1–34.

King, M.B. (1991). The natural history of eating pathology in attenders to primary medical care. *International Journal of Eating Disorders*, **10**, 379–387.

Kreipe, R.E. and Piver Dukarm, C. (1996). Outcome of anorexia nervosa related to treatment utilizing an adolescent medicine approach. *Journal of Youth and Adolescence*, **25**, 483–497.

Kreipe, R.E., Churchill, B.H., and Strauss, J. (1989). Long-term outcome of adolescents with anorexia nervosa. *American Journal of Diseases of Children*, **143**, 1322–1327.

Lacey, J.H. (1992). Long-term follow-up of bulimic patients treated in integrated behavioural and psychodynamic treatment programmes. In *The course of eating disorders: Long-term follow-up studies of anorexia and bulimia nervosa*. (ed. W. Herzog, H-C. Deter, and W. Vandereycken,), pp. 150–173. Springer-Verlag, Berlin.

Le Grange, D., Eisler, I., Dare, C., and Russell, G.F.M. (1992). Evaluation of family treatments in adolescent anorexia nervosa: A pilot study. *International Journal of Eating Disorders*, **12**, 347–357.

Lesser, L.I., Ashenden, B.J., Debushey, M., and Eisenberg, L. (1960). Anorexia nervosa in children. *American Journal of Orthopsychiatry*, **30**, 572–580.

Martin, F.E. (1985). The treatment and outcome of anorexia nervosa in adolescents: a prospective study and five year follow-up. *Journal of Psychiatric Research*, **19**, 509–514.

Mitchell, J.E., Pyle, R.L., Hatsukami, D., Goff, G., Glotter, D., and Harper, J. (1989). A 2–5 year follow-up study of patients treated for bulimia. *International Journal of Eating Disorders*, **8**, 157–165.

Mitchell, J.E., Raymond, N., and Specker, S. (1993). A review of the controlled trials of pharmacotherapy and psychotherapy in the treatment of bulimia nervosa. *International Journal of Eating Disorders*, **14**, 229–247.

Morgan, H.G. and Russell, G.F. M. (1975). Value of family background and clinical features as predictors of long-term outcome in anorexia nervosa: Four-year follow-up study of 41 patients. *Psychological Medicine*, **5**, 355–371.

Morgan, H.G., Purgold, J., and Welbourne, J. (1983). Management and outcome in anorexia nervosa—a standardized prognostic study. *British Journal of Psychiatry*, **143**, 282–287.

Norring, C.E.A. and Sohlberg, S.S. (1993). Outcome, recovery, relapse and mortality across six years in patients with clinical eating disorders. *Acta Psychiatrica Scandinavica*, **87**, 437–444.

Nussbaum, M., Shenker, I.R., Baird, D., and Saravay, S. (1985). Follow-up investigation in patients with anorexia nervosa. *Journal of Pediatrics*, **106**, 835–840.

Patton, G.C. (1988). Mortality in eating disorders. *Psychological Medicine*, **18**, 947–951.

Pierloot, R.A., Wellens, W., and Houben, M.E. (1975). Elements of resistance to a combined medical and psychotherapeutic program in anorexia nervosa. *Psychotherapie und Psychosomatik*, **26**, 101–117.

Pope, H.G., Hudson, J.I., Jonas, J.M., and Yurgelun-Todd, D. (1985). Antidepressant treatment of bulimia. A two-year follow-up study. *Journal of Clinical Psychopharmacology*, **5**, 320–327.

Råstam, M., Gillberg, I.C., and Gillberg, C. (1995). Anorexia nervosa 6 years after onset. 2. Comorbid psychiatric problems. *Comprehensive Psychiatry*, **26**, 70–76.

Rathner, G. (1992). Aspects of the natural history of normal and disordered eating and some methodological considerations. In *The course of eating disorders: Long-term follow-up studies of anorexia and bulimia nervosa*, ed. W. Herzog, H-C. Deter, and W. Vandereycken, pp. 273–303. Springer-Verlag, Berlin.

Ratnasutiya, R.H., Eisler, J., Szmukler, G.I., and Russell, F.F.M. (1991). Anorexia nervosa: Outcome and prognostic factors after 20 years. *British Journal of Psychiatry*, **158**, 495–502.

Remschmidt, H., Wienand, W., and Wewetzer, W. (1990). The long-term course of anorexia nervosa. In *Anorexia nervosa*, ed. H. Remschmidt and M.H. Schmidt, pp. 127–136. Hogrete and Huber, Toronto.

Robin, A.L., Siegel, P.T., Koepke, T., Moye, A.W., and Tice, S. (1994). Family therapy versus individual therapy of adolescent females with anorexia nervosa. *Journal of Developmental and Behavioral Pediatrics*, **15**, 111–116.

Robin, A.L., Siegel, P.T., and Moye, A.W. (1995). Family versus individual therapy for anorexia: Impact on family conflict. *International Journal of Eating Disorders*, **17**, 313–322.

Rollins, N. and Blackwell, A. (1968). The treatment of anorexia nervosa in children and adolescents. Stage, I. *Journal of Child Psychology and Psychiatry*, **9**, 81–91.

Rosenvinge, J.H. and Mouland, S.O. (1990). Outcome and prognosis of anorexia nervosa—A retrospective study of 41 subjects. *British Journal of Psychiatry*, **156**, 92–97.

Russell, G.F.M. (1979). Bulimia nervosa: An ominous variant of anorexia nervosa. *Psychological Medicine*, **9**, 429–448.

Russell, G.F. M. (1992). Anorexia nervosa of early onset and its impact on puberty. In *Feeding problems and eating disorders in children and adolescents*, ed. P.J. Cooper and A. Stein, pp. 85–112. Harwood Academic Publishers, Chur.

Russell, G.F.M., Szmukler, G.I., Dare, C., and Eisler, I. (1987). An evaluation of family therapy in anorexia nervosa and bulimia nervosa. *Archives of General Psychiatry*, **44**, 1047–1056.

Santonastaso, P., Panarotto, L., and Silvestri, A. (1991). A follow-up study on anorexia nervosa: Clinical features and diagnostic outcome. *European Psychiatry*, **6**, 177–185.

Schork, E.J., Eckert, E.D., and Halmi, K.A. (1994). The relationship between psychopathology, eating disorder diagnosis, and clinical outcome at 10-year-follow-up in anorexia nervosa. *Comprehensive Psychiatry*, **35**, 113–123.

Seidensticker, J. and Tzagournis, M. (1968). Anorexia nervosa—clinical features and long-term follow-up. *Journal of Chronic Diseases*, **21**, 366–367.

Smith, C., Feldman, S.S., Nasserbakht, A., and Steiner, H. (1993). Psychological characteristics and DSM-III-R diagnoses at 6-year follow-up of adolescent anorexia nervosa. *Journal of the American Academy of Child and Adolescent Psychiatry*, **32**, 1237–1245.

Sohlberg, S., Norring, C., Holmaren, S., and Rosmark, B. (1989). Impulsivity and long-term prognosis of psychiatric patients with anorexia nervosa/bulimia nervosa. *Journal of Nervous and Mental Disease*, **177**, 249–258.

Steiner, H., Mazer, C., and Litt, I.F. (1990). Compliance and outcome in anorexia nervosa. *Journal of Western Medicine*, **157**, 133–139.

Steinhausen, H-C. and Boyadjieva, S. (1996). The outcome of adolescent anorexia nervosa: Findings from Sofia. *Journal of Youth and Adolescence*, **25**, 473–481.

Steinhausen, H-C. and Glanville, K. (1983). A long-term follow-up of adolescent anorexia nervosa. *Acta Psychiatrica Scandinavica*, **68**, 1–10.

Steinhausen, H-C. and Glanville, K. (1984). Der langfristige Verlauf der Anorexia nervosa. *Nervenarzt*, **55**, 236–248.

Steinhausen, H-C. and Seidel, R. (1993a). Outcome in adolescent eating disorders. *International Journal of Eating Disorders*, **14**, 487–496.

Steinhausen, H-C. and Seidel, R. (1993b). Short-term and intermediate-term outcome in adolescent eating disorders. *Acta Psychiatrica Scandinavica*, **88**, 169–173.

Steinhausen, H-C., Rauss-Mason, C., and Seidel, R. (1991). Follow-up studies of anorexia nervosa: A review of four decades of outcome research. *Psychological Medicine*, **21**, 447–451.

Striegel-Moore, R.H., Silberstein, L.R., French, P., and Rodin, F. (1989). A prospective study of disordered eating among college students. *International Journal of Eating Disorders*, **8**, 523–532.

Sturzenberger, S., Cantwell, D.P., Burroughs, J., Salkin, B., and Green, J.K. (1977). A follow-up study of adolescent psychiatric inpatients with anorexia nervosa: The assessment of outcome. *Journal of the American Academy of Child and Adolescent Psychiatry*, **16**, 703–715.

Sunday, S.R., Reeman, I.M., Eckert, E., and Halmi, K.A. (1996). Ten-year outcome in adolescent onset anorexia nervosa. *Journal of Youth and Adolescence*, **25**, 533–544.

Swift, W.J., Ritholz, M., Kalin, N.H., and Kaslow, N. (1987). A follow-up study of thirty hospitalized bulimics. *Psychosomatic Medicine*, **49**, 45–55.

Theander, S. (1970). Anorexia nervosa. A psychiatric investigation of 94 female patients. *Acta Psychiatrica Scandinavica* (Suppl 214), 1–194.

Theander, S. (1996). Anorexia nervosa with an early onset: Selection, gender, outcome, and results of a long-term follow-up study. *Journal of Youth and Adolescence*, **25**, 419–429.

Tolstrup, K. (1965). Die Charakteristika der jüngeren Fälle von Anorexia nervosa. In Anorexia nervosa. (ed. J.E. Meyer and H Feldman, pp. 51–9. Thieme, Stuttgart.

Toner, B.B., Garfield, P.E., and Garner, D.M. (1986). Long-term follow-up of anorexia nervosa. *Psychosomatic Medicine*, **48**, 520–529.

van der Ham, T., van Strien, D.C., and van Engeland, H. (1994). A four-year prospective follow-up study of 49 eating-disordered adolescents: differences in course of illness. *Acta Psychiatrica Scandinavica*, **90**, 229–235.

Vandereycken, W. and Pieters, G. (1992). A large-scale longitudinal follow-up study of patients with eating disorders: Methodological issues and preliminary results. In *The course of eating disorders: Long-term follow-up studies of anorexia and bulimia nervosa*, ed. W. Herzog, H-C. Deter, and W. Vandereycken, pp. 182–197. Springer-Verlag, Berlin.

Walford, G. and McCune, N. (1991). Long-term outcome in early-onset anorexia nervosa. *British Journal of Psychiatry*, **9**, 27–40.

Walsh, T. (1995). Pharmacotherapy of eating disorders. In *Eating disorders and obesity. A comprehensive handbook.*, ed. K.D. Brownell and C.G. Fairburn, pp. 313–317. Guilford Press, New York.

Warren, W. (1968). A study of anorexia nervosa in young girls. *Journal of Child Psychology and Psychiatry and Allied Disciplines*, **9**, 27–40.

WHO (1992). *The ICD-10 classification of mental and behavioural disorders. Clinical descriptions and diagnostic guidelines*. World Health Organization, Geneva.

Willi, J. and Hagemann, R. (1976). Langzeitverläufe von Anorexia nervosa. *Schweizerische Medizinische Wochenschrift*, **106**, 1459–1465.

Willi, J., Limacher, B., Helbling, P., and Nussbaum, P. (1989). 10-Jahres-Katamnese der 1973–1975 im Kanton Zürich erstmals hospitalisierten Anorexie-Fälle. *Schweizerische Medizinische Wochenschrift*, **119**, 147–155.

Wonderlich, S.A., Fullerton, D., Swift, W.J., and Klein, M.H. (1994). 5-Year outcome from eating disorders—relevance of personality disorders. *International Journal of Eating Disorders*, **15**, 233–244.

Yager, J., Landsverk, J., and Edelstein, C.K. (1987). A 20-month follow-up study of 628 women with eating disorders. I. Course and severity. *American Journal of Psychiatry*, **144**, 86–94.

Yager, J., Rorty, M., and Rossotto, E. (1995). Coping styles differ between recovered and nonrecovered women with bulimia nervosa, but not between recovered women and non-eating-disordered control subjects. *Journal of Nervous and Mental Disease*, **183**.

Ziolko, H.U. (1978). Zur Katamnese der Pubertätsmagersucht. *Archiv für Psychiatrie und Nervenkrankheiten*, **225**, 117–125.

14 Somatoform disorders and chronic physical illness

M. Elena Garralda and Luiza A.D. Rangel

In this chapter we discuss two groups of problems: somatoform disorders and chronic physical illness started in childhood. The first part of the chapter deals with risk factors and outcome of childhood somatoform disorders. Risk and prognostic factors for psychiatric disorders in children suffering from chronic physical illnesses and their long-term effects are discussed in the second part.

Somatoform disorders

Clinical picture

Classification

The somatoform disorders, as defined in current classification systems, apply across the age range to children and to adults. In ICD-10 (WHO 1994) they are characterized by repeated presentation of physical symptoms together with persistent requests for medical investigations in spite of consistently negative findings and reassurance by doctors that the symptoms have no physical basis. If any physical disorders are present, they do not explain the nature and extent of symptoms or the distress and preoccupation of the patients.

The main subcategories of somatoform disorders are as follows.

- *Somatization* disorder: here the main features are *multiple, recurrent* and frequently changing physical symptoms of at least 2 years duration. The disorder has a chronic and fluctuating cause and is often associated with disruption of social and interpersonal behaviour.
- *Hypochondriacal* disorder: the essential feature is *persistent preoccupation* with the possibility of having one or more serious and progressive physical disorders.
- Somatoform *autonomic dysfunction*: symptoms are presented by the patient as if they were due to physical disorder of a system or organ that is largely or completely under autonomic innervation, e.g. palpitations, sweating, flushing.
- Persistent somatoform *pain disorder:* here the predominant complain is persistent, severe, and distressing pain.

Other disorders classified elsewhere in ICD-10 also present with physical symptoms and share some of the main features of somatoform disorders. These disorders include

- *neurasthenia*, better known now as chronic fatigue syndrome, characterized by complaints of fatigue after effort and often associated with some decrease in coping efficiency in daily tasks.

- *dissociative disorders* with partial or complete loss of control of bodily movements; paralysis and anaesthesia may also develop closely in time with traumatic events, insoluble and intolerable problems, or disturbed relationships.

Persistent pain, dissociative disorders, and chronic fatigue syndrome are seen in children, but hypochondriacal and autonomic dysfunction somatoform disorders are probably rare. Somatization disorder as an ICD-10 diagnosis is controversial in children in that it requires the presence of at least six functional physical symptoms: due to children's comparatively limited repertoire of illness and physical symptoms it would seem less likely to be diagnosed than in adults. However, it is not rare for children with functional symptoms to have more than one physical complaint at any one time and the recent development of questionnaires for use specifically in childhood including comprehensive lists of physical symptoms should help clarify the frequency and associations of childhood somatization disorder.

Research on childhood presentations suggestive of these disorders tends not to use formal and rigorous criteria such as ICD-10 or the closely related DSM. There is usually insufficient information on the handicap caused by the symptoms, associated physical and psychiatric disorders, and patterns of medical consultation. The common denominator is normally the presence of recurrent physical symptoms without adequately explanatory physical disorder. This is close enough to the somatoform disorders to allow extrapolation of the findings and work on functional (or non-organic) physical symptoms in children will be drawn on in this chapter.

Prevalence

In the epidemiological survey by Offord *et al.* (1987) parents were asked whether their 12–16 year old children and adolescents reported somatic symptoms or seemed to them sickly: this was reported for 11% of girls and 4% of boys. In line with this, 10% of adolescents in general population studies describe frequent or persistent physical symptoms, this being more common in girls than in boys, with headaches and poor sleep being most prominent (Aro 1987). Population rates of aches and pains in children inevitably vary in different studies but there is considerable consistency to the finding that they are present in about 10% (Goodman and McGrath 1991). Many children and adolescents present to primary care and paediatric clinics with functional symptoms (8–10% in the survey by Starfield *et al.* 1980).

Most epidemiological research has focused on the presence of specific functional symptoms, particularly abdominal pains and headaches. It shows that more than 10% of children in the general population report recurrent abdominal pains severe enough to affect their daily activities (Apley and Naish 1958, Faull and Nicol 1986, Golding and Butler 1986, Zuckerman *et al.* 1987). Occasional headaches are present in as many as 50% of schoolchildren (Hockaday 1982) but migraine is less common (5–10% of 12 year olds: Bille 1962, Oster 1972, Zuckerman *et al.* 1987, Abu-Arefeh and Russell 1994).

It is not uncommon for several symptoms to occur concurrently. In an US study of schoolchildren and adolescents, 50% reported at least one somatic symptom over the previous 2 weeks, 15% had had 4 or more, and 1% more than 12 (Garber *et al.* 1991). Eminson *et al.*

(1996) have found higher rates (8%) of children with 13 symptoms or more, but this was based on 'lifetime' prevalence.

Chronic fatigue as a symptom is believed to be common in adolescence (23% of children and adolescents reported low energy levels in Garber *et al.*'s epidemiological survey) but there are no satisfactory epidemiological studies of chronic fatigue syndrome in this age group. Dissociative disorders are probably very rare and seen only in small percentages of children attending child psychiatry clinics (1–2% of referrals in the study by Leslie 1988). They are likely to be more frequent in paediatric clinics, but this has not been documented.

Clinical symptoms

Earlier reviews have shown convergence in the nature of the psychological and social factors associated with functional somatic symptoms in children and adolescents whether presenting with aches and pains, fatigue, or motor dysfunction, and whether presenting in general population settings or among children consulting medical services (Garralda 1992, 1996). Commonly a physical illness or ailment precipitates the physical complaint and may even coexist with it. Most children with symptoms suggestive of somatoform disorder do not have associated psychiatric disorders, but a third to a half may have comorbid anxiety or depressive disorders. Personality features are seen as probably contributing to the development of somatoform disorders. Children tend to be described as conscientious and obsessional, sensitive, insecure, and anxious. Family factors are also thought to be relevant, through high levels of health problems and preoccupation with illness which are likely to anxiously sensitize both children and parents to the experience of physical symptoms and lead to seeking assurance from medical services. Other features are noted in these families, including high academic and behavioural expectations. It is also suggested that a combination of emotional distance in relationships, unusually high togetherness around health issues, and anomalies in social relationships affecting intimacy are relevant factors (Garralda, 1996). Stressful events probably contribute to the onset and maintenance of somatization in children: the combination of certain child and family features may affect children's ability to modulate their response to stresses, particularly those involving threatened or actual losses.

Intervention studies

There has been little research into the treatment of functional symptoms in childhood. The few attempts at systematic evaluation of interventions have commonly been based on small numbers of children and have involved a combination of several treatment components, so that it is difficult to tease out the essential therapeutic elements. Treatments for specific problems such as abdominal pains and headaches have been devised for use in community, school, primary care, and outpatient paediatrics settings. Non-specific advice by primary care doctors tends not to be seen as helpful by mothers of children with recurrent abdominal pains (Faull and Nicol 1986), but helping parents to understand the links between psychological and physical pain is found helpful (Wasserman *et al.* 1988). Apley (1975) noted improvements in the majority of children with recurrent abdominal pains seen in paediatric outpatient clinics and managed with psychotherapeutically informed interventions aimed at identifying specific anxieties in parents and children and pointing out the associations between pain and stress.

More resolution of symptoms and fewer recurrences were reported in treated than in non-treated children.

Comparable results have been reported in small studies using behavioural techniques. Finney *et al.* (1989) treated children with recurrent abdominal pains referred to primary based paediatric psychology services by a combined therapy including self-monitoring of pain, limiting the attention given to the symptom, use of relaxation, dietary fibre supplementation, and encouragement to the child to participate in routine activities. The results indicated improvements in pain symptoms and reduced school absences. Sanders *et al.* (1989) used a comparable treatment in children with recurrent abdominal pains referred by paediatricians, family physicians, or self-referrals. They found that the treatment group tended to improve more quickly than a non-treatment group. Sanders *et al.* (1994) described the results of a controlled clinical trial involving 44 7–14 year old children with recurrent abdominal pains who were randomly allocated either to a behavioural family intervention or to standard paediatric care. Both treatment conditions resulted in significant improvements on measures of pain intensity and pain behaviour, but children under psychological intervention had a higher rate of complete elimination of pain, lower levels of relapse at 6–12 month follow-up, and less interference with their activities as a result of pain. Parents reported more satisfaction with the treatment. After controlling for pretreatment levels of pain, children's active self-coping, and mothers' care-giving strategies were significant independent predictors of pain behaviour at post-treatment.

Work carried out in school settings and paediatric outpatient clinics for adolescents with migraine and functional headaches has shown that tension headaches can be substantially improved by relaxation training. In some studies of adolescents this is superior to attention placebo control treatment and as effective whether administered at the clinic or as a home-based self-administered treatment (Larsson and Mellin 1988). McGrath *et al.* (1988) failed to report a superiority of relaxation over placebo discussions on psychological topics in young adolescents with headaches severe enough to lead to referral to migraine paediatric neurology clinics. It seems from this study that attending a clinic and receiving brief assurance and assistance was sufficient to bring relief in a number of cases, but further reports suggest that self-help relaxation treatments may be superior to a credible placebo control in reducing migraine attacks (Larsson 1992).

Accounts outlining what is regarded as clinically effective psychiatric treatment of children with conversion disorder emphasize the importance of close liaison between child psychiatrists and paediatricians and moving the emphasis from the physical to the psychological at a pace with which the family can cope (Leslie 1988, Grattam-Smith *et al.* 1988). This is frequently combined with physiotherapy and family work. Sherry *et al.* (1991) reported a favourable outcome in most children with psychosomatic musculoskeletal pain seen at a major paediatric rheumatology referral centre and treated with intensive physical and occupational therapy along with individual or family psychotherapy; 78% became symptom free or fully functional.

The importance of engaging the family in treatment seems paramount. In Vereker's (1992) small sample of children with chronic fatigue syndrome, better outcome was suggested for families who had taken up psychiatric treatment. Feder *et al.* (1994) described an intervention which they felt was successful in treating children with fatigue syndrome. This included demystifying the problem, acknowledging that the fatigue is real, providing symptomatic relief, modifying stress, decreasing secondary gain (for example extra attention from worried parents and being allowed to remain home rather than attend school), encouraging outside activities and normal functioning, and maintaining follow-up.

There is thus evidence that treatment can improve functional symptoms of various levels of severity in children in the short term. More work is required, however, to identify the most efficient treatment ingredients for different symptoms and levels of severity using methodologically strong designs. Little is known about the benefits of psychiatric treatment for adult outcome. Again, further treatment studies and their effects on long-term follow-ups are needed.

Short term and long term outcome

Short-term outcome

There is evidence for waxing and waning of functional symptoms in children. However, most studies have not examined the effects of interventions and most of what we know about outcome is from work on children who may or may not have had a variety of treatments.

Work from epidemiological general populations studies indicates that the frequency of abdominal pains increases gradually from 3 to 9 years of age and then decreases steadily up to adolescence. There are also age changes in headache frequency (Bille 1962, Oster 1972). Less severe headaches are reported for 3% of 3 year olds but as many as 20% of schoolchildren (Zuckerman et al. 1987, Bille 1962, Borge et al. 1994). Bille reported migraine in 1% of 7 year olds but in 4 times this rate (4–5%) of 12 year olds. In Oster's study the peak prevalence for headaches was at 12 years of age, 3 years later than for abdominal pains. A considerable proportion (a third to a half) of the children with headaches become symptom-free in follow-up studies.

Most evidence available from children who have been under medical care is from short-term follow-up studies. Wasserman et al. (1988) for example carried out an 8–15 month follow-up of a group of adolescents with recurrent abdominal pains. Most patients continued to have at least one episode of pain during follow-up but three-quarters of the mothers volunteered that the pain had become less intense and more manageable with the child's understanding of its nature and associations and attributed the better understanding to the psychiatric evaluation. Stickler and Murphy (1979) carried out a longer (5–10 year) follow-up of inpatient children with recurrent abdominal pains. They noted that three-quarters of their sample of 161 had recovered, mostly within a few months of admission. That left a small group running a protracted course with multiple medical investigations. Definite pathology was eventually diagnosed in 3 out of the 161 patients: 1 had anorexia nervosa and 2 had inflammatory bowel disease. This had already been strongly suspected on clinical grounds during the assessment while in hospital.

Short-term follow-up studies are available for childhood hysteria. In the study by Leslie (1988), children seen for psychiatric assessment and treatment had a particularly good outcome with symptom resolution in 85% within 3 months of starting treatment; Grattan-Smith et al. (1988) reported improvement following discharge from psychiatric treatment in 60%. Kotsopoulos and Snow (1986) reported improvements in 70% of their sample of children with a variety of conversion-like presentations, though some developed psychiatric disorders.

Similarly, short-term outcome studies are available for chronic fatigue states in childhood. In a follow-up of 55 patients 2–6 years after outpatient paediatric evaluation, 65% reported resolution of symptoms and 29% improvement, with 6% remaining unchanged. (Feder *et al.* 1994). Rangel *et al.* (1996) have documented recovery in two-thirds of severely affected patients.

In conclusion, about two-thirds of patients with functional symptoms and probable somatoform disorders seen in medical services recover in the short term (and a third to a half of all those with functional symptoms in general population epidemiological studies).

Long-term outcome

Little is known about the long-term outcome into adulthood of somatoform conditions, although it seems that it may be rather unfavourable with indications that a number of children continue to have symptoms into adulthood or experience recurrences. It is therefore possible that shorter-term follow-up gives too optimistic a picture of outcome. In a 30 year follow-up study of children with abdominal pains, Christensen and Mortensen (1975) noted that pains recurred in adult life after a pain-free period in adolescence. Half the adults with a childhood history of abdominal pains reported gastrointestinal symptoms in adulthood, with pictures consistent with 'irritable bowel syndrome' (IBS), gastritis, and, in a minority of patients, ulcers. Interestingly there was an excess of abdominal pains amongst these subjects' children.

Continuity versus discontinuity

The study of children with chronic abdominal pains by Christensen and Mortensen (1975) discussed above suggests continuities in symptomatology into adulthood, since about half those with a child history of abdominal pain continued to have gastrointestinal symptoms in adulthood. The reverse of this approach is to consider the childhood prevalence of abdominal symptoms in adults with functional gastrointestinal conditions. Again evidence of continuity is derived from the fact that histories of abdominal pain in childhood are more common amongst adult patients with IBS than amongst controls (Jones and Lydeard 1992). IBS is a somatoform-like condition. It consists of recurrent abdominal pain or discomfort associated with changes in bowel motility, frequency, and consistency. It is estimated that 20% of adults in the industrialized world suffer this syndrome: if half the children with recurrent abdominal pains (5% of the general population) go on to develop adult gastrointestinal functional conditions then about 25% of adult disorders such as IBS may have started in childhood.

Studies examining the family history of children with abdominal pains similarly demonstrate a link between childhood and adult functional pain. Thus a family history of ill health including gastrointestinal symptoms is a frequently noted feature in children with abdominal pains (Routh and Ernst 1984, Wasserman *et al.* 1988). It is difficult to know to what extent this reflects a common biological predisposition to experience gastrointestinal complaints, or whether it indicates that pain is learnt behaviour, a family means of expressing distress ,and an underlying factor for biographical and intergenerational symptom continuity. The work by Walker and Green (1989) and Walker *et al.* (1993) has confirmed high rates of family abdominal problems among children with chronic abdominal pain when compared with well children and with those with emotional disorders. The latter suggests a specificity in the relationship which cannot be explained by the coexistence of associated emotional disorders in children with recurrent pain.

Work addressing somatization disorders has demonstrated that children of affected parents have an excess of somatic complaints and days off school (Dura and Beck 1988, Livingstone 1993). The continuation of somatic problems into adulthood is further highlighted by the work of Craig *et al.* (1993). The authors found that patients presenting to general practitioners with somatization were more likely to report illness in childhood than other groups of patients with psychological problems. Little information is available on the childhood history of adults with fatigue states or conversion disorders.

The evidence quoted so far shows continuities between childhood and adult symptoms. There is insufficient evidence to know whether somatoform-type disorders in childhood are precursors for other types of psychiatric disorders. However, what seems to be clear from follow-up studies is that the symptoms are rarely explained by the development of new physical diseases. Evidence from a study of children with chronic fatigue syndrome severe enough to lead to referral to tertiary paediatric clinics suggests an excess of anxiety states in children after recovery from the fatigue state (Rangel *et al.* 1996) but this is not sufficient to conclude that the physical disorders were a precursor or manifestation of anxiety states.

Risks and prognostic factors

Do the factors thought to increase the risk for the development of somatoform disorders in childhood contribute to their continuation in childhood? This is an issue requiring further research. Prominent amongst factors deserving further enquiry are the role of child personality features, life stresses, and family physical symptoms and/or concerns that may reinforce illness behaviour in the child (Garralda 1996). Similarly, little is known about the risk factors which determine the persistence of disorder into adulthood. Most work addresses the short-term outcome of abdominal pains in children but additional information can be derived from the studies of adults which have looked back at possibly related factors present during these patients' childhood. The evidence so far suggests that in addition to severity of the problem much the same factors which contribute to the development of the disorders (e.g. child social competence, negative life events, parental somatic symptoms, beliefs regarding the physical nature of the problem, and avoidant coping strategies) play a part for their continuation.

Borge *et al.* (1994) showed a trend for 4 year olds with more frequent abdominal pain to have a worse prognosis in later childhood. Walker and Green (1991) examined the relation between negative life events and both symptom severity and symptom reduction in a follow-up study of children with recurrent abdominal pains compared with a control group of subjects with pain of organic origin. More events predicted poorer resolution of pain, but only in the functional group: in these children negative life events were also associated with continuation of anxiety symptoms. In a subsequent report Walker *et al.* (1994) examined potential moderating variables from a 1 year follow-up survey on 197 paediatric patients with abdominal pain. The moderating variables studied were child social and academic competence on the Harter questionnaire, parental somatic symptoms, and child's gender. Having fathers with high levels of somatic symptoms predicted continuation of symptoms in the child at follow-up, regardless of the presence of associated life stresses.

The relevance of mediating factors was documented as follows: high levels of negative events at follow-up were associated with more somatic symptoms but only in children low in social competence and in families with high levels of life events. Boys with mothers with many somatic symptoms also had more somatic symptoms at follow-up. This would seem to indicate that lower self-esteem and the severity of the stress increase the risk for the continuation of functional abdominal pains in children exposed to a variety of life events. Having parents with high levels of somatic symptoms would have an effect independent of life events. The indications from the adult literature are that the style of responding to life stresses is of relevance for somatization. Craig *et al.* (1994) found adult somatising patients to report more life events likely to produce symptoms of 'secondary gain' from physical illness than patients with no somatic symptoms and to be less likely than depressed patients to adopt 'neutralizing' efforts to cope with such a crisis.

The continuation of chronic fatigue syndrome at 2 year follow-up in adults has been found to be linked to the strength of the belief in a solely physical cause for symptoms, to untreated psychological distress, and to the use of avoidant coping strategies (such as reducing activity and/or dietary, social, and other restrictions) (Joint Working Group 1996). In line with this there are indications that for children with fatigue states acceptance of psychiatric treatment may be linked to a good outcome (Vereker 1992).

Over and above the tendency for symptoms to persist in a considerable number of children, little is known about the general psychiatric and social adjustment of children with somatoform disorders. Many severely affected children can clearly recover and lead full normal lives in late adolescence, but little is known about their adult adjustment.

Conclusions

It may be concluded that in spite of fluctuations there is evidence of considerable continuity into adulthood of childhood symptoms suggestive of somatoform disorders. This is demonstrated by the high percentages of affected children still having similar symptoms in adulthood and by the familial aggregation of symptoms. Psychiatric treatment has positive effects in the short term but little is known about its potential benefits for adult outcome. Life stresses, family aggregation, and the child's view of him- or herself probably contribute to the continuation of symptoms.

Chronic physical illness

Chronic physical illness in children, defined as a physical disorder which last at least 1 year and is associated with persistent or recurrent handicap of some kind, is present in about 5% of all children in western countries (Rutter *et al.* 1970, McAnerney 1985, Pless and Nolan 1991) the most common problems being asthma, eczema, and epilepsy. A number of studies have examined whether chronic physical illness affects the quality of child and family life by investigating whether it carries a high risk for psychiatric disturbance. Results have not always been consistent, but it is possible to draw some general conclusions when due note is taken of illness-related sampling and measurement issues. Other aspects of the child's emotional and social adjustment have also been addressed (i.e. self-esteem, relationships, educational progress) (McAnnerney 1985, Eiser 1990).

When assessing psychiatric adjustment a commonly used research strategy is to compare children with different physical problems. The group of conditions that have been shown convincingly to be linked to increased psychiatric risk are disorders with brain involvement and epilepsy. Breslau (1990) summarized the evidence from epidemiological surveys showing that any increase in psychiatric risk for children with chronic physical illness is to a large extent accounted for by disorders with brain involvement and epilepsy.

Clinical picture

The course of chronic illness is often punctuated by stresses and deterioration which may involve increased medical contacts, hospitalization, family disruption, and subjective distress and discomfort for child and the family. Surveys that have examined child psychiatric adjustment in relation to temporary stressful illness changes have documented a deterioration in psychiatric status at times such as when diabetes is first diagnosed, when starting dialysis treatment in children with chronic renal failure, or after transfer to adult units in youngsters with cystic fibrosis (Wass *et al.* 1977, Kovacs *et al.* 1985, Shaw 1991). Transient adjustment reactions may be the most common type of psychiatric disorder in chronically ill children.

Although there is no clear answer to the question of whether severity of physical illness influences psychiatric risk, the balance of evidence generally favours a link, with more problems in psychiatric adjustment in the more severely affected children with conditions such as eczema, diabetes, cystic fibrosis, and chronic renal failure (Steinhausen *et al.* 1983, Garralda *et al.* 1988, Pless and Nolan 1991, Daud *et al.* 1993). However, some surveys have documented an excess of behaviour problems and mood changes *specifically in school* in the *less severely affected* children (Pless and Nolan 1991). This may be a function of teachers being universally aware of illness and making allowances for more severely affected children but not for ill children with less obvious problems.

There are indications that rather than antisocial behaviour, children with non-neurological physical illness are particularly prone to develop emotional symptoms (Rutter *et al.* 1970, Pless and Nolan 1991, Daud *et al.* 1993). This may be linked to the fact that physical illness in the child can generate family and social changes known to be risk factors for the development of childhood emotional disorders. These factors include mood disorders in parents, possibly overinvolved overprotected parenting, life stresses, and general adversity (Reynolds *et al.* 1998). The reasons why many ill children develop only minor as opposed to frank emotional disorders may be partly related to the comparably lesser severity and greater versatility of stresses in ill children compared with the stresses of children who develop emotional disorders. Increased rates of minor psychiatric mobility for example are reported in parents of ill children but these can be reversed following improvement in the child's physical state (Reynolds *et al.* 1991). Moreover, heightened protective and involved parenting may be psychologically adaptive for children under stress and with special developmental needs.

In fact, given the stresses involved in childhood chronic physical illness, the good overall adjustment in the majority of children may seem surprising. Over and above the issues discussed so far, it seems highly plausible that illness mobilizes factors which are psychologically protective and contribute to the child's favourable adjustment (Eiser 1990). It has been shown that as well as increasing family stress, chronic illness in the child enhances support in a number of social areas (Reynolds *et al.* 1988). In some surveys as many parents report that the illness results in greater support as in increased stress for their marriage. However, marital breakdown is overall not increased in the families of children with chronic illness (Sabbeth and Leventhal 1984). Chronic illness may lead to heightened parental empathy and sympathy towards the child, and in young children it does not appear to affect the security of parent–child attachments in the absence of repeated potentially stressful separations (Daud *et al.* 1993). In addition, distressing experiences, if adequately handled, may promote or at any rate not adversely affect coping.

Intervention studies

Virtually all children with chronic physical illness surviving into adulthood have had repeated contacts with paediatric units and this often involves attention to psychosocial issues. In the longitudinal population study by Pless *et al.* (1989), subjects who had been chronically physically ill had received medical treatment for emotional disorders significantly more often than the rest of the population. Being known to medical services would have increased the chance of emotional problems being recognized and of having access to psychiatric help. In the study by Morton *et al.* (1994), 47% of adult renal survivors compared with 17% healthy controls reported psychiatric problems in childhood or adolescence and, in line with this, treatment for psychological problems was significantly more common amongst the renal group (27% versus 2%). In contrast, although significantly more *adult* patients were taking psychotropic medication, particularly night sedation when admitted to hospital, they had not had more contact with psychiatric services than healthy controls in adulthood. In the work by Mayou *et al.* (1991), higher hospital admission rates in a diabetic sample were associated with more psychiatric disorder and worse glycaemic control, again suggesting high likelihood of recognition and attention to psychiatric problems amongst ill subjects.

Long-term outcome

A significant increase in knowledge has accrued over recent years on long-term adult outcome as opposed to short-term outcome of childhood chronic illness has, and this forms the basis of the following discussion.

Despite the diverse nature of chronic physical illnesses in childhood it has been widely assumed that overall they have the potential for causing significant and permanent interference with physical and emotionally growth and development. As discussed above, chronic physical illness in childhood does affect psychiatric health and it is reasonable to assume that the accumulation of stress reactions in childhood should lead to increased psychiatric morbidity in adulthood.

The existing evidence in fact suggests that the adult adjustment of children surviving chronic physical illness is not compromised. Pless *et al.* (1989) reported a population-based longitudinal study of children with physical disorders. A total birth cohort was followed up for 36 years. Out of a total of 5362 children, 10% had had a chronic physical illness and nearly 500 with childhood chronic illness were identified in adulthood. As adults they were significantly more likely than other adults to have been in hospital with a seriously incapacitating illness for a minimum of 28 consecutive days or away from work or seriously incapacitated for a period of 3 weeks. Even so they accounted for a relatively small proportion (about a fifth) of incapacitating illness in adult life. Although between 15 and 26 years of age they had reported more emotional problems than other cohort members, psychiatric research interviews at 36 years of age revealed no significant increase of emotional problems in this group.

The findings were confirmed in a Finnish study by Kokkonen and Kokkonen (1993): psychiatric disorder was not significantly increased in young adults with a history of chronic illness in childhood when compared with healthy controls. It was noted, however, that patients with chronic disease had *more severe* psychiatric disorders and those with the more severe physical illness were the ones more likely to have psychiatric disorders.

Discontinuities in psychiatric adjustment and better outcome in adulthood than in childhood is further suggested by work on adults who have had surgical correction for congenital heart disease in childhood (Utens *et al.* 1994) and from a study in early adulthood of 45 survivors of childhood end-stage chronic renal failure (ESCRF) (Morton *et al.* 1994). When compared with age- and sex-matched community healthy controls, young adult ESCRF survivors reported significantly more episodes of psychiatric disturbance before (including illness-related problems such needle phobias and other problems of adjustment to dialyses) but not after 17 years of age. Most patients had had successful transplants and were in relatively good health but they had a number of factors implying risks for psychiatric disorder including an excess of psychiatric problems in childhood, long experience of severe physical illness, lower self-esteem in adulthood, and reduced social and work achievement. The authors noted a trend in the renal group for more severe depressive disorders and suicidal behaviour (the rates for major depressive disorder were twice those of controls and comparable to those from studies of adult patients with ESCRF) as well as a tendency to attribute psychological problems to events related to the physical condition.

High rates of depressive disorder have also been found in survivors of other childhood illnesses (Kokkonen and Kokkonen 1993). Life with chronic illness is not uncommonly punctuated by discouraging recurrences and complications, and by having to cope with the death of others with a similar condition: understandably, this could lead to periods of profound despair in a minority of subjects. However, illness may have had a protective effect towards some behaviours such as alcohol and other substance abuse (Pless *et al.* 1993, Morton *et al.* 1994). This suggests both risk and protective aspects of chronic illness in relation to adult psychiatric morbidity. In concluding that psychiatric adjustment is better in adulthood than in childhood it must be noted that a number of children do not survive and those may have been most severely affected in childhood, both physically and psychologically.

Closer continuities between childhood and adult psychiatric adjustment have been reported for children with chronic illnesses characteristically affecting the brain. Breslau and Marshall (1985) carried out a 5 year follow-up of 255 children with physical disabilities who had been 6–18 years of age at first assessment. Children with cystic fibrosis followed a trend toward better adjustment in contrast with children with conditions involving the brain. The majority of the latter who had been classified as psychologically severely impaired remained at this level of impairment 5 years later. The outcome may, however, be more favourable with longer follow-up. In a long-term outcome study of children with temporal lobe seizures, the majority of whom had had associated psychiatric disorders in childhood, Lindsay *et al.* (1979) found an increased risk for schizophrenia (10%) but 70% of those survivors who were not gravely mentally retarded were psychiatrically healthy.

In the follow-up study by Mayou *et al.* (1991), psychiatric disorder and subthreshold psychological distress were greater among young adults with insulin-dependent diabetes (most probably starting in childhood) than in comparable general population surveys. In this study 12% of men and 19% of women had psychiatric disorders of mild to moderate severity and diabetic control was significantly worse in subjects with higher levels of psychological distress. There was, however, no study comparison group and it is not clear therefore whether psychiatric outcome is less favourable in young adults with diabetes than in those with other disorders.

Considerable interest has been directed at the study of the social adjustment of adults with a history of chronic illness in childhood. Pless *et al.* (1993) found a remarkably good social prognosis in their chronically physically ill sample. The majority of patients had very similar chances of marriage and of becoming parents as those who had been healthy in childhood and they differed little on such indicators as everyday social life, contacts with friends, going out, and belonging to clubs. Social adversity was linked to unfavourable outcome, and ill children from lower social groups had a greater chance of childhood mortality, significantly reduced educational achievement at school, employment opportunities, and chances of home ownership.

In the study by Reynolds *et al.* (1993), young adult renal patients were less socially mature than healthy controls: more of them lived with their parents, fewer had an intimate relationship outside the family, they had fewer school qualifications and more unemployment. Early start of illness and current health problems were associated with poorer social outcome. The majority of patients, however, were in employment and the level of subjective stress and support derived from most social areas explored was comparable in renal patients and in controls. Having a close relationship with a member of the opposite sex was the only domain for which renal patients reported more stress than controls. The authors concluded that a life long history of renal failure leads to suboptimal or delayed social functioning on conventional indicators, but this does not imply increased subjective distress by patients and quality of life does not appear to be substantially impaired. This would suggest that patients develop during childhood appropriate, realistic expectations with regard to social and personal life which may be different from those of their age peers.

In terms of educational performance, patients had entered adult life with fewer educational qualifications. This was not due to premature school leaving, as more patients than controls had gone on to further education. It was more likely to be due to poor school performance, since most patients felt their schooling had been affected by illness or treatment and by the difficulties in keeping up with the work. Emphasizing the importance of school attendance in ill children can minimize school absence (Sturge *et al.* 1997) but in addition it seems important to actively promote ways of optimizing children's educational performance.

Problems in social adjustment have been found to be linked to difficulties caused by the illness and to psychiatric adjustment in some studies (Mayou *et al.* 1991, Morton *et al.* 1994, Kokkonen 1995) but the associations between social maturity and physical handicap may become less pronounced as patients get older (Beck *et al.* 1986).

Follow-up of patients with cystic fibrosis (Walters *et al.* 1993) indicates that most adults live fulfilling lives in spite of some qualitative differences in social functioning from the norm, with for example fewer middle-range but more higher-level educational qualifications, less marriage in men and more employment. In Walter *et al.*'s ill sample, employed subjects had had less than 2 weeks' sick leave a year but half of those not employed gave ill health as a reason for their unemployment. Many patients said that they never revealed their cystic fibrosis at job interviews and those who did were less likely to be employed, though this may be accounted for by those with less severe conditions being able to disguise their disease more easily.

Ross *et al.* (1992) carried out a 22 year follow-up study of patients with wheezing in childhood. They showed asthmatic subjects to be comparable in a number of social indicators to those who had wheezed only in the presence of upper respiratory tract infections and to a comparison group who had had no respiratory symptoms as children. Social indicators included educational attainment, employment, housing, and eventual social class. However, the majority of children had had asthma of only mild or moderate intensity and the results might not have apply to more severely affected subjects.

Eiser and Havermans (1994) described the long-term social adjustment of childhood cancer. On the whole the results were positive. Survivors had a good adjustment and generally achieved life goals comparable to those in the general population. Educational level seemed similar or slightly above population levels, but males may have been rejected from military service more and fewer women were married. Survivors treated for central nervous symptoms tumours may have more problems in social areas. It was noted that many youngsters reported changes in academic plans and in career goals and some reported job discrimination. The authors noted that survivors and their families may revise their views about what is important in life and adapt their lives accordingly.

Continuity and discontinuity

The studies quoted above suggest continuities in the *type* of psychiatric disorders associated with chronic illness, with trends for more depressive and anxiety disorders in adult survivors than in healthy controls in line with the suggested increases of emotional disorders in ill children (Pless *et al.* 1989, Mayou *et al.* 1991, Morton *et al.* 1994, Garralda 1994).

As discussed above there is considerable discontinuity in *levels* of psychiatric disturbance amongst adult survivors of chronic physical childhood illness, except perhaps for those with conditions affecting the brain, but there is probably continuity in the types of disorders when present (mood disorders and illness-related problems).

Risks and prognostic factors

It seems likely that severity of the physical disorder and brain involvement are risk factors not only for the development of psychiatric disorders in ill children but also for the continuation of psychiatric morbidity in adult survivors. Pless *et al.* (1989) for example found that the proportion with psychiatric problems was greatest for those with severe disabilities. In young adults with juvenile arthritis, links have been shown between feelings of depression and severity of disability (David *et al.* 1994). Young adults who have had surgical correction for congenital heart disease in childhood have if anything a better psychological outcome than healthy controls, but the degree to which health is affected following the surgical repair in childhood is not always clear (Utens *et al.* 1994). In the study by Breslau and Marshall (1985), children with physical disabilities and conditions involving the brain (i.e. cerebral palsy, myelodysplasia, and multiple physical handicaps) maintained high scores particularly in domains addressing behaviour and isolation. The latter was directly related to level of mental retardation but the authors found that brain involvement conferred a risk for social isolation quite independently of retardation. In Lindsay *et al.*'s (1979) follow-up of children with temporal lobe seizures, patients 'escaping psychiatric illness' were found to be notably extroverted and successful.

Further information on risk factors is provided by the study by Morton *et al.* (1994) of young adult survivors of ESCRF. No significant associations were found within the renal group between psychiatric disorder and treatment status (i.e. transplant or dialysis), age at onset of symptoms or of renal replacement therapy, final height achieved, or stigmatizing physical signs, though in many cases (18/21) psychiatric disorder appeared to be directly precipitated or influenced by renal disease and treatment. The minority of patients with multiple psychiatric disorders differed from other ESCRF survivors by having increased social dysfunction (for example fewer educational qualifications and more problems in relationships) and decreased self-esteem, and in addition the majority (5/7) had had psychological problems in childhood or adolescence. These may be risk factors for severe psychiatric disorders in adulthood.

In contrast with the generally favourable psychiatric adjustment of adult survivors of childhood chronic illness, a number of reports indicate difficulties in the area of self-esteem. In the follow-up study by Morton *et al.* (1994) renal patients had scores on the Rosenberg scales indicating significantly decreased self-esteem. Stepwise discriminant statistical analysis showed the main predictors of self-esteem to be lack of educational achievement, early onset of symptoms of renal disease, unemployment, living with parents, recollections of lack of maternal care in childhood and a history of more than one psychiatric disorder since age 17. Current treatment status—whether on dialysis or post-transplant—did not contribute. Self-esteem is seen as linked to a sense of having control over the direction of one's life. Living with an illness such as renal failure challenges the sense of control, but in this sample it would seem that this had a significant effect only if the problem had started early in childhood, if it had affected education substantially, and if there had been psychiatric problems in childhood.

Beck *et al.* (1986) found a trend towards lower self-esteem amongst ESCRF patients with more visible handicaps (cushingoid appearance, transplant scars, atypical height and proportions) but visibility of handicap may have been confounded by other factors such as illness severity, prognosis, duration, and age, and Morton *et al.* (1994) did not find a contributory effect for growth problems or physical stigma. The work by Beck *et al.* suggests the beneficial effects of time and age. They found that older patients and those with longer elapsed time since transplant had higher self-esteem and were less anxious than younger patients. Several patients remarked that although they had been self-conscious earlier, particularly during their adolescent years, they had grown used to their appearance and were not bothered as much by peoples' reactions to them. Some had compensated by excelling academically or sharing their feelings with other patients, and some drew upon their religious beliefs. Similar attitudes and achievement orientation may have contributed to the particularly favourable outcome in terms of self-esteem reported by adults with a history of surgical correction for heart disease in childhood (Utens *et al.* 1994).

Conclusions

It may be concluded that although psychiatric disorders—particularly adjustment disorders to illness-related stresses—are increased in ill children, the psychiatric adjustment of adult survivors is not substantially compromised. There is in fact some evidence for better adjustment with older age in adults. There may be an increased risk for adult depression but a decreased risk for substance abuse. Childhood illness may increase the chances that emotional problems are attended to but it is not known whether and how this contributes to the generally favourable psychosocial adjustment of adult survivors of childhood illness. Brain involvement and severity of the physical condition are probably risk factors for psychiatric morbidity in adulthood. In spite of qualitative differences in the social adjustment of adult survivors of illness when compared with population norms, most present as subjectively well adjusted with preserved quality of life

References

Abu-Arefeh, I. and Russell, G. (1994). Prevalence of headache and migraine in schoolchildren. *British Medical Journal*, **309**, 765–769.

Apley, J. (1975). *The child with abdominal pains*. Blackwell Scientific, Oxford.

Apley, J. and Naish, N. (1958). Recurrent abdominal pains: a field survey of 11,000 school children. *Archives of Disease in Childhood*, 33, 165–170.

Aro, H. (1987). Life stress and psychosomatic symptoms among 14–16 year of Finnish adolescents. *Psychological Medicine*, 17, 191–201.

Beck, A.L., Nethercut, G.E., and Crittenden, M.R (1986). Visibility of handicap, self-concept, and social maturity among young adult survivors of end-stage renal disease. *Development and Behavioural Pediatrics*, **7**, 93–96.

Bille, B. (1962). Migraine in children. *Acta Paediatrica*, **51** (Suppl. 136).

Borge, A.I.H., Nordhagen, R., Moe, B., Botten, G., and Bakketeig, L.S. (1994). Prevalence and persistence of stomach and headache among children. Follow-up of a cohort of Norwegian children from 4 to 10 years of age. *Acta Paediatrica*, **83**, 433–437.

Breslau, N. (1990). Chronic physical illness. In *Handbook of studies on child psychiatry*, ed. B.J. Tonge, G. Burrows, and J.S. Werry, Elsevier, Amsterdam.

Breslau, N. and Marshall, I.A. (1985). Psychological disturbance in children with physical disabilities: continuity and change in a 5-year follow-up. *Journal of Abnormal Child Psychology*, **13**, 199–216.

Christensen, M.F. and Mortensen, O. (1975). Long-term prognosis in children with recurrent abdominal pain. *Archives of Disease in Childhood*, **50**, 110–114.

Craig, T.K.J., Boardman, A.P., Mills, K., Daly-Jones, O., and Drake, H. (1993). The South London Somatisation study I: longitudinal course and the influence of early life experiences. *British Journal of Psychiatry*, **163**, 579–588.

Craig, T.K.L., Drake, H., Mills, K., and Boardman, A.P. (1994). The South London Somatisation study II: influence of stressful life events and secondary gain. *British Journal of Psychiatry*, **165**, 248–258.

Daud, L.R., Garralda, M.E., and David, T.J. (1993). Psychosocial adjustment in pre-school children with atopic dermatitis. *Archives of Disease in Childhood*, **69**, 670–676.

David, J., Cooper, C., Hickey, L., Lloyd, J., Dore, C., McCullough, C., Woo, P. (1994). The functional and psychological outcomes of juvenile chronic arthritis in young adulthood. *British Journal of Rheumatology*, **33**, 876–881.

Dura, J.R. and Beck, S.J. (1988). A comparison of family functioning when mothers have chronic pain. *Pain*, **35**, 79–89.

Eminson, M., Benjamin, S., Shortall, A., and Woods, T. (1996). Physical symptoms and illness attitudes in adolescents: an epidemiological study. *Journal of Child Psychology and Psychiatry*, **37**, 519–528.

Eiser, C. (1990). *Chronic illness disease: an introduction to psychological theory and research.* Cambridge University Press, Cambridge.

Eiser, C. and Havermans, T. (1994). Long term social adjustment after treatment for childhood cancer. *Archives of Disease in Childhood*, **70**, 66–70.

Faull, C. and Nicol, A.R. (1986). Abdominal pain in six-year-olds: an epidemiological study in a new town. *Journal of Child Psychology and Psychiatry*, **27**, 251–260.

Feder, H., Dworkin, P., and Orkin, C. (1994). Outcome of 48 pediatric patients with chronic fatigue; a clinical experience. *Archives of Family Medicine*, **3**, 1049–1055.

Finney, J.W., Lemanek, K.L., Cataldo, M.F. Katz., H.P., and Fuqua, R.W. (1989). Pediatric psychology in primary health care: brief targeted therapy for recurrent abdominal pain. *Behavioural Therapy*, **20**, 283–291.

Garber, J., Walker, L.S., and Zeman, J. (1991). Somatisation symptoms in a community sample of children and adolescents: further validation of the childrens somatisation inventory. *Journal of Consulting and Clinical Psychology*, **3**, 588–595.

Garralda, M.E., Jameson, R.A., and Reynolds, J.M. (1988). Psychiatric adjustment in children with chronic renal failure. *Journal of Child Psychology and Psychiatry*, **29**, 79–90.

Garralda, M.E. (1992). A selective review of child psychiatric syndromes with a somatic presentation. *British Journal of Psychiatry*, **161**, 759–773.

Garralda, M.E. (1994). Chronic physical illness and emotional disorder in childhood. *British Journal of Psychiatry*, **164**, 8–10.

Garralda, M.E. (1996). Somatization in children. *Journal of Child Psychology and Psychiatry*, **37**, 13–33.

Golding, J. and Butler, N.R. (1986). Headaches and stomach aches. In *From birth to five*, ed. N.R. Butler and J. Golding, Chapter 9. Pergamon Press, Oxford.

Goodman, J.E. and McGrath, P.J. (1991). The epidemiology of pain in children and adolescents: a review. *Pain*, **46**, 247–264.

Grattan-Smith, P., Fairley, M., and Procopis, P. (1988). Clinical features of conversion disorder. *Archives of Disease in Childhood*, **63**, 408–414.

Hockaday, J.M. (1982). Headache in children. *British Journal of Hospital Medicine*, **27**, 383–391.

Joint Working Group (1996). *Chronic fatigue syndrome*. Report, Royal College of Physicians, London.

Jones, R. and Lydeard, S. (1992). Irritable bowel syndrome in the general population. *British Medical Journal*, **304**, 87–90.

Kokkonen, J. (1995). The social effects in adult life of chronic physical illness since childhood. *European Journal of Pediatrics*, **154**, 676–681.

Kokkonen, J. and Kokkonen, E-R. (1993). Prevalence of mental disorders in young adults with chronic physical disease since childhood as identified by the Present State Examination and the CATEGO program. *Acta Psychiatrica Scandinavica*, **87**, 239–243.

Kotsopoulos, S. and Snow, B. (1986). Conversion disorders in children: a study of clinical outcome. *Psychiatric Journal of the University of Ottawa*, **11**, 134–139.

Kovacs, M., Feinberg, T.L., Paulauskas, S., Finkelstein, R., Pollock, M., Crouse-Novak, M. (1985). Initial coping responses and psychosocial characteristics of children with insulin-dependent diabetes mellitus. *Journal of Pediatrics*, **106**, 827–834.

Larsson, B. (1992). Behavioural treatment of somatic disorders in children and adolescents. *European Child and Adolescent Psychiatry*, **1**, 68–81.

Larsson, B. and Mellin, L. (1988). The psychological treatment of recurrent headache in adolescents-short term outcome and its prediction. *Headache*, **28**, 187–195.

Leslie, S.A. (1988). Diagnosis and treatment of hysterical conversion reactions. *Archives of Disease in Childhood*, **63**, 506–511.

Lindsay, J., Ounsted, C., and Richards, P. (1979). Long-term outcome in children with temporal lobe seizures. iii: psychiatric aspects in childhood and adult life. *Development Medicine and Child Neurology*, **21**, 630–636.

Livingstone, R. (1993). Children of people with somatisation disorder. Journal of American Child Adolescent Psychiatry, 32: 536–544.

Mayou, R., Peveler, R., Davies, B., Mann, J., and Fairburn, C. (1991). Psychiatric morbidity in young adults with insulin-dependent diabetes mellitus. *Psychological Medicine*, **21**, 639–645.

McAnarney, E.R. (1985). A challenge for handicapped and chronically ill adolescents. *Journal of Adolescent Health Care*, 6, 90–101.

McGrath, P.J., Humphreys, P., Goodman, J.T., Keene, D., Firestone, P., Jacob, P., and Cunningham, S.J. (1988). Relaxation prophylaxis for childhood migraine a randomised placebo-controlled trial. *Development Medicine and Child Neurology*, **30**, 626–631.

Morton, M.J.S., Reynolds, J.M., Garralda, M.E., Postlethwaite, R.J., and Goh, D. (1994). Psychiatric adjustment in end stage renal disease: a follow-up study of former paediatric patients. *Journal of Psychosomatic Research*, **38**, 293–303.

Offord, D.R., Boyle, M.H., Szatmari, P., Rae-Grant, N.I., Links, P.S., Cadman, D.T., Byles, J.A., Crawford, J.W., Munroe, B.H., Byrne, C., Thomas, H., and Woodward, C.A. (1987). Ontario child health study. II. Six-month prevalence of disorder and rates of service utilization. *Archives of General Psychiatry*, **44**, 833–836.

Oster, J. (1972). Recurrent abdominal pain, headache and limb pains in children and adolescents. *Pediatrics*, **50**, 429–436.

Pless, I.B. and Nolan, T. (1991). Revision, replication and neglect—research on maladjustment in chronic illness. *Journal of Child Psychology and Psychiatry*, **22**, 347–365.

Pless, I.B., Cripps, H.A., Davies, M.J.C., and Wadsworth, M.E.J. (1989). Chronic physical illness in childhood: psychological and social effects in adolescence and adult life. *Development Medicine and Child Neurology*, **31**, 746–755.

Pless, I.B., Power, C., and Peckham, C.S. (1993). Long-term psychosocial sequelae of chronic physical disorders in childhood. *Pediatrics*, **91**, 1131–1136.

Rangel, L. Garralda, M.E., Levin, M., Roberts, H. (1996). A follow-up study of children and adolescents with fatigue syndrome. Paper presented at 43rd Annual Meeting of the American Academy of Child and Adolescent Psychiatry, Philadelphia, P.A.

Reynolds, J.M., Garralda, M.E., Jameson, R.A., and Postlethwaite, R.J. (1988). How parents and families cope with chronic renal failure. *Archives of Disease in Childhood*, **63**, 821–826.

Reynolds, J.M., Garralda, M.E., Postlethwaite, R., and Goh, D. (1991). Changes in psychosocial adjustment following renal transplantation. *Archives of Disease in Childhood*, **66**, 508–513.

Reynolds, J.M., Morton, M.J.S., Garralda, M.E., Postlethwaite, R.J., and Goh, D. (1993). Psychosocial adjustment of adult survivors of a paediatric dialysis and transplant programme. *Archives of Disease in Childhood*, **68**, 104–110.

Ross, S., Godden, D., McMurray, D., Douglas, A., Oldham, D., Friend, J., Legge, J., and Douglas, G. (1992). Social effects of wheeze in childhood: 25 year follow up. *British Medical Journal*, **305**, 545–548.

Routh, D.K. and Ernst, A.R. (1984). Somatization disorder in relatives of children and adolescents with functional abdominal pain. *Journal of Pediatric Psychology*, **9**, 427–437.

Rutter, M., Tizard, J., and Whitmore, K. (1970). *Education, health and behaviour*. Longman, London.

Sabbeth, B. and Leventhal, J. (1984). Marital adjustment to chronic childhood illness: a critique of the literature. *Pediatrics*, **73**, 762–768.

Sanders, M.R., Rebgetz, M., Morrison, M., Bor, W., Gordon, G., and Dadds, M. (1989). Cognitive-behavioural treatment of recurrent nonspecific abdominal paIn an analysis of generalisation, maintenance, and side effects. *Journal of Consulting and Clinical Psychology*, **57**, 294–300.

Sanders, M.R., Shepherd, R.W., Cleghorn, G., and Woodford, H. (1994). Treatment of recurrent abdominal pain in children: a controlled comparison of cognitive behavioural family intervention and standard paediatric care. *Journal of Consulting and Clinical Psychology*, **62**, 306–314.

Shaw, J. (1991). Psychosocial adjustment in patients with cystic fibrosis. MPhil thesis, University of Manchester.

Sherry, D.D., McGuire, T., Mellins, E., Salmonson, K., Wallace, C.A., and Nepom, B. (1991). Psychosomatic musculoskeletal pain in childhood: clinical and psychological analyses of 100 children. *Pediatrics*, **88**, 1093–1099.

Starfield, B., Gross, E., Wood, M., Pantell, R., Allen, C., Gordon, B., Moffatt, P., Drachman, R., and Katz, H. (1980). Psychosocial and psychosomatic diagnoses in primary care of children. *Paediatrics*, **66**, 159–167.

Steinhausen, H., Schindler, H., Stephen, H. (1983). Correlates of psychopathology in sick children: an empirical model. *Journal of the American Academy of Child Psychiatry*, **22**, 559–564.

Stickler, G.B. and Murphy, D.B. (1979). Recurrent abdominal pain. *American Journal of Diseases of Children*, **133**, 486–489.

Sturge, C., Garralda, M.E., Boissin, M., Dore, C.J., Woo, P. (1997). School attendance and juvenile chronic arthritis. *British Journal of Rheumatology*, **36**, 1218–1223.

Utens, E.M.W.J., Verhulst, F.C., Erdman, R.A.M., Meijboom, F.J., Duivenvoorden, H.J., Bos, E., Roelandt, J.R.T.C., and Hess, J. (1994). Psychosocial functioning of young adults after surgical correction for congenital heart disease in childhood: a follow-up study. *Journal of Psychosomatic Research*, **38**, 745–758.

Vereker, M. (1992). Chronic fatigue syndrome: a joint paediatric–psychiatric approach. *Archives of Disease of Childhood*, **67**, 505–555.

Walker, L.S. and Greene, J.W. (1989). Children with recurrent abdominal pain and their parents: more somatic complaints, anxiety, and depression than other patient families? *Journal of Pediatric Psychology*, **14**, 231–243.

Walker, L.S., and Greene, J. (1991). Negative life events and symptom resolution in pediatric abdominal pain patients. *Journal of Pediatric Psychology*, **16**, 341–360.

Walker, L.S., Garber, J., and Greene, J.W. (1993). Psychosocial correlates of recurrent childhood pain—a comparison of pediatric patients with recurrent abdominal pain, organic illness and psychiatric disorders. *Journal of Abdominal Psychology*, **102**, 248–258.

Walker, L.S., Garber, J., and Greene, J.W. (1994). Somatic complaints in pediatric patients: a prospective study of the role of negative life events, child social and academic competence and parental somatic symptoms. *Journal of Consulting and Clinical Psychology*, **62**, 1213–1221.

Walters, S. Brittion, J., and Hodson, M.E. (1993). Demographic and social characteristics of adults with cystic fibrosis in the United Kingdom. *British Medical Journal*, **306**, 549–552.

Wass, V.J., Barratt, T.M., Howart, R.V., Marshall, W.A., Chantler, C., Ogg, C.S., Cameron, J.S. Baillod, R.A., and Moorhead, J.F. (1977). Home dialysis in children. *Lancet*, **i**, 242–246.

Wasserman, A.L. Whittington, P.F., and Rivara, F. (1988). Psychogenic basis for abdominal pain in children and adolescents. *Journal of American Academy of Child and Adolescent Psychiatry*, **27**, 179–184.

WHO (1994). *Pocket guide to the ICD-10 classification of mental and behavioural disorders with glossary and diagnostic criteria for research: ICD-10: DCR-10*. Churchill Livingstone, London.

Zuckerman, B., Stevenson, J., and Bailey, V. (1987). Stomach aches and headaches in a community sample of preschool children. *Pediatrics*, **79**, 677–682.

15 Autism spectrum disorders

Christopher Gillberg

Clinical picture

Autism has proved to be a valid phenomenological description of a developmental disorder that is recognizable across the life-span and across different cultures. At the same time, it is a heterogeneous syndrome, co-occurring with a variety of abilities and disabilities. Several subcategories of autism spectrum disorders—or, to use the terminology of DSM-IV (APA 1994) and ICD-10 (WHO 1992), 'pervasive developmental disorders'—exist, including autistic disorder, Asperger syndrome, and disintegrative disorder.

All autism spectrum disorders are characterized by symptoms from the so-called triad of social, communication, and imagination impairments (Wing and Gould 1979). The impairment in reciprocal social interaction is severe and affects peer relationships, ability to share with others, and social and emotional reciprocity. The impairment in reciprocal communication affects verbal and non-verbal functions. The restriction of imaginative abilities results in concrete thinking, a restriction of the behavioural repertoire with motor stereotypies, narrow interest patterns, and ritualistic behaviours of various kinds. Abnormal responses to sensory stimuli, hyperactivity, self-injurious behaviours, eating disorders, and sleep problems are all common, but are not included among the diagnostic criteria.

The symptom pattern in classic *autistic disorder* is seen most clearly in children with mild–moderate mental retardation. About half of this group have no speech and usually do much better on performance than on verbal tasks at neuropsychological testing. Those who do speak usually start late and show prolonged periods of echolalia. Motor stereotypies are often very pronounced. The full syndrome is usually well recognized before the child's third birthday. Some children are clearly deviant from the beginning of life, but others appear to have normal or almost normal development during the first 18–24 months (Volkmar and Cohen 1989). The frequency of autistic disorder appears to be around 1 in 1000 children (Gillberg 1995).

The DSM-IV (APA 1994) and ICD-10 (WHO 1992) criteria for autistic disorder are very similar. The diagnostic criteria for autistic disorder/infantile autism have changed several times in the last 20 years. It is not clear how these changes may be reflected in outcome variation, but it is clear that the overlap between DSM-III (APA 1980), DSM-III-R (APA 1987), and DSM-IV (APA 1994) criteria is nowhere near complete (Sponheim *et al.* 1996).

Children with *Asperger syndrome* are usually of low normal, normal, or superior general intelligence and have similar but more subtle abnormalities. They may be perceived as relatively normal early on, even though completely normal social and language development is the exception. Verbal competencies are often better than perceptual abilities. It is more common than autistic disorder, possibly around 3–4 in 1000 children (Ehlers and Gillberg 1993).

The Gillberg and Gillberg (1989) criteria were the first published operationalized criteria for Asperger syndrome, based specifically on Asperger's own descriptions of his syndrome. The DSM-IV-concept (APA 1994) does not identify Asperger's 'autistic psychopathy' as outlined by the man behind the syndrome (Miller and Ozonoff 1997). The major issues under debate is (a) whether Asperger syndrome and autistic disorder are completely separate—for instance in terms of early social and language development—and (b) whether a diagnosis of one can later be changed to the other.

Disintegrative disorder is symptomatically similar to autistic disorder, but onset of clinically striking problems is after age 3 years. It is very rare, and appears to occur in fewer than 2 in 100 000 children (Burd *et al.* 1989).

In other disorders on the autism spectrum (including 'atypical autism' (WHO 1992), 'other autistic-like condition' (Nordin and Gillberg 1997), and 'pervasive developmental disorder not otherwise specified' (APA 1994)), the symptom pattern is atypical and full criteria for any of the aforementioned categories are not met.

Studies of natural course

There have been several studies of the natural course of autistic disorder, but only a handful of such studies in the field of other disorders on the autism spectrum. Autism, like other developmental disorders, shows changes with age in respect of prevailing symptomatology (Rutter 1978, Waterhouse and Fein 1984, Frith 1989, Wing 1989, Gillberg *et al.* 1990, Frith 1991, Wing 1996).

Analysis of videotapes from the first birthday have demonstrated subtle abnormalities in social behaviours in children with autism compared to those with subsequent normal development (Osterling and Dawson 1992). In the majority of cases, children with autism can be distinguished from normal and also from related developmental disorders around 2 years of age (Dahlgren and Gillberg 1989, Gillberg *et al.* 1990, Baron-Cohen *et al.* 1992, Lord 1995). In these young children, there might be an overlap in symptomatology between autism and other communication disorders and global mental retardation. Also, there might be transient patterns of autism in normal children and in those with severe brain pathology, e.g. as described by Chess (1977) in her follow-up of children with rubella embryopathy.

The pattern of classical autism is most often recognized in children during the preschool years, especially in children who also have global mental retardation. The standard diagnostic criteria might not be met at a young mental age, because a certain developmental level is needed for some behaviours to emerge. This results in diagnostic challenges in cases of autism combined with severe mental retardation, where it sometimes takes until the age of 4–5 years for the clinical picture to be clear. Later, developmental changes occur that may give rise to new diagnostic difficulties. Therefore, for older children and adolescents, it is often helpful to review the characteristics and behaviours that occurred around the ages of 4–5 years (Le Couteur *et al.* 1989).

In some children with normal intellectual ability, autism spectrum problems may not be obvious until the age of 6–8 years or even later. For these children also, subsequent development further increases the difficulty of reaching a correct diagnosis. There is a certain risk that the underlying developmental disorder will never be identified in these children with a more atypical autism pattern, including those with Asperger syndrome.

Wing (1983, 1987) has outlined three major subtypes of individuals who were once diagnosed with childhood autism: the aloof group, the passive group, and the active but odd group.

Empirical support for this subgrouping has been provided by studies of adolescents and young adults in Göteborg and Umeå, Sweden (Gillberg and Steffenburg 1987, von Knorring and Hägglöf 1993) and, recently, in reports on preschool children (Waterhouse *et al.* 1996). Incidentally, even though not formally delineated, there were clear indications in Kanner's writings that this subtyping would have been relevant among his cases also (Kanner 1971).

- The *aloof group* comprises those individuals who retain characteristics of autistic aloneness. They appear to prefer to be left alone and even to withdraw actively from the proximity of other human beings. It may not be as obviously apparent in adult age, but the aloofness shows in the company of others in that the individual with autism does not readily react to other people's questions or approaches. Adult people with autism in this group cause problems mostly if demands are made. They may be quite easy to 'handle' if they are left completely to themselves. On the other hand, leaving them alone quickly leads to the deterioration of acquired and self-help skills.

- The *passive group* may also appear aloof. However, approaches by both strangers and well-known people are accepted in a quite friendly manner. They may have 'automatic' imitation skills enabling them to participate in some social activities without appearing extremely odd, just as long as reciprocal social interaction is not demanded. Change of routines may be very upsetting to this group, as well as to the aloof and active groups. Because of the overall friendly attitude of passive people with autism, disturbed behaviour in connection with change may be especially alarming. Unless those living with or caring for these individuals are well informed, tragic mistakes may be made, such as expulsion from a secure group or admission for psychiatric treatment in an emergency ward.

- In the *active but odd group*, behaviour problems are common. On the surface, grown-ups in this group appear to be totally unlike those in the other two groups, but they share the lack of reciprocity. The active group tends to approach other people with physical touching if mute, or constant repetitive questioning if speaking. Endless monologues or questioning may seem rather harmless, but anyone who has been confronted with this behaviour for any length of time, and learned that answering leads to even further repetitions of the same questions, knows how wearing and frustrating it is.

Within these three groups there is, of course, considerable variation. Some people may show characteristics of more than one subtype. Personality differences naturally play an essential role in all cases. The dominating pattern of behaviour may emerge in situations with special demands of social interaction, e.g. for children in situations of unstructured play. Lorna Wing has described changes from one type of social interaction to another in some individuals. The most typical changes seem to be from the aloof group to the passive or to the active but odd group. Rarely, individuals with autism become less interactive, i.e. more aloof, with the years.

Waterhouse *et al.* (1996) looked at the Wing subtypes and other diagnostic differences among preschool children with social impairment. They found two overlapping patterns. One group included most of the aloof cases. This group had high scores on diagnostic instruments, little or no speech, and severe developmental impairment. The other group included the majority of cases with active but odd social interaction. This group often had a diagnosis of 'other pervasive developmental disorder' (i.e. less severe or atypical forms of autism spectrum disorders), higher IQ, and better adaptive functioning but more repetitive and ritualistic behaviours than the first group. The passive type of social interaction was found in both groups. The sample has been followed up well into school age and the data suggests that there is stability with regard to subtype in this perspective.

Intervention studies

Given the serious implications of a diagnosis of autism, it is slightly surprising that intervention studies have been relatively few and far between.

Special education and behavioural modification have proved themselves to be worthwhile features of several intervention programmes (Keel *et al.* 1997, Howlin 1997). Improvements in the areas of behaviour problems and communication, although not dramatic, are usually clearly evident with a psychoeducational approach such as that advocated by proponents of the TEACCH (Treatment and Education of Autistic and Communication handicapped CHildren) philosophy. Behaviour modification is moderately effective, at least in the short to intermediate term (Howlin and Rutter 1987). Some studies (e.g. Lovaas 1989) have indicated major gains with rigorous behaviour therapy.

Some medications (e.g. haloperidol) ameliorate some symptoms of autism (Campbell 1989), but are not extensively used in clinical practice because of a high risk of extrapyramidal and other side-effects (Gillberg 1997a,b). Many newer drugs—including the atypical neuroleptics and selective serotonin reuptake inhibitors (SSRIs)—are being evaluated in autistic disorder and Asperger syndrome, but little is known about their role in treatment of autism spectrum disorders at the time of going to press with this book.

When children are diagnosed or suspected of having autism at an early age, e.g. 2 years, then subsequent development to normal or to another related disorder is not exceedingly rare (discussed in the section on symptom patterns). Conversely, some children with autism and severe cognitive disorders may have been missed at initial screening. Therefore, when judging results of follow-up and intervention studies, the age of the sample at diagnosis is an important factor (Tossebro 1990).

Participants in the TEACCH programme had better academic performances than a comparable sample 15–20 years earlier (Venter *et al.* 1992). Better structured and more continuous education was thought to be the reason for this improvement. However, the pupils with autism in this recent study did not show results that were in level with their IQ, e.g. problems with reading comprehension were noted. One report mentioned some increase of IQ as a result of one preschool year of intensive educational intervention (Harris *et al.* 1991). The same degree of IQ change has been found in children with other types of developmental disorders, e.g. developmental language disorders (Field *et al.* 1990). In an epidemiological study there was an average 15-point discrepancy in IQ between children from two geographical regions; one possible explanation could be fewer services available for children under 5 years old in the population with lower IQ (Bryson 1996). The study by Lovaas (1989) indicated major therapeutic gains after intensive training of relatively high-functioning preschool children with autism, but, so far, this spectacular result has not been replicated by other groups, and it is uncertain whether the findings are applicable in the low-functioning group of individuals with the disorder. Further studies are needed to demonstrate clear and lasting effects of early interventions. One aspect of interest is the risk of secondary deprivation from environmental stimuli because of the child's disabilities, and the possibility to counteract this by early start of services.

A small fraction of all persons with autism develop into rather normal grown-ups. In most follow-up studies (Gillberg 1991) they constitute no more than a small percentage of all cases with autism. Among over 700 children with autism seen over a 20 year period in the Department of Child and Adolescent Psychiatry in Göteborg, we have followed at least a dozen, who, under age 5 years, showed all the characteristics of Kanner autism, but 10 years later were only a little odd, had some peculiarities of spoken language, and had one or more age peers. Cases such as these are often regarded as related to 'cures' of various kinds rather than as examples of different developmental pathways. However, there is not enough evidence to suggest that any intervention can so dramatically alter the course of autism that it is reasonable to speak of a cure. Some positive aspects can be found in most programmes (Howlin 1997). The most successful intervention programmes are built on knowledge of autism, and they are realistic and have long-term goals. Treatment is individualized and based on support for, and cooperation with, families.

Short-and long-term outcomes

A lot is known about outcome—both in the shorter- and longer-term perspective—in autistic disorder, and there is a small literature on disintegrative disorder and other autistic-like conditions. Little study has so far been devoted to the long-term outcome of representative groups of individuals with Asperger syndrome.

Adolescence

Symptom aggravation and deterioration

Several authors (Brown 1969, Rutter 1970, Kanner 1971, Gillberg and Schaumann 1981, Gillberg and Steffenburg 1987, von Knorring and Hägglöf 1993) have described cases of autism who show clear deterioration in adolescence. According to these studies, 12–22% of children with autism can be expected to show cognitive and behavioural deterioration in puberty accompanied by a regression and reappearance of many of the symptoms typical of the preschool period (Gillberg 1991). Unfortunately, so far, prospective neurobiological studies of deteriorating autism cases have not been reported. Gillberg and Schaumann (1981) and Gillberg and Steffenburg (1987) have suggested that low IQ, epilepsy, female sex, and a family history of affective disorders might increase the risk of deterioration in puberty in autism.

In the cases without clear deterioration, there is also often a period with aggravation of symptoms at the onset of puberty, or a year before or after. Self-destructiveness, explosive changes of mood, aggressiveness, restlessness, and hyperactivity may be found. In the Göteborg studies (Gillberg and Steffenburg 1987), such aggravation has been observed in about half of all cases with classic autism or autistic-like conditions. There is a tendency for periodicity, in some cases with a return to 'normal' for at least weeks or months and then new periods of exacerbation of negative behavioural symptoms. This seems to be particularly common if there is a family history of affective disorder (see below).

The pubertal symptom aggravation, whether accompanied by deterioration or not, very often prompts some kind of medication. In one study, before puberty, less than 1 in 4 children with autism was on medication affecting the nervous system, whereas at age 16–23 years, 3 out of 4 were given such treatment (Gillberg and Steffenburg 1987). Although most medications prescribed in the pubertal period appear to do little to alter the negative course, our clinical impression has been that lithium can sometimes be effective in controlling pubertal behavioural/ 'mood' swings in autism (Campbell 1989). There are case histories where SSRIs or haloperidol have been of help. There is large interindividual variation in the effectivity of medication; no standard treatment can be described; long-term sequelae (e.g. of haloperidol treatment) must be taken into consideration.

It is important to point out that some of the 'pubertal symptom aggravation' may also be the effect of the sheer physical growth in size and strength of the person with autism. Teachers and parents come to realize that the behaviours and problems shown by the child with autism will probably continue into adult life and will stand out as even more deviant in an adolescent or adult than in a child.

Improvement

Many children with autism go through their teens without more behaviour problems than are usually associated with puberty in normal children (Gillberg and Steffenburg 1987). Some children improve perceptibly during the teenage period (Kanner 1972). These are usually children with relatively good cognitive abilities, who have also shown positive development during the early school years (Szatmari *et al.* 1989). In a study from Japan, Kobayashi *et al.* (1992) found that 43% of a group of about 200 individuals with autism had clear improvement during the teenage period, mostly between 10 and 15 years of age (however, in 32% there was deterioration).

Szatmari *et al.* (1989) commented on the positive development that often occurred in late adolescence. The parents of the subjects in their study with good outcome had worked very hard for their children, e.g. to avail themselves and their children of resources for education and recreation, but the data did not allow conclusions on the significance of these efforts for the positive prognosis.

Inactivity

The marked overactivity seen in many young children with autism is often followed by a state of 'underactivity' in adolescence (Wing 1996). There may sometimes be an extreme degree of 'psychomotor retardation' and a total or almost total lack of initiative and yet no clear indications of depressive feelings (Rutter 1970). When growing up, people with autism—like other individuals—often lose their interest in playing with objects, doing puzzles, and having playful motor activities. They have more problems than usual in finding new hobbies and new ways of getting exercise, so the risk of inactivity is high.

Changes in physical appearance

Among children with autism and mental retardation or borderline intellectual functioning, physical changes sometimes occur, so that pretty, bright-looking children may come out of puberty looking more deviant and 'dull'. This can, very occasionally, be due to an underlying medical disorder such as tuberous sclerosis or neurofibromatosis, which may produce skin problems and other physically visible changes only after infancy and childhood (Gillberg and Coleman 1992).

Problems associated with sexual maturation

For most individuals with autism, puberty is not associated with serious problems connected with sexual maturation. Many parents of girls with autism worry about what might happen in connection with the onset of menstruation. Often these changes are accepted by the child in a very matter of fact way (Wing 1980). The growth of sexual drive, as a rule, is not accompanied by a corresponding growth in the field of social 'know-how', and this may lead to embarrassing behaviours. This appears to be particularly true of moderately and severely retarded boys with autism, who may expose themselves or masturbate in public (Gillberg 1984). Sometimes the sexual behaviour is 'interpreted' in quite sophisticated terms: however, one simple explanation for what we consider inappropriate sexual behaviour is that the young boy with autism is doing one of the few pleasurable things he knows how to do in life. The social and planning deficits associated with autism preclude the planning of such activities in ways which will be socially acceptable to other people. It is usually easy to diminish the extent to which the person with autism masturbates by introducing other interesting activities as a substitute.

Some people with autism may be involved unintentionally in homo- or heterosexual contacts (Haracopos 1988) for the simple reason that they may be lacking in reticence and suspiciousness to such an extent that they may be taken advantage of sexually.

Depression and periodicity

Feelings of unhappiness and/or depression are often reported, and may be particularly likely to occur in high-functioning autism or Asperger syndrome (Wing 1981, Tantam 1988). These better-functioning individuals may become painfully aware that they are different from other adolescents. A few develop a strong desire for friendship, but may be totally unable to establish social relationships because they lack the necessary skills. Social skills groups, role-playing, and videotape feedback followed by systematic training may be useful when trying to teach youngsters with autism the requirements of social interaction and conversation. Such measures may help alleviate depressive feelings. Sometimes, individual supportive psycho-therapy also is indicated. Medication is rarely used, but tricyclic antidepressants and SSRIs can sometimes contribute to reducing depressive symptoms in autism.

There are several clinical accounts (Coleman 1976, Wing 1983, Gillberg 1984) and a few systematic studies (Gillberg and Steffenburg 1987) acknowledging a periodic intensification of symptoms in the autistic syndromes. This periodicity may be particularly prominent in puberty (Komoto et al. 1984). However, after thorough interviewing of the parents it is often evident that it has been present from the onset in infancy or early childhood.

In children of families with affective disorder, there is sometimes a typical episode of major depression associated with autism. This might represent a more primary depressive disorder. There is now accumulating evidence that autism may be associated with a family history of affective disorder (Lotter 1967, DeLong and Dwyer 1988, DeLong and Nohria 1994, Smalley *et al.* 1995). Early authors generally tended to attribute conditions such as recurrent depression in the parents to reactions against the situation with the handicapped child. Later writers have considered genetic factors instead. It is likely that a hereditary trait of periodicity exists in some cases of autism in which parents and other relatives have shown major affective disorders.

Catatonia

Wing and Shah (1994) and Wing (1996) have drawn attention to a group of relatively high-functioning individuals with autism or Asperger syndrome who develop pronounced catatonic features in late adolescence. In a follow-up study currently in progress of individuals diagnosed in early childhood as suffering from autism or autistic-like condition, at least 3 out of 46 cases showed moderate to severe catatonia at age 28–35 years (Gillberg 1996, unpublished). A young German woman with classic childhood autism and severe catatonia recently published an autobiography, originally written in Norwegian, but translated into Swedish (Schäfer 1996).

Epilepsy and other medical conditions

There are idiopathic' cases of autism and cases described in connection with a variety of other neurological/medical disorders. The chain of cause and effect is seldom clear. The comorbid conditions may

- be part of the pathogenetic process (as important causes of brain dysfunction or as modifying factors)
- have the same background as autism, i.e. be parallel manifestations, or
- occur at random.

For children with autism and a medical disorder, the general outcome will depend—to a greater or lesser extent—on the art and course of that disorder. For example, it is clear that outcomes in autism with Angelman syndrome or tuberous sclerosis are different from those of autism associated with the fragile X syndrome (Gillberg 1991). Medical investigations and treatment can seldom radically change the prognosis for subjects with autism. Nevertheless, it is important to consider the potential benefits of medical intervention in all cases and use the same principles as in other neurological and neurodevelopmental disorders, i.e. individualized programmes, regular follow-up, and renewed investigations when needed. Impairment of vision and hearing must be detected.

Children with autism quite often have epilepsy, either from their first years of life or with onset during childhood and adolescense. It seems that around 20–30% of all people with autism develop epilepsy before age 30 years (Rutter 1970, Gillberg and Steffenburg 1987, Olsson *et al.* 1988, Volkmar and Nelson 1990, Rossi *et al.* 1995). The risk of epilepsy is highest among people with the combination of autism and severe mental retardation, but the rate is increased in those of normal intelligence also (Gillberg and Steffenburg 1987, Olsson *et al.* 1988, Goode *et al.* 1994).

Developmental disorders such as autism and/or language dysfunction and co-occurring epilepsy often have a common background in brain dysfunction. In some cases, epileptic processes in themselves seem to be the cause of behavioural and developmental disorders

(Deonna 1993, Tuchman 1994). Epileptic discharges without clinical seizures may under certain circumstances be of pathogenetic importance. In many but not all of these complex cases, it is possible to improve the situation by medical treatment.

In the past there has been much controversy as to whether to include children with obvious brain dysfunction in the category of autism or not. Some would still argue for the exclusion of those with major neurological impairment. The onset of epilepsy in adolescents with autism who previously demonstrated no signs of neurological dysfunction demonstrates the impossibility of such a position. At the present time, there is no way of predicting in early childhood (the time when autism is most often diagnosed) just who will experience seizures later in life.

Mortality

According to a review of the outcome literature in autism, mortality in the age group 2–30 years may be significantly increased (Gillberg 1991). Even though it is hard to compare mortality rates across western countries, it appears that mortality after the first year of life up until about age 30 years might be increased from about 0.6% in the general population to almost 2% in autism. The higher rate in autism could be accounted for by the association of autism with severe mental retardation and certain severe medical conditions, such as epilepsy (Goode *et al.* 1994).

Continuity versus discontinuity

Ideally, outcome studies should be prospective, longitudinal, and population-based. There should be clear descriptions of comorbid conditions (in the case of autism these should include mental retardation, language deficits, affective disorders, obsessive–compulsive disorders, and medical syndromes). The long-term effects of the different conditions and their possible interactions need to be evaluated.

Several follow-up studies reporting on the overall outcome for children diagnosed as suffering from autism, childhood psychosis, or autistic-like conditions have been published. The outcome studies published up to the mid 1970s were closely examined by Lotter (1978). Only a few of these studies presented enough detail to allow conclusions. They all yielded remarkably consistent results, in spite of the fact that only one was population-based (Lotter 1974). In the 1980s only one more population-based follow-up study was published (Gillberg and Steffenburg 1987). A further follow-up study of a population-based cohort was reported in the early 1990s (von Knorring and Hägglöf 1993). These reports also showed results which corroborated the findings from the previous studies. In all the studies published, a poor or very poor outcome with regard to social adjustment, and with a high degree of stability of the diagnosis of autism, was seen in 60–75% of the cases followed up to preadolescence or early adult life. A good outcome with near normal or normal social life and acceptable functioning at work or school in spite of certain difficulties in social relationships and oddities in behaviour—and few, if any clear symptoms of autism—was seen in 5–15% of the cases. In the studies mentioned, 40–55% of the people with autism/childhood psychosis had been placed in institutions at follow-up.

Risks and prognostic factors

General cognitive level

Possibly the single best predictor of outcome is IQ rating at the time of diagnosis in childhood (Rutter 1970, Lotter 1978, Gillberg and Steffenburg 1987, Gillberg 1991). On the whole, IQ remains as stable throughout childhood for children with autism as for normal or mentally retarded children (Rutter 1983, Lord and Schopler 1989, Freeman et al. 1991).

Those who have an IQ of less than 50 before age 5–6 years are likely to have a poor, or very poor, prognosis regarding social functioning. In those with higher IQ it is much more difficult to make a reliable prediction of outcome. Findings of poor social outcome are to be expected in populations with severe mental retardation, with or without autism. Almost no one with an IQ under 50 can be expected to live independently. The prognosis need not be as 'bad' when looking at other factors (such as personal wellbeing and meaningful tasks in daily life). Therefore, there is a need for more specific instruments in order to differentiate outcome. Van Bourgondien *et al.* (1989) from the TEACCH program have compared adults with autism and mental retardation to those with the same degree of redardation but no autism. The former group had higher frequency of ritualistic behaviours and need for sameness, a greater likelihood of becoming anxious, more odd behaviours, greater difficulties entertaining themselves, and more isolation from others.

The few published follow-up studies (all clinic-based) focusing specifically on high-functioning people with autism (Szatmari *et al.* 1989, Rumsey and Hamburger 1988, Venter *et al.* 1992) suggest that outcome is considerably better than in children with autism and low IQ. Quite a number of such cases actually have a fair prognosis and may be able to hold on to qualified jobs, live independent lives, and even marry and raise children (Wing 1981, Szatmari *et al.* 1989). Even so, the prognosis for this group is severely restricted as compared with people without autism. The Vineland Adaptive Behavior Scale (VABS; Sparrow *et al.* 1984) has been used in recent studies to characterize social and adaptive development. In the Szatmari *et al.* study (1989), 12 out of 16 (75%) individuals with autism and childhood IQ in excess of 65 had a Vineland Social Development Quotient of 70 or greater at ages 17–34 years. In contrast, Venter *et al.* (1992) found only 3 of 22 (14%) individuals with autism and IQ in the low normal or normal range had a Vineland Quotient in the same range at ages 18–37 years. This is surprising given that a prerequisite for entry into the latter study was availability of adequate schooling and being raised in a family setting. One reason for the discrepant findings is the high rate of attrition in the study by Szatmari. Another possible reason is that both studies included clinical rather than epidemiological cohorts, with all the variability in clinical severity that may stem from this.

Schatz and Hamdan-Allen (1995) compared IQ and VABS scores in children with autism and/or mental retardation. With increasing IQ level, children with mental retardation but no autism also had correspondingly higher social skills according to the VABS. For children with autism, higher IQ did not mean the same increase in VABS score. Thus, the discrepancy between IQ and social quotient tends to be small or non-existent in children with autism combined with severe mental retardation and larger when children have autism without general intellectual dysfunction.

Church and Coplan (1995) described in detail the course of 15 children with autism and IQ over 70; initially all cases met the DSM-III-R criteria for autism. The course was highly variable, but there was improvement concerning the obvious autistic traits in all children (at follow-up no child met the full criteria for autism). All had persistent problems, often school-related and centred around social skill deficits and 'labelling'. Many subjects were misunderstood and did not get the most adequate help at school, when they no longer had the 'label' of autism. The authors concluded from the parent reports that early services had been important for the children's progress

A number of cases in this group have major psychiatric problems. However, conclusions are rendered difficult because of the clinical nature of the samples studied.

Communication

All the follow-up studies agree that the absence of communicative speech at age 5–6 years is indicative of a worse long-term overall outcome. There is a clear covariation between IQ and level of communication, but probably there is some prognostic factor in language development apart from this. In follow-up of subjects with severe receptive language difficulties, many of them show social deficits in adult life (but not of the same magnitude as in autism) (Rutter *et al.* 1992).

Speech as a prognostic indicator is useful for group effects but not always for individual children. Even in those who show no intelligible speech at 5 years of age (about half the group with classical autism) there may later be major speech development and a fair overall outcome. Occasionally one comes across a child who unexpectedly starts to talk or communicate at age 10 or even later.

Efforts have been made to find what variables are most important for a subsequent development of speech. Signs of social responsiveness as well as the capacities to produce phonemes and imitate words are of interest (Windsor *et al.* 1994). Mundy *et al.* (1990) demonstrated, in a small sample of children with autism, that non-verbal joint attention skills were a predictor of language development.

Neuropsychological deficits

Measures of flexibility and cognitive shifting abilities tended to be good predictors of social outcome in a few studies (Szatmari *et al.* 1989, Berger *et al.* 1993), and it is possible that in the future more refined neuropsychological tests will help us develop better prognostic instruments in autism spectrum disorders.

Ozonoff and McEvoy (1994) found stable deficiencies in both executive function and theory of mind tests in individuals with autism during a 3 year period; a comparison group with learning disabilities matched on IQ had improvement of test results in relation to increase in mental age. Ozonoff and Miller (1995) studied the effect of a program to teach theory of mind to a small group of adolescents with autism and normal IQ. A meaningful increase of test results was demonstrated. No change was found in broader ratings of social competence. Further studies of longer duration are needed to assess the generalization of the abilities.

Difficulties in understanding affective states and sharing emotions with other people are important components of the communicative and social deficits. Stability of individual patterns of responsiveness to affects of other people has been demonstrated in studies of children with autism tested during the preschool period and then after 5 years' follow-up (Dissanayake *et al.* 1996). At all periods, the responsiveness and empathy ratings were related to the cognitive level of the individual child.

A study by Klin *et al.* (1995) showed concordance between the neuropsychological profiles of subjects (at least a subgroup) with Asperger syndrome and subjects with the non-verbal learning disability syndrome, a condition which has much in common with developmental learning disabilities caused by right hemisphere damages. Findings like this underscore the importance of detailed neuropsychological testing so that specific deficits and capacities may be discovered and serve as a basis for intervention. Such intervention has proved to be of help for individuals with non-verbal learning disabilities (Rourke 1989).

Other autism spectrum disorders

It is reasonable to assume that the Asperger group, often of average or above average intelligence, would have a considerably better outcome than those with classic autism. It is also clear that many have excellent outcomes, at least if the ability to intuitively reciprocate in social interaction is disregarded. Some individuals have a poor outcome, with a variety of psychiatric, and more sociologically derived, diagnostic labels applied to them in adult age. It seems that suicidal acts, atypical depression, and alcoholism may all occur at increased rates in Asperger syndrome (Wing 1981, Wolff 1995, Gillberg and Ehlers 1998).

Individuals who have autistic-like conditions and mental retardation at levels similar to those encountered in autism seem to have outcomes that correspond to those seen in classic autism.

Conclusions

For the most part, we must retain a cautious attitude when discussing outcome in autism with parents. The majority of children with autism will show deviance and socially or psychiatrically handicapping conditions throughout life, but others will improve enough to make it possible to lead an (almost) independent adult life. The level of mental retardation and other comorbid conditions (such as medical syndromes and other neuropsychiatric disorders) are important, but in the young child there is no certain way of knowing to which of these two broad outcome groups the child will later belong.

There is a continued need for prospective, longitudinal studies of children with autism spectrum disorders. The role of interventions of various kinds needs to be addressed in such studies. We do not yet know to what extent any of the currently used interventions may alter ultimate outcome. Nevertheless, short- and intermediate-term benefits have been documented after specific treatments.

What is perhaps most needed in future follow-up studies is a measure of quality of life, and not just of whether an individual has improved with regard to the basic impairments. There is no clear correlation between the severity of symptoms and personal experiences (in autism or in other dysfunctions). The reactions among people in and around the family and the availability of services will determine the degree of handicap for the individual and the family. For individuals with normal or near normal intellectual ability, a diffuse notion of 'something wrong' might lead to more suffering than would a straightforward outline of objective deficits and abilities.

References

APA (1980). *Diagnostic and statistical manual of mental disorders*, 3rd edn. American Psychiatric Association. Washington, D.C.

APA (1987). *Diagnostic and statistical manual of mental disorders*, 3rd edn, revised. American Psychiatric Association, Washington, D.C.

APA (1994). *Diagnostic and statistical manual of mental disorders*, 4th edn. American Psychiatric Association, Washington, D.C.

Baron-Cohen, S., Allen, J., and Gillberg, C. (1992). Can autism be detected at 18 months? The needle, the haystack and the CHAT. *British Journal of Psychiatry*, **161**, 839–843.

Berger, H., van Spaendonck, K., Horstink, M., and Buytenhuijs, E. (1993). Cognitive shifting as a predictor of progress in social understanding in high-functioning adolescents with autism: a prospective study. *Journal of Autism and Developmental Disorders*, **23**, 341–359.

Brown, W.T. (1969). Adolescent development of children with infantile psychosis. *Seminars in Psychiatry*, **1**, 79–89.

Bryson, S. (1996). Brief report: Epidemiology of autism. *Journal of Autism and Developmental Disorders*, **26**, 165–167.

Burd, L., Fisher, W., and Kerbeshian, J. (1989). Pervasive disintegrative disorder: are Rett syndrome and Heller dementia infantilis subtypes? *Developmental Medicine and Child Neurology*, **31**, 609–616.

Campbell, M. (1989). Pharmacotherapy in autism: An overview. In *Diagnosis and treatment of autism*, ed. C. Gillberg, pp. 203–218. Plenum, New York.

Chess, S. (1977). Follow-up report on autism in congenital rubella. *Journal of Autism and Childhood Schizophrenia*, **7**, 68–81.

Church, C.C. and Coplan, J. (1995). The high-functioning autistic experience: birth to preteen years. *Journal of Pediatric Health Care*, **9**, 22–29.

Coleman, M. (ed.) (1976). *The Autistic Syndromes*. North-Holland, Amsterdam.

Dahlgren, S.O. and Gillberg, C. (1989). Symptoms in the first two years of life. A preliminary population study of infantile autism. *European Archives of Psychiatry and Neurological Sciences*, **238**, 169–174.

DeLong, G.R. and Dwyer, J.T. (1988). Correlation of family history with specific autistic subgroups: Asperger s syndrome and bipolar affective disease. *Journal of Autism and Developmental Disorders*, **18**, 593–600.

DeLong, R. and Nohria, C. (1994). Psychiatric family history and neurological disease in autism spectrum disorders. *Developmental Medicine and Child Neurology*, **36**, 441–448.

Deonna, T. (1993). Annotation: cognitive and behavioural correlates of epileptic activity in children. *Journal of Child Psychology and Psychiatry*, **34**, 611–620.

Dissanayake, C., Sigman, M., and Kasari, C. (1996). Long-term stability of individual differences in the emotional responsiveness of children with autism. *Journal of Child Psychogy and Psychiatry*, **25**, 415–433.

Ehlers, S. and Gillberg, C. (1993). The epidemiology of Asperger syndrome. A total population study. *Journal of Child Psychology and Psychiatry*, **34**, 1327–1350.

Field, M., Fox, N., Radcliffe, J. (1990). Predicting IQ changes in preschoolers with developmental delay. *Journal of Developmental and Behavioural Pediatrics*, **11**, 184–189.

Freeman, B.J., Rahbar, B., Ritvo, E.R., Bice, T.L., Yokota, A., and Ritvo, R. (1991). The stability of cognitive and behavioral parameters in autism: A twelve-year prospective study. *Journal of the American Academy of Child and Adolescent Psychiatry*, **30**, 479–482.

Frith, U. (1989). *Autism: explaining the enigma*. Basil Blackwell, Oxford.

Frith, U. (ed.) (1991). *Autism and asperger syndrome*. Cambridge University Press, Cambridge.

Gillberg, C. (1984). Autistic children growing up: problems during puberty and adolescence. *Developmental Medicine and Child Neurology*, **26**, 125–129.

Gillberg, C. (1991). Outcome in autism and autistic-like conditions. *Journal of the American Academy of Child and Adolescent Psychiatry*, **30**, 375–382.

Gillberg, C. (1995). The prevalence of autism and autism spectrum disorders. In *The epidemiology of child and adolescent psychopathology*, ed. F.C. Verhulst and H.M. Koot, pp. 227–257. Oxford University Press, Oxford.

Gillberg, C. (1997a). Neuroleptikabehandling av barn och ungdomar. *SBU rapport—Behandling med neuroleptika*. Volym 1, kapitel 10, sid. 193–208. (In Swedish)

Gillberg, C. (1997b). Neuroleptikabehandling vid utvecklingsstörning. *SBU rapport—Behandling med neuroleptika*. Volym 1, kapitel 11, sid. 209–217. (In Swedish)

Gillberg, C. and Coleman, M. (1992). *The biology of the autistic syndromes*, 2nd edn. MacKeith Press, London.

Gillberg, C., and Ehlers, S. (1998). High-functioning people with autism and Asperger syndrome. A literature review. In Schopler, E., Mesibov, G., and Kunce, L. (Eds.) *Asperger syndrome or high functioning autism?* pp. 79–106. New York, Plenum.

Gillberg, I.C. and Gillberg, C. (1989). Asperger syndrome—some epidemiological considerations: a research note. *Journal of Child Psychology and Psychiatry*, **30**, 631–638.

Gillberg, C. and Schaumann, H. (1981). Infantile autism and puberty. *Journal of Autism and Developmental Disorders*, **11**, 365–371.

Gillberg, C. and Steffenburg, S. (1987). Outcome and prognostic factors in infantile autism and similar conditions: a population-based study of 46 cases followed through puberty. *Journal of Autism and Developmental Disorders*, **17**, 273–287.

Gillberg, C., Ehlers, S., Schaumann, H., Jakobsson, G., Dahlgren, S.O., Lindblom, R., Bågenholm, A., Tjuus, T., and Blidner, E. (1990). Autism under age 3 years: a clinical study of 28 cases referred for autistic symptoms in infancy. *Journal of Child Psychology and Psychiatry*, **31**, 921–934.

Goode, S., Rutter, M., and Howlin, P. (1994). A 20-year follow-up of children with autism. Paper presented at the 13th Biennial Meetings of ISSBD, Amsterdam.

Haracopos, D. (1988). *Hvad med mig?* Andonia, Svendborg, Denmark.

Harris, S.L., Handleman, J.S., Gordon, R., Kristoff, B., and Fuentes, F. (1991). Changes in cognitive and language functioning of preschool children with autism. *Journal of Autism and Developmental Disorders*, **21**, 281–290.

Howlin, P. (1977). Prognosis in autism? Do specialist treatments affect long-term outcome? *European Child and Adolescent Psychiatry*, **6**, 55–72.

Howlin, P. and Rutter, M. (1987). *Treatment of autistic children*. Wiley, London.

Kanner, L. (1971). Follow-up study of eleven children originally reported in 1943. *Journal of Autism and Childhood Schizophrenia*, **1**, 119–145.

Kanner, L. (1972). How far can children with autism go in matters of social adaptation? *Journal of Autism and Childhood Schizophrenia*, **2**, 9–33.

Keel, J.H., Mesibov, G.B., and Woods, A.V. (1997). TEACCH-supported employment program. *Journal of Autism and Developmental Disorders*, **27**, 3–9.

Klin, A., Volkmar, F.R., Sparrow, S.S., Cichetti, D.V., and Rourke, B.P. (1995). Validity and neuropsychological characterization of Asperger syndrome: convergence with nonverbal learning disabilities syndrome. *Journal of Child Psychology and Psychiatry*, **36**, 1127–1140.

Kobayashi, R., Murata, T., and Yoshinaga, K. (1992). A follow-up study of 201 children with autism in Kyushu and Yamaguchi areas, Japan. *Journal of Autism and Developmental Disorders*, **22**, 395–411.

Komoto, J., Udsui, S., Otsuki, S., and Terao, A. (1984). Infantile autism and Duchenne muscular dystrophy. *Journal of Autism and Developmental Disorders*, **14**, 191–195.

Le Couteur, A., Rutter, M., Lord, C., Rios, P., Robertson, S., Holdgrafer, M., and McLennan, J. (1989). Autism diagnostic interview: a standardized investigator-based instrument. *Journal of Autism and Developmental Disorders*, **19**, 363–387.

Lord, C. (1995). Follow-up of two-year-olds referred for possible autism. *Journal of Child Psychology and Psychiatry*, **36**, 1365–1382.

Lord, C. and Schopler, E. (1989). The role of age at assessment, developmental level, and test in the stability of intelligence scores in young autistic children. *Journal of Autism and Developmental Disorders*, **19**, 483–499.

Lotter, V. (1967). Epidemiology of autistic conditions in young children. II. Some characteristics of the parents and children. *Seminars in Psychiatry*, **1**, 163–173.

Lotter, V. (1974). Factors related to outcome in autistic children. *Journal of Autism and Childhood Schizophrenia*, **4**, 263–277.

Lotter, V. (1978). Follow-up studies. In *Autism: A reappraisal of concepts and treatment*, ed. M. Rutter and E. Schopler, pp. 475–495. Plenum, New York.

Lovaas, I., Calouri, K., and Jada, J. (1989). The nature of behavioural treatment and research with young autistic persons. In *Diagnosis and treatment of autism*, ed. C. Gillberg, pp. 285–305. Plenum, New York.

Miller, J.N. and Ozonoff, S. (1997). Did Asperger's cases have Asperger disorders? A research note. *Journal of Child Psychology and Psychiatry*, **38**, 247–251.

Mundy, P., Sigman, M., and Kasari, C. (1990). A longitudinal study of joint attention and language development in autistic children. *Journal of Autism and Developmental Disorders*, **20**, 115–128.

Nordin, V. and Gillberg, C. (1998). The long-term course of autistic disorders: update on follow-up studies. *Acta Psychiatrica Scandinavica*, **97**, 99–108.

Olsson, I., Steffenburg, S., and Gillberg, C. (1988). Epilepsy in autism and autistic-like conditions: a population-based study. *Archives of Neurology*, **45**, 666–668.

Osterling, J. and Dawson, G. (1992). Early recognition of children with autism: a study of first birthday home videotapes. *Journal of Autism and Developmental Disorders*, **24**, 247–259.

Ozonoff, S. and McEvoy, R.E. (1994). A longitudinal study of executive function and theory of mind development in autism. *Development and Psychopathology*, **6**, 415–431.

Ozonoff, S. and Miller, J.N. (1995). Teaching theory of mind: A new approach to social skills training for individuals with autism. *Journal of Autism and Developmental Disorders*, **25**, 415–433.

Rossi, P.G., Parmeggiani, A., Bach, V., Santucci, M., and Visconti, P. (1995). EEG features and epilepsy in patients with autism. *Brain and Development*, **17**, 169–174.

Rourke, B. (1989). *Nonverbal learning disabilities: the syndrome and the model.* Guilford, New York.

Rumsey, J.M. and Hamburger, S.D. (1988). Neuropsychological findings in high-functioning men with infantile autism, residual state. *Journal of Clinical and Experimental Neuropsychology*, **10**, 201–221.

Rutter, M. (1970). Autistic children: infancy to adulthood. *Seminars in Psychiatry*, **2**, 435–450.

Rutter, M. (1978). Diagnosis and definition. In *Autism. A reappraisal of concepts and treatment*, ed. M. Rutter and E. Schopler, pp. 1–25. Plenum, New York.

Rutter, M. (1983). Cognitive deficits in the pathogenesis of autism. *Journal of Child Psychology and Psychiatry*, **24**, 513–531.

Rutter, M., Mawhood, L., and Howlin, P. (1992). Language delay and social development. In *Specific speech and language disorders in children*, ed. R. Fletcher and D. Hall, pp. 63–78. Whurr, London.

Schatz, J. and Hamdan-Allen, G. (1995). Effects of age and IQ on adaptive behavior domains for children with autism. *Journal of Autism and Developmental Disorders*, **25**, 51–60.

Schäfer, S. (1996). *Stjärnor, linser och äpplen. Att leva med autism.* Cura, Stockholm. (In Swedish).

Smalley, S.L., McCracken, J., and Tanguay, P. (1995). Autism, affective disorders, and social phobia. *American Journal of Medical Genetics (Neuropsychiatric Genetics)*, **60**, 19–26.

Sparrow, S.S., Balla, D.A., and Cicchetti, D.V. (1984). *The Vineland Adaptive Behavior Scales.* American Guidance Service, Circle Pines, M.N.

Sponheim, E. (1996). Changing criteria of autistic disorders: A comparison of the ICD-10 research criteria and DSM-IV with DSM-III-R., CARS., and ABC. *Journal of Autism and Developmental Disorders*, **26**, 513–525.

Szatmari, P., Bartolucci, G., Brenner, R., Bond, S., and Rich, S. (1989). A follow-up study of high-functioning autistic children. *Journal of Autism and Developmental Disorders*, **19**, 213–225.

Tantam, D. (1988). Asperger's syndrome. *Journal of Child Psychology and Psychiatry*, **29**, 245–255.

Tossebro, J. (1990). Utviklingsprognose ved autism—en advarsel mot mirakelkurer. *Glasskulen*, **17**, 15–26 (In Norwegian).

Tuchman, R.F. (1994). Epilepsy, language, and behaviour: clinical models in childhood. *Journal of Child Neurology*, **9**, 95–102.

van Bourgondien, M.E., Mesibov, G., and Castelloe, P. (1989). Adaptation of clients with autism to group home settings. Paper presented at the National Conference of the Autism Society of America. Seattle, WA.

Venter, A., Lord, C., and Schopler, E. (1992). A follow-up study of high-functioning autistic children. *Journal of Child Psychology and Psychiatry*, **33**, 489–507.

Volkmar, F.R., and Cohen, D.J. (1989). 'Disintegrative disorder or "late onset" autism?' *Journal of Child Psychology and Psychiatry*, **30**, 717–724.

Volkmar, F.R. and Nelson, D.S. (1990). Seizure disorders in autism. *Journal of the American Academy of Child and Adolescent Psychiatry*, **29**, 127–129.

Volkmar, F.R., Cicchetti, D.V., Bregman, J., and Cohen, D.J. (1992). Three diagnostic systems for autism: DSM-III., DSM-III-R., and ICD 10. *Journal of Autism and Developmental Disorders*, **22**, 483–492.

von Knorring, A.-L. and Hägglöf, B. (1993). Autism in Northern Sweden. A population based follow-up study: Psychopathology. *European Child and Adolescent Psychiatry*, **2**, 91–97.

Waterhouse, L. and Fein, D. (1984). Developmental trends in cognitive skills for children diagnosed as autistic and schizophrenic. *Child Development*, **55**, 236–248.

Waterhouse, L., Morris, R., Allen, D., Dunn, M., Fein, D., Feinstein, C., Rapin, I., and Wing, L. (1996). Diagnosis and classification in autism. *Journal of Autism and Developmental Disorders*, **26**, 59–86.

WHO (1992). *The ICD-10 Classification of Mental and Behavioural Disorders. Diagnostic Criteria for Research*. World Health Organization, Geneva.

Windsor, J., Doyle, S.S., and Siegel, G.M. (1994). Language acquisition after mutism: A longitudinal case study of autism. *Journal of Speech and Hearing Research*, **37**, 96–105.

Wing, L. (1980). *Early childhood autism*. Pergamon, Oxford.

Wing, L. (1981). Asperger's syndrome: a clinical account. *Psychological Medicine*, **11**, 115–129.

Wing, L. (1983). Diagnosis, clinical description and prognosis. In *Early childhood autism*, ed. L. Wing. Pergamon Press, Oxford.

Wing, L. (1989). The diagnosis of autism. In *Diagnosis and treatment of autism*, ed. C. Gillberg, pp. 5–22. Plenum, New York.

Wing, L. (1996). *The autism spectrum*. Constable, London.

Wing, L. and Attwood, A. (1987). Syndromes of autism and atypical development. In *Handbook of autism and pervasive developmental disorders*, ed. D.J. Cohen and A.M. Donnellan, pp. 3–19. Wiley, New York.

Wing, L. and Gould, J. (1979). Severe impairments of social interaction and associated abnormalities in children: epidemiology and classification. *Journal of Autism and Developmental Disorders*, **9**, 11–29.

Wing, L. and Shah, A. (1994). Catatonic features in autism. Paper given at the Autism on the Agenda Conference, Leeds, UK, 8–10 April.

Wolff, S. (1995). *Loners. The life path of unusual children*. Routledge, London.

16 Schizophrenic psychosis

Jon M. McClellan and John S. Werry

Schizophrenia is a neurodevelopmental disorder with deficits in cognition, affect, and social relatedness. It is often a chronic condition, with significant long-term morbidity and functional impairment. Given the longevity of symptoms, coupled with the inherent social and occupational dysfunction, schizophrenia consumes an enormous amount of therapeutic and social resources. It therefore remains a significant area of public health concern.

Although schizophrenia is primarily considered an adult disorder, its occurrence in children has been described since the time of Kraepelin (Werry and Taylor 1994). Historically, however, as the concept of childhood psychoses evolved, autism and pervasive developmental disorders were historically grouped underneath the rubric of 'childhood schizophrenia'. Therefore, owing to this shift in nosology, there are only a small number of studies available that have adequately distinguished childhood schizophrenia from autism.

Research examining these nosologic issues demonstrated that autism was a discrete disorder, distinct from schizophrenia (Kolvin *et al.* 1971, Rutter 1972). Thus, beginning with ICD-9 (World Health Organization 1978) and DSM-III (APA 1980), childhood schizophrenia was again diagnosed using the adult criteria. Subsequent research has generally validated this decision (Beitchman 1985, Werry 1992).

The research examining schizophrenia in youth remains sparse. Treatment studies, and research examining schizophrenia in adolescence, are especially lacking. Methodological problems within the literature include retrospective designs, lack of standardized assessment tools such as diagnostic interviews, small subject pools, and lack of comparison groups (McClellan and Werry 1994).

Schizophrenia in children under age 13 years has often been described as 'prepubertal'. However, this term has been defined by age rather than physical development. To avoid ambiguity, we have proposed that early onset schizophrenia (EOS) be defined as onset prior to 18 years of age, with a subgroup of very early onset schizophrenia (VEOS) defined as onset before age 13 years. We will use these terms in this chapter.

Clinical picture

Schizophrenia is diagnosed in children and adolescents using the same criteria as for adults. The two major diagnostic systems, DSM-IV (APA 1994) and ICD-10 (WHO 1990) both include positive and negative symptoms as diagnostic criteria. Positive symptoms consist of hallucinations, delusions, and disorganized thinking and behavior. Negative symptoms consist of paucity of speech, paucity of thought content, apathy, avolition, and flat affect

(Andreasen *et al.* 1990). The two diagnostic systems differ in their duration criteria. ICD-10 requires a duration of 1 month. DSM-IV requires a total duration of 6 months, during which time active symptoms are present for at least a 1 month period. These two sets of criteria were found to have high diagnostic agreement in a study of hospitalized psychotic adolescents (Armenteros *et al.* 1995).

Although the same criteria are used as for adults, some specific developmental characteristics associated with EOS have been noted and we outline these below.

Premorbid functioning

EOS generally has an insidious onset, with a life-long history of developmental and personality abnormalities (McClellan and Werry 1994). An age of onset before age 12 years is associated with highest rates of premorbid problems (Alaghband-Rad *et al.* 1995). The abnormalities most frequently described are symptoms of being socially withdrawn, odd, and isolated. Also noted are behavioral disorders and multiple developmental delays, including lags in cognitive, motor, sensory, and social functioning. Autism and pervasive developmental disorders have been reported (Watkins *et al.* 1988, Cantor et. al. 1982).

It is important to differentiate between these premorbid features, and a diagnosis of schizophrenia. Many children are considered odd, or have multiple developmental problems. However, most will not have the prerequisite psychotic symptoms required to make the diagnosis of schizophrenia (McKenna *et al.* 1994).

Symptomatology in EOS

Hallucinations, thought disorder, and flattened affect have all been consistently found in EOS. Systematic delusions and catatonic symptoms are described less frequently (Remschmidt *et al.* 1991, Werry *et al.* 1991, Green *et al.* 1992, Russell 1994). Developmental differences in language and cognition potentially influence the spectrum and quality of symptom presentation (Cantor *et al.* 1982, Watkins *et al.* 1988, Werry 1992, Volkmar 1996). Children tend to have less complex delusions, with the content reflecting childhood themes (Russell 1994). In both psychotic and non-psychotic children, positive symptoms increase linearly with age, whereas negative symptoms occur more frequently in early childhood and late adolescence (Bettes and Walker 1987). Children with high IQs (greater than 85) have more positive symptoms than those with low IQs (less than 85) (Bettes and Walker 1987).

Most hallucinations in children lack the requisite persistence and associated symptomatology required for schizophrenia (Garralda 1984a,b, 1985). These diagnostic issues have led to high rates of misdiagnosis, especially in children (McKenna *et al.* 1994). A child's report of hallucinations may represent imagination, misinterpretation of normal intrapsychic experiences, misunderstanding of the clinician's question, developmental phenomena, dissociative phenomena, factitious symptoms, or symptoms of another psychotic illness (i.e. a mood disorder). These issues must be examined prior to diagnosing a child with schizophrenia, given its long-lasting treatment and prognostic ramifications.

Significant rates of formal thought disorder have been reported in children with schizophrenia, other psychotic disorders, and those at risk for psychosis by virtue of having a psychotic mother (Kolvin 1971, Cantor *et al.* 1982, Arboleda and Holzman 1985, Watkins *et al.* 1988, Caplan *et al.* 1989). Caplan *et al.* (1989) reliably differentiated children with schizophrenia from normal controls using a measure of illogical thinking and loose associations. It is important, however, to differentiate the thought disorder of psychosis from that of either developmental delays or language disorders.

Rapidity of onset

VEOS generally has an insidious onset (Kolvin 1971, Green *et al.* 1992, Asarnow *et al.* 1994a, Russell *et al.* 1994). Conversely, reports of onset in early adolescence describe both high rates of acute or subacute onset, defined as less than 1 year (Eggers 1978, Werry *et al.* 1991) whereas others found a predominance of insidious onset (Kolvin 1971).

Schizophrenic subtypes

Both DSM-IV and ICD-10 describe different subtypes of schizophrenia, including paranoid, disorganized or hebephrenic, catatonic, undifferentiated, and residual. ICD-10 also uses the subtypes simple and postschizophrenic depression, which are not found in DSM-IV. In EOS, reports vary as to whether the paranoid subtype (Eggers 1978) or the undifferentiated subtype (Werry *et al.* 1991, McClellan *et al.* 1993) is more common. We do not currently have sufficient evidence to justify categorizing EOS as a separate diagnostic group (Werry 1992).

Cognitive and language dysfunction

Approximately 10–20% of youth with EOS have low IQs (Kolvin 1971, Eggers 1978, Asarnow and Ben-Meir 1988, Werry *et al.* 1991, Green *et al.* 1992, McClellan *et al.* 1993). Language and communication deficits are common (Baltaxe and Simmons 1995, Caplan *et al.* 1996). Children with schizophrenia have deficits in their information processing capacities, a finding also noted in adults (Asarnow *et al.* 1994b).

Assessing a child with severely impaired language for psychotic symptoms can be a diagnostic challenge (Werry and Taylor 1994). The standard presentations of hallucinations and delusions involve language. In a child with severely impaired language and/or cognition, the clinician is dependent on observations of behavior. Caution must be used in making a diagnosis of schizophrenia in such children. However, psychotic symptoms may be identified when their emergence is associated with a deterioration in mental status and global functioning.

Differential diagnosis

It is important to recognize other disorders which may present as schizophrenia. The following is an abbreviated discussion: for further details see McClellan and Werry (1994).

Schizoaffective disorder

Early onset schizoaffective disorder has not been well studied. Eggers (1989) found that 28% of his EOS sample at follow-up had schizoaffective psychoses, an ICD-9 diagnosis that overlaps with DSM-IV diagnoses of bipolar disorder and schizoaffective disorder. Other follow-up studies of psychotic youth have found that the diagnosis of schizoaffective disorder (DSM-III-R) occurred rarely and was felt to be unreliable (Werry *et al.* 1991, McClellan *et al.* 1993).

Psychotic mood disorders

Both schizophrenia and psychotic mood disorders (especially bipolar disorder) typically present with a variety of affective and psychotic symptoms (Joyce 1984, Carlson 1990, Werry *et al.* 1991, McClellan *et al.* 1993). This overlap in symptomatology increases the likelihood of misdiagnosis at the time of onset. Longitudinal reassessment is therefore needed to ensure accuracy of diagnosis. Family psychiatric history may also be a helpful differentiating factor, although it is important to note that studies also have found an increased family history of depression in schizophrenic youth (Werry 1992). The use of standardized diagnostic measures improves accuracy (Carlson *et al.* 1994).

Autism/pervasive developmental disorders

Children with pervasive developmental disorders lack the required positive psychotic symptomatology, i.e. hallucinations and delusions, required for a diagnosis of schizophrenia (Kolvin 1971, Green *et al.* 1986, McClellan and Werry 1994). Pervasive developmental disorders usually have a younger age of onset and lack a normal period of development. However, some schizophrenic children also have a lifelong history of developmental delays (Watkins *et al.* 1988). Since early brain injury has been associated with both schizophrenia and autism, it is possible that both illnesses may occasionally coexist, linked by a common central nervous system deficit that occurred early in development. However, if this occurs, the onset of schizophrenia will be later then that of autism, generally after 5 years of age.

Other behavioral and/or emotional disorders (including personality disorders)

Youth with conduct disorders and other non-psychotic emotional disorders may report psychotic-like symptoms (Garralda 1984a,b, Del Beccaro *et al.* 1988, Volkmar 1996). When compared to psychotic children, these children have lower rates of delusions and thought disorder (Garralda 1985). At follow-up, an increase in personality dysfunction, including personality disorders, but not psychotic disorders, has been found (Garralda 1984a,b, Lofgren *et al.* 1991, McClellan *et al.* 1993). When there is a history of abuse or neglect, the psychotic-like symptoms may represent dissociative symptoms (Nurcombe 1990).

Organic conditions

The list for potential organic etiologic agents causing psychosis is exhaustive (Cummins 1985). Conditions which must be considered include:

- delirium
- VEOS
- seizure disorders
- central nervous system lesions (e.g. brain tumors, congenital malformations, head trauma)

- neurodegenerative disorders (e.g. huntington's chorea, lipid storage disorders)

- metabolic disorders (e.g. endocrinopathies, wilson disease)

- toxic encephalopathies (e.g. abuse of substances such as amphetamines, cocaine, hallucinogens, phencyclidine, and solvents; prescribed medications such as stimulants, corticosteroids or anticholinergic agents, and other toxins such as heavy metals)

- infectious diseases (e.g. encephalitis, meningitis and/or human immunodefiency virus (HIV) related syndromes.

Given the significant rates of comorbid substance abuse with schizophrenia (as high as 50% comorbidity in some studies), it is not uncommon for a history of drug abuse to be obtained at the first onset of psychoses (McClellan *et al.* 1993). If the psychotic symptoms persist for longer than a few weeks despite documented detoxification, a primary psychotic disorder diagnosis must be considered.

Studies of natural course

Epidemiology

It has been estimated that 0.1–1% of all schizophrenic disorders present before age 10 years, with 4% occurring prior to 15 years of age (Remschmidt *et al.* 1994). However, the research examining juvenile populations is inadequate. In an study examining young adults during their first episode of schizophrenia ($n = 232$), 47% had displayed the first sign of their illness before age 21 years (Häfner and Nowotny 1995). However, only 21% developed psychotic symptoms prior to this age.

Clinical experience suggests that schizophrenia with onset prior to age 12 years is rare. The rate of onset than increases sharply during adolescence, with the peak ages of onset generally ranging from 15 to 30 years (Häfner and Nowotny 1995). There are reported cases of onset prior to age 6 years (Russell 1994), but evidence for the illness in children this young must be carefully scrutinized.

EOS, especially with onset prior to age 13 years, occurs predominantly in males (McClellan and Werry 1994). As age increases, this ratio tends to even out. Since the adult literature suggests that the age of onset in males is 5 years earlier than that in females (Loranger 1984, Häfner and Nowotny 1995), the male predominance in EOS appears to be a cross-sectional effect.

Studies of natural course

There are few studies examining the course of EOS. Most are retrospective, and none factor out the influence of treatment. The adult literature suggests that schizophrenia is a phasic disorder (Werry and Taylor 1994). The recognition of these phases is important for making diagnostic and therapeutic decisions. However, it is also important to note that there is a great deal of individual variability in regards to clinical presentation and course of illness. The phases are as follows.

Prodrome

Prior to the overt development of psychotic symptoms, most patients will experience some degree of functional deterioration. This may include social withdrawal, odd or schizotypal preoccupations, deteriorating academic performance, worsening hygiene and self-care skills, dysphoria, and/or idiosyncratic or bizarre behaviors. Some youth will also experience a behavioral deterioration, with an increase in acting-out, aggressive behaviors, or other conduct problems, including substance abuse (McClellan *et al.* 1993). These symptoms may confuse the diagnostic picture.

The prodrome may represent a marked change from baseline functioning, or alternatively, a worsening of premorbid personality/behavioral characteristics. The prodromal phase varies greatly in time, from an acute change (days to weeks) to chronic impairment (months to years) (Werry and Taylor 1994). Many youth, especially those with VEOS, have an insidious onset (Werry *et al.* 1991, McClellan *et al.* 1993, Russell 1994). In such cases it may be difficult to distinguish between the premorbid personality/cognitive abnormalities, and the onset of the disorder.

Acute phase

During the acute phase positive symptoms predominate (i.e. hallucinations, delusions, thought disorder, and disorganized behavior). These symptoms are usually associated with a marked deterioration in mental status and in functioning. This phase generally lasts 1–6 months, although it may persist for over a year (Werry and Taylor 1994). The length of this phase is in part determined by treatment response. Remschmidt *et al.* (1991) found that symptoms tended to shift from positive to negative over the course of treatment.

Recuperative/recovery phase

As the acute psychosis remits, there is generally a period lasting several months where the patient continues to experience a significant degree of impairment (Werry and Taylor 1994). This is most often due to negative symptoms (flat affect, anergia, social withdrawal), although it is common for some positive symptoms to persist (Remschmidt *et al.* 1991). In addition, some patients will develop a postschizophrenic depression (ICD-10) characterized by dysphoria and flat affect.

Residual phase

As they recover, youth with EOS may have prolonged periods (several months or more) without active positive symptoms. However, during this phase most patients will continue to experience some degree of impairment due to negative symptoms.

Chronically ill patients

A small number of patients will remain chronically symptomatic, despite adequate treatment, over a period of many years (Eggers 1978, Werry *et al.* 1991, McClellan *et al.* 1993, Asarnow *et al.* 1994a). These patients are among the most severely impaired, and require the most intensive treatment resources. The advent of the atypical antipsychotic agents offers some promise for these individuals, since clozapine has been effective for treatment refractory schizophrenia (Meltzer *et al.* 1994).

The longitudinal course of schizophrenia often follows a pattern whereby increasing deterioration occurs after each cycle until, after about 10 years, the disorder tends to burn itself out, leaving a residual state of varying disability characterized predominately by negative symptoms (Werry and Taylor 1994). There are insufficient data to determine whether this long-term pattern holds for EOS. Some youth with schizophrenia may only have one cycle, although this is not common (Eggers 1978, Werry *et al.* 1991, McClellan *et al.* 1993, Asarnow *et al.* 1994a). Recovery is incomplete in approximately 80% of cases where youth have had more than one episode (Werry and Taylor 1994).

Intervention studies

The treatment of EOS has not been well researched so much of the treatment recommendations are extrapolated from the adult literature, which is extensive. The treatment of EOS requires comprehensive multimodal interventions which incorporate both psychopharmacologic and psychosocial therapies (McClellan and Werry 1994). Specific interventions are tailored to the developmental characteristics of the patient, the needs of their family, and the different stages of the disorder. An array of therapeutic resources are needed, including inpatient/daypatient psychiatric units, medication management, psychoeducational services, intensive case management, family interventions, vocational and rehabilitative assistance, and in some cases, residential programs (McClellan and Werry 1994). Appropriate special education services are also an important component of treatment.

Psychopharmacology

The efficacy of antipsychotic medication as a specific treatment for schizophrenia has been firmly established (APA 1997). However, there are few studies with adolescents and children (Campbell and Cueva 1995). In children with schizophrenia, haloperidol (0.02–0.12 mg/kg) was found to be superior to placebo in reducing symptoms of thought disorder, hallucinations, and persecutory ideation (Spencer *et al.* 1992). Loxitane was superior to placebo in a study of adolescents with schizophrenia (Pool *et al.* 1976). Youth can experience the same side-effects noted in adults, e.g. extrapyramidal symptoms, sedation, tardive dyskinesia, and neuroleptic malignant syndrome (McClellan and Werry 1994). Their use of these drugs therefore needs to be closely monitored. The long-term use of neuroleptics in EOS has not been studied (Campbell and Cueva 1995).

The most significant advance in the pharmacotherapy of schizophrenia is the advent of the novel antipsychotic agents, including clozapine, risperidone, olanazpine and melperone. These agents are considered atypical since they are not primary D_2 (dopamine) antagonists (like traditional neuroleptics), but instead are serotonergic antagonists, with some D_1 activity (Meltzer *et al.* 1994). Clozapine is more effective than traditional neuroleptics in reducing both positive and negative symptoms. However, its use is limited by the potential for neutropenia and/or seizures. Although the other atypical agents need to be further studied, they all have a lower risk for extrapyramidal symptoms, and may be more effective for negative symptoms

(Meltzer *et al.* 1994). These agents will probably replace traditional neuroleptics as the primary medication for treating schizophrenia.

There are few studies examining the use of atypical agents in youth. Clozapine has been found to effectively treat EOS (Birmaher *et al.* 1992, Blanz and Schmidt 1993, Gordon *et al.* 1994, Towbin *et al.* 1994). In 21 youth (mean age 14.0 ± 2.3 years) with childhood onset schizophrenia, clozapine (mean dose 176 mg ± 149 mg/day) was superior to haloperidol (16 ± 8 mg/day) for treating both positive and negative symptoms. However, while on clozapine, five youth developed significant neutropenia (this resolved spontaneously in three of subjects), and two had seizures. Therefore, although the efficacy of clozapine is encouraging, the possible increased rate of adverse reactions in youth raises concerns. The other atypical agents have not been studied with this age group, although there are positive case reports describing the use of risperidone (Quintana and Keshavan 1995). Further research is needed.

Other medications have been used as adjuncts to antipsychotic agents, including lithium, benzodiazepines, and anticonvulsants (APA 1997). However, their use in youth with schizophrenia has not been examined.

There are some general guidelines for the psychopharmacologic management of schizophrenia. For a more detailed discussion, see McClellan and Werry (1994). Prior to initiating a medication trial, an adequate psychiatric evaluation is needed which includes documentation of targeted symptoms. The patient and his or her family should be provided with adequate information regarding diagnosis, medication options, and side-effects. The antipsychotic therapy should be implemented for a period of no less than 4–6 weeks, using adequate dosages, before efficacy of the medication choice is determined. Long-term monitoring is needed to determine adequate dosing needs, and monitoring for side-effects.

Psychosocial therapies

In the adult literature, most traditional psychotherapies have not been found to be specifically helpful for treating schizophrenia (Goldstein 1989). However, psychoeducational therapies have been shown to decrease relapse rates (Goldstein 1989). Psychoeducational interventions are generally directed at family functioning, problem-solving and communication skills, and relapse prevention (Falloon *et al.* 1984, Goldstein 1989).

The family interventions stem in part from research regarding expressed emotion. Expressed emotion refers to attributes of overprotectiveness or criticism expressed towards the patient. The relapse rates for patients with schizophrenia are higher when living in families characterized as having high expressed emotion (Leff and Vaughn 1985). Family intervention programs, in conjunction with medication therapy, have been shown to significantly decrease schizophrenia relapse rates over the first year of treatment (Goldstein 1989).

Another important psychoeducational modality is social skills training. These programs focus on improving the patient's strategies for dealing with conflict and avoidance, identifying the correct meaning, content, and context of verbal messages within their families, and enhancing their socialization and vocational skills. The combination of family treatment, social skills training, and medication therapy has also been shown to decrease relapse rates (Hogarty *et al.* 1986).

Rund *et al.* (1994) compared the effectiveness of a psychoeducational treatment program to the standard community treatment, in a sample of adolescents with schizophrenia (12 subjects per group). The psychoeducational treatment program included parent seminars, problem-solving sessions, milieu therapy (while the subjects were hospitalized), and networks (reintegrating the subjects back into their schools and communities). These interventions were used in conjunction with medication therapy. The standard treatment group received a mixture of individual psychotherapy, milieu therapy, and medications. Outcome was assessed after 2 years. Those receiving the psychoeducational treatment program had lower rates of rehospitalization. Subjects with poor premorbid psychosocial functioning benefited the most from the psychoeducational program. Clinical improvement was associated with the families expressed emotion ratings changing from high to low. Furthermore, the psychoeducational program was more cost-effective. More research is needed in this area. However, in children and adolescents with schizophrenia, family treatment and social skills training should be considered helpful adjuncts to medication treatment.

Short-term and long-term outcomes

There are very few studies examining long-term outcome in EOS. Most are retrospective. Assessing outcome in schizophrenia is complicated by two factors:

- Since schizophrenia is a phasic disorder, the outcome will vary dependent on the phase during which the assessment occurs.

- Historically other disorders have been misdiagnosed as schizophrenia, particularly bipolar disorder, so outcome studies may be influenced by diagnostic errors (Eggers 1989, Werry *et al.* 1991).

Short-term outcome is invariably predicted by premorbid characteristics, treatment response, and adequacy of therapeutic resources. Remschmidt *et al.* (1991) found that, in 113 adolescents and young adults (mean age 18.3 ± 3 years) with schizophrenia, only 14% had a complete remission of symptoms during the index hospitalization. The same authors also reported on a cohort of 64 individuals with schizophrenia (ages 12–22 years) who entered a special rehabilitation program. This sample was followed at 3 month intervals over a 1 year period. Significant improvement was noted in symptomatology and cognitive functioning. Subjects with higher levels of cognitive abilities and premorbid functioning did better at outcome.

There are some differences between studies which have examined outcome over approximately a 5 year period. In two retrospective studies of youth with primarily adolescent onset schizophrenia (Werry *et al.* 1991, McClellan *et al.* 1993), the majority of subjects displayed moderate to severe impairment at outcome: 80–90% had two or more episodes during the follow-up period, whereas only a few had a complete remission (Werry *et al.* 1994). Outcome was best predicted by premorbid and intellectual functioning (Werry *et al.* 1992).

Asarnow *et al.* (1994a) followed 18 children with VEOS over a 2–7 year period. In their sample, 44% showed minimal improvement, or a deteriorating course. After 1 year, only two children displayed no evidence of symptoms. However, between 2 and 7 years, one-third of the sample no longer met criteria for either schizophrenia or schizoaffective disorder. Four youth had no psychiatric disorders at outcome. The children in this study received extensive pharmacologic and psychosocial treatment, which may have influenced the findings.

There are two long-term outcome studies. Maziade *et al.* (1996a,b) followed up on 40 subjects with EOS (mean follow-up period 14.8 years, mean age of onset 14.0 years). Only two subjects had a complete recovery. The majority (74%) were moderately to severely impaired. Outcome was best predicted by premorbid functioning, and the severity of positive and negative symptoms during acute episodes (Maziade *et al.* 1996a).

Eggers (1978, 1989) followed 57 patients with childhood schizophrenia (onset between 7 and 13 years of age) over a mean follow-up period of 16 years. At outcome, 28% had schizo-affective disorder (Eggers 1989). Overall, 50% of the sample were significantly impaired at outcome, 30% had good to satisfying social adaptation, and 20% had a complete remission (Eggers 1979). Those with schizoaffective disorder had a more favorable course (Eggers 1989). They also tended to have fewer premorbid difficulties, which was also a significant prognostic factor. Onset before age 10 (*n* = 11) was uniformly associated with a poor outcome.

Within this same sample, 44 subjects were reassessed after a mean follow-up period of 42 years (Eggers and Bunk 1997). The outcome ratings were similar: 25% had complete remission; 25% partial remission, and 50% chronic impairment. An insidious onset (over more than a 4 week period) and an age of onset before age 12 years were both associated with greater disability at outcome.

In general, the results of these studies are consistent with the adult literature. There are few studies which have compared EOS to adult onset schizophrenia. Yang *et al.* (1995) found that onset before 15 years of age was associated with higher ratings of negative symptoms in adulthood, and Häfner and Nowotny (1995) reported greater social impairment in patients with onset before age 21 years. These two studies support the clinical observations that EOS may have a more insidious and chronic course, with less favorable outcome.

Continuity versus discontinuity

EOS is generally a continuous disorder. In long-term outcome studies, the disorder persists in most youth. However, a few children with EOS have no psychiatric illnesses at follow-up (Asarnow *et al.* 1994a). In others the diagnosis changes. A significant proportion of youth originally diagnosed with schizophrenia either have bipolar disorder (Carlson 1990, Werry *et al.* 1991, McClellan *et al.* 1993), or schizoaffective disorder (Eggers 1989) at outcome.

The evidence to date suggests that schizophrenia in youth is essentially the same hetero-geneous disorder as in adults (Beitchman 1985, Werry 1992). This is based on the similarities between symptomatology, course, treatment response, outcome, and family history (Werry 1992). The differences between EOS and adult onset disease appear to be more quantitative and developmental, rather than representing fundamentally different disorders. Therefore, the current practice of using the adult criteria, and not classifying EOS as a distinct disorder (or subgroup), is justified.

Risks and prognostic factors

Schizophrenia is associated with a multitude of psychosocial problems; including difficulties with interpersonal relationships, self-care skills, school failure, joblessness, homelessness, poverty, violence, and incarceration (APA 1997). In follow-up studies of EOS, only a small minority of patients at outcome were in full time education or employment; and less than one-third were living independently (age-adjusted) (Werry *et al.* 1994).

Patients with schizophrenia also have an increase risk for depression, substance abuse, and general medical problems, and have a higher mortality rate than the general population (APA 1997). The overall risk of suicide or accidental death directly due to psychosis in youth with EOS appears to be approximately 5% (Eggers 1978, Werry *et al.* 1991). In adults, the lifetime suicide risk is estimated at 10% (APA 1997).

Substance abuse adds to the morbidity of the disorder, and increases the risk for treatment failure and suicide. In adults with schizophrenia, estimated rates of concurrent substance abuse disorders range from 40 to 60% (APA 1997). In outcome studies of EOS, some have found high rates of comorbid substance abuse disorders (over 50%) (McClellan *et al.* 1993), although others have not (Werry *et al.* 1991). The reported rates are predictably higher in samples where the subjects are predominately adolescents or young adults (versus children).

In studies of adults with schizophrenia, good prognostic factors include female gender, good premorbid functioning, acute onset with precipitating factors, a family history of mood disorders, higher IQ, and symptoms that are predominately positive, not negative, or disorganized (APA 1997). In youth with EOS, a better outcome is predicted by good premorbid functioning, higher intellectual functioning, and degree of recovery from the first episode (Eggers 1989, Werry and McClellan 1992). Other potential prognostic factors include treatment availability and response, comorbid conditions, and psychosocial supports/family issues (Asarnow *et al.* 1994). VEOS is felt to have a worse prognosis. This may be because prognosis is predicted in part by premorbid functioning, including IQ (Werry and McClellan 1992). Children with VEOS are more likely to have a history of premorbid abnormalities, including an insidious onset, with significant cognitive and/or language difficulties (McClellan and Werry 1994).

Conclusions

Schizophrenia occurs quite rarely before the age of 12 years, with the incidence than rising after the onset of puberty. Clinical characteristics include an increased prevalence in males, high rates of premorbid abnormalities (including social and neurodevelopmental problems), and an increased family history of schizophrenia. EOS is usually a phasic illness, with significant morbidity and social/occupational impairment. The long-term prognosis is generally mixed to poor, although some patients do recover.

Treatment response appears to be similar to that reported for adults, although research in this area is greatly lacking. Recent important advances in treatment efficacy include the atypical antipsychotic agents, and the incorporation of psychoeducational curricula into comprehensive treatment programs.

Schizophrenia remains a major public health challenge. Further research is greatly needed, especially in regards to treatment modalities and etiology. Since schizophrenia appears to be a neurodevelopmental disorder (Weinberger 1987), the study of youth with schizophrenia may provide important information as to how the disorder evolves in a developmental context. The timing of the onset of the disorder may have varying consequences on cognitive, language, and social development. Identifying such factors may provide important clues to the potential underlying etiological mechanisms.

References

Alaghband-Rad, J., McKenna, K., Gordon, C.T., Albus, K.E., Hamburger, S.D., Rumsey, J.M., Frazier, J.A., Lenane, M.C., and Rapoport, J.L. (1995). Childhood-onset schizophrenia: the severity of premorbid course. *Journal of the American Academy of Child and Adolescent Psychiatry*, **34**, 1273–1283.

APA (1980) *Diagnostic and statistical manual of mental disorders*, 3rd edn. American Psychiatric Association, Washington, DC.

APA (1994) *Diagnostic and statistical manual of mental disorders*, 4th edn. American Psychiatric Association, Washington, DC.

APA (1997) Practice guideline for the treatment of patients with schizophrenia. *American Journal of Psychiatry*, Supplement, 154, 1–63.

Andreasen, N.C., Flaum, M., Swayze, V.W. *et al.* (1990) Positive and negative symptoms in Schizophrenia. *Archives of General Psychiatry*, **47**, 615–621.

Arboleda, C. and Holzman, P.S. (1985). Thought disorder in children at risk for psychosis. *Archives of General Psychiatry*, **42**, 1004–1013.

Armenteros, J.L., Fennelly, B.W., Hallin, A., Adams, P.B., Pomerantz, P., Michell, M., Sanchez, L.E., and Campbell, M. (1995). Schizophrenia in hospitalized adolescents: clinical diagnosis, DSM-III-R, DSM-IV, and ICD-10 criteria. *Psychopharmacology Bulletin*, **31**(2), 383–387.

Asarnow, J.R. and Ben-Meir, S. (1988). Children with schizophrenia spectrum and depressive disorders: a comparative study of premorbid adjustment, onset pattern and severity of impairment. *Journal of Child Psychology and Psychiatry*, **29**, 477–488.

Asarnow, J.R., Tompson, M.C., and Goldstein, M.J. (1994a). Childhood onset schizophrenia: a follow-up study. *Schizophrenia Bulletin*, **20**(4), 647–670.

Asarnow, R., Asamen, J., Granholm, E., Sherman, T., Watkins, J.M., and Williams, M.E. (1994b). Cognitive/neuropsychological studies of children with a schizophrenic disorder. *Schizophrenia Bulletin*, **20**(4), 647–670.

Baltaxe, C.A.M. and Simmons III, J.Q., (1995). Speech and language disorders in children and adolescents with schizophrenia. *Schizophrenia Bulletin*, **21**(4), 677–692.

Beitchman, J.H. (1985) Childhood schizophrenia: a review and comparison with adult-onset schizophrenia. *Psychiatric Clinics of North America*, **8**, 793–814.

Bettes, B. and Walker, E. (1987). Positive and negative symptoms in psychotic and other psychiatrically disturbed children. *Journal of Child Psychology and Psychiatry*, **28**, 555–567.

Birmaher, B., Baker, R., Kapur, S., *et al.* (1992). Clozapine for the treatment of adolescents with schizophrenia. *Journal of the American Academy of Child and Adolescent Psychiatry*, **31**, 160–164.

Blanz, B. and Schmidt, M.H. (1993). Clozapine for schizophrenia (letter). *Journal of the American Academy of Child and Adolescent Psychiatry*, **32**, 223–224.

Bradbury, T.N. and Miller, G.A. (1985). Season of birth in schizophrenia: a review of evidence, methodology and etiology. *Psychological Bulletin*, **98**, 569–594.

Campbell, M and Cueva, J.E. (1995). Psychopharmacology in child and adolescent psychiatry: a review of the past seven years. Part II. *Journal of the American Academy of Child and Adolescent Psychiatry*, **34**(10), 1262–1272.

Cantor, S., Evans, J., Pearce, J. *et al.* (1982) Childhood schizophrenia, present but not accounted for. *American Journal of Psychiatry*, **139**, 758–762.

Caplan, R., Guthrie, D., Gish, B., Tanguay, P., and David-Lando, G. (1989). The Kiddie Formal Thought Disorder Scale: clinical assessment, reliability, and validity. *Journal of the American Academy of Child and Adolescent Psychiatry*, **28**, 408–416.

Caplan, R., Guthrie, D., and Komo, S. (1996). Conversational repair in schizophrenic and normal children. *Journal of the American Academy of Child and Adolescent Psychiatry*, **35**(7), 950–958.

Carlson, G.A., Fennig, S., and Bromet, E.J. (1994). The confusion between bipolar disorder and schizophrenia in youth: where does it stand in the 1990s. *Journal of the American Academy of Child and Adolescent Psychiatry*, **33**, 453–460.

Carlson, G.A. (1990). Child and adolescent mania: diagnostic considerations. *Journal of Child Psychology and Psychiatry*, **31**, 331–342,

Cummings, J.L. (1985). *Clinical neuropsychiatry*. Grune and Stratton, Orando, FL.

Del Beccaro, M.A., Burke, P., and McCauley, E. (1988). Hallucinations in children, a follow-up study. *Journal of the American Academy of Child and Adolescent Psychiatry*, **27**, 462–465.

Eggers, C. (1978). Course and prognosis in childhood schizophrenia. *Journal of Autism and Childhood Schizophrenia*, **8**, 21–36.

Eggers, C. (1989). Schizo-affective psychosis in childhood: a follow-up study. *Journal of Autism and Developmental Disorders*, **19**, 327–334.

Eggers, C. and Bunk, D. (1997). The long-term course of early-onset schizophrenia. *Schizophrenia Bulletin*, **23**, 105—118.

Falloon, I.R.H., Boyd, J.L., and McGill, G.W. (1984*). Family care for schizophrenia: a problem-solving approach to mental illness*. Guilford New York.

Garralda, M.E. (1984a). Hallucinations in children with conduct and emotional disorders: I. The clinical phenomena. *Psychological Medicine*, **14**, 589–596.

Garralda, M.E. (1984b). Hallucinations in children with conduct and emotional disorders: II. the follow-up study. *Psychological Medicine*, **14**, 597–604.

Garralda, M.E. (1985). Characteristics of the psychoses of late onset in children and adolescents (a comparative study of hallucinating children). *Journal of Adolescence*, **8**, 195–207,

Goldstein, M.J. (1989). Psychosocial treatment of schizophrenia. In *Schizophrenia: scientific progress*, ed. S.C. Schulz and C.A. Tamminga, pp. 318–324. Oxford University Press, New York.

Gottesman, I. and Bertelson, A. (1989). Confirming unexpressed genotypes for schizophrenia. *Archives of General Psychiatry*, **46**, 867–872.

Green, W.H., Padron-Gayol, M., Hardesty, A.S., and Bassiri, M. (1992). Schizophrenia with childhood onset: a phenomenological study of 38 cases. *Journal of the American Academy of Child and Adolescent Psychiatry*, **31**, 5968–5976.

Häfner, H. and Nowotny, B. (1995). Epidemiology of early-onset schizophrenia. *European Archives of Psychiatry and Clinical Neurosciences*, **245**, 80–92.

Hanson, D.R. and Gottesman, I.I. (1976). The genetics, if any, of infantile autism and childhood schizophrenia. *Journal of Autism and Childhood Schizophrenia*, **6**, 209–234.

Hogarty, G.E., Anderson, C.M., Reiss, D.J. *et al.* (1986). Family psychoeducation, social skills training, and maintenance chemotherapy in the aftercare treatment of schizophrenia. I. One-year effects of a controlled study on relapse and expressed emotion. *Archives of General Psychiatry*, **43**, 633–642.

Kane, J.M. (1987). Treatment of schizophrenia. *Schizophrenia Bulletin*, **13**, 133–156.

Kolvin, I. (1971). Studies in the childhood psychoses. *British Journal of Psychiatry*, **6**, 209–234.

Leff, J. and Vaughn, C. (1985). *Expressed emotion in families: its significance for mental illness.* Guilford,New York.

Lofgren, D.P., Bemporad, J., King, J., Lindem, K.,and O'Driscoll, G. (1991). A prospective follow-up study of so called borderline children. *American Journal of Psychiatry*, **148**, 1541–1547.

Maziade, M., Bouchard, S., Gingras, N., Charron, L., Cardinal, A., Roy, M., Gauthier, B., Tremblay, G., Cote, S., Fournier, C., Boutin, P., Hamel, M., Merette, C., and Martinez, M. (1996a). Long-term stability of diagnosis and symptom dimensions in a systematic sample of patients with onset of schizophrenia in childhood and early adolescence. II: positive/negative distinction and childhood predictors of adult outcome. *British Journal of Psychiatry*, **169**, 371–378.

Maziade, M., Gingras, N., Rodrigue, C., Bouchard, S., Cardinal, A., Gauthier, B., Tremblay, G., Cote, S., Fournier, C., Boutin, P., Hamel, M., Roy, M., Martinez, M., and Merette, C. (1996b). Long-term stability of diagnosis and symptom dimensions in a systematic sample of patients with onset of schizophrenia in childhood and early adolescence. I: nosology, sex and age of onset. *British Journal of Psychiatry*, **169**, 361–370.

McClellan, J.M. and Werry, J.S. (1992). Schizophrenia. In *Psychopharmacologic treatment of childhood psychiatric disorders*, ed. D. Shaffer, *North American Clinics of Psychiatry*, **15**(1), 131–148.

McClellan, J.M. and Werry, J.S. (1994). Practice parameters for the assessment and treatment of children and adolescents with schizophrenia. *Journal of the American Academy of Child and Adolescent Psychiatry*, **33**(5), 616–635.

McClellan, J.M. and Werry, J.S. (1997). Practice parameters for the assessment and treatment of children and adolescents with bipolar disorder. *Journal of the American Academy of Child and Adolescent Psychiatry*, **36**, 138–156.

McClellan, J.M., Werry, J.S., and Ham, M. (1993). A follow-up study of early onset psychosis: comparison between outcome diagnoses of schizophrenia, mood disorders and personality disorders. *Journal of Autism and Developmental Disorders*, **23**, 243–262.

McKenna, K., Gordon, C.T., Lenane, M., Kaysen, D., Fahey, K., and Rapoport, J. (1994). Looking for childhood onset schizophrenia: the first 71 cases screened. *Journal of the American Academy of Child and Adolescent Psychiatry*, **33**(5), 636–644.

Meltzer, H.Y., Lee, M.A., and Ranjan, R. (1994). Recent advances in the pharmacotherapy of schizophrenia. *Acta Psychiatrica Scandinavica*, **90** (Suppl 384), 95–101.

Nurcombe, B. (1990). Dissociative hallucinosis and allied conditions. Institute on Psychosis in Childhood and Adolescence, Annual Congress of the American Academy of Child and Adolescent Psychiatry, Chicago, IL.

Pool, D., Bloom, W., Mielke, D.H. *et al.* (1976). A controlled evaluation of loxitane in seventy-five adolescent schizophrenia patients. *Current Therapeutic Research Clinical and Experimental*, **19**, 99–104,

Quintana, H. and Keshavan, M. (1995). Case study: risperidone in children and adolescents with schizophrenia. *Journal of the American Academy of Child and Adolescent Psychiatry*, **34**, 1292–1296.

Remschmidt, H., Martin, M., Schulz, E., Gutenbrunner, C., and Fleischhaker, C. (1991). The concept of positive and negative schizophrenia in child and adolescent psychiatry. In *Positive versus negative schizophrenia*, ed. A. Marneros, N.C. Andreasen, and M.T. Tsuang, pp. 219—242. Springer-Verlag, Berlin.

Remschmidt, H.E., Schulz, E., Martin, M., Warnke, A., and Trott, G-E. (1994). childhood onset schizophrenia: history of the concept and recent studies. *Schizophrenia Bulletin*, **20**, 727–745.

Russell, A.T. (1994). The clinical presentation of childhood-onset schizophrenia. *Schizophrenia Bulletin*, **20**(4), 631–647.

Rutter, M. (1972). Childhood schizophrenia reconsidered. *Journal of Autism and Childhood Schizophrenia*, **2**, 315–337.

Spencer, E.K., Kafantaris, V., Padron-Gayol, M.V., Rosenberg, C., and Campbell, M. (1992). Haloperidol in schizophrenic children: early findings from a study in progress. *Schizophrenia Bulletin*, **28**(2), 183–186.

Towbin, K.E., Dykens, E.M., and Pugliese, R.G. (1994). Clozapine for early developmental delays with childhood-onset schizophrenia: protocol and 15-month outcome. *Journal of the American Academy of Child and Adolescent Psychiatry*, **33**, 651–657.

Volkmar, F.R. (1996). Child and adolescent psychosis, a review of the past 10 years. *Journal of the American Academy of Child and Adolescent Psychiatry*, **35**(7), 843–885.

Watkins, J.M., Asarnow, R.F., and Tanguqy, P. (1988). Symptom development in childhood onset schizophrenia. *Journal of Child Psychology and Psychiatry*, **29**, 865–878.

Weinberger, D. (1987). Implications of normal brain development for the pathogenesis of schizophrenia. *Archives of General Psychiatry*, **44**, 660–669.

Werry, J.S. (1979). Psychoses. In *Psychopathological disorders of childhood*, 2nd edn, ed. H.C. Quay and J.S. Werry. Wiley, New York.

Werry, J.S. (1992). Child and adolescent (early onset) schizophrenia: A review in light of DSM-III-R. *Journal of Autism and Developmental Disorders*, **22**, 601–624.

Werry, J.S. and McClellan, J (1992). Predicting outcome in child and adolescent (early-onset) schizophrenia and bipolar disorder. *Journal of the American Academy of Child and Adolescent Psychiatry*, **31**, 147–150.

Werry, J.S. and Taylor, E. (1994). Schizophrenic and allied disorders. In *Child and adolescent psychiatry, modern approaches*, ed. M. Rutter, E. Taylor, and L.Hersov, pp. 594–615. Blackwell Scientific, Oxford.

Werry, J.S., McClellan, J. and Chard, L. (1991). Early-onset schizophrenia, bipolar and schizoaffective disorders: a clinical and follow-up study. *Journal of the American Academy of Child and Adolescent Psychiatry*, **30**, 457–465.

Werry, J.S., McClellan, J., Andrews, L., and Ham, M (1994). Clinical features and outcome of child and adolescent schizophrenia. *Schizophrenia Bulletin*, **20**, 619–630.

WHO (1978). *International Classification of Diseases (ICD-9)*. World Health Organization, Geneva.

WHO (1992). *The ICD-10 Classification of Mental Health and Behavioural Disorders: Clinical Descriptions and Diagnostic Guidelines*. World Health Organization, Geneva.

Yang, P.C., Liu, C.Y., Chiang, S.Q., Chen, J.Y., Lin, T.S. (1995). Comparison of adult manifestations of schizophrenia with onset before and after 15 years of age. *Acta Psychiatrica Scandinavica*, **91**, 209–212.

17 Tic disorders and Tourette's syndrome

Youngshin Kim and James F. Leckman

Since George Gilles de la Tourette described nine cases of chronic motor and phonic tics in his 1885 paper, efforts to understand the etiology and pathogenesis of Tourette syndrome (TS) have focused on neurological, psychodynamic, and psychopharmacological aspects of the syndrome (Gilles de la Tourette 1885). More recent formulations have built upon advances in epidemiology, genetics, developmental neuroscience, neuroimmunology, and *in vivo* neuroimaging. Integrative, multidisciplinary efforts are needed to take full advantage of our expanding knowledge base and advances in related areas. Based on cumulative findings, a working model of the pathogenesis of TS has emerged over the past decade (Leckman *et al.* 1997). The key feature of this model includes reciprocal interaction of genes and the environment occurring during the course of central nervous system (CNS) development.

In the following sections, we review various studies of the pathogenesis of TS and their findings in the areas of the clinical picture, natural course, intervention studies, outcome studies, continuity and discontinuity, and risk and prognostic factors. We begin with an examination of the available clinical data concerning phenomenological characteristics and the course of the syndrome.

Clinical picture

Tics are sudden, rapid, recurrent, non-rhythmic, stereotyped movements or vocalizations. A tic occurs as a spontaneous movement, or in response to a premonitory urge, which transiently relieves the sensation. In contrast to other movement disorders, tics are generally not continuous, but occur in a bout-like fashion. Tics are further divided into simple and complex tics according to the involvement of muscle groups and tic manifestations (APA 1994). Simple motor tics involve an individual muscle group and produce an instantaneous eye blink, neck jerk, facial grimace, or shoulder shrug. Complex motor tics involve either a purposive appearing cluster of simple motor tics, or a coordinated pattern of movements such as facial gestures, touching, smelling an object, jumping, stamping, or copropraxia (obscene gesture). Vocal tics, which are produced by moving air through the nose, mouth, or throat, may be simple sounds, such as throat clearing, grunting, sniffing, snorting, and barking, or may be complex, for example, words, phrases or sentences out of context, coprolalia (use of socially unacceptable words, frequently obscene), palilalia (repeating one's own sounds or words), or echolalia (repeating the last-heard sound, word, or phrase).

DSM-IV classifies tic disorders into four categories:

- Transient Tic Disorder
- Chronic Motor or Vocal Tic Disorder (CTD)
- Tourette's Disorder
- Tic Disorder Not Otherwise Specified,

according to duration of tics (transient–less than 1 year, chronic–more than 1 year) and types of tics (presence of motor tics, vocal tics, or combined multiple motor tics and more than one vocal tic) (APA 1994). The *International Classification of Disease*, 10th edition (ICD-10; WHO 1992) classifies tic disorders into five categories based on the same criteria of duration and types of tics:

- Transient Tic Disorder
- Chronic Motor or Vocal Tic Disorder
- Combined Vocal and Multiple Motor Tic Disorder (de la Tourette's Syndrome)
- Other Tic Disorder
- Tic Disorder Unspecified.

There has been an ongoing effort to understand whether TS and CTD are etiologically related disorders. Family genetic studies and cross-sectional clinical studies suggest that CTD may be a mild form of TS. This conclusion is based on the findings of a high rate of CTD in biological relatives of TS (Kidd *et al.* 1980, Pauls *et al.* 1991). In addition, TS and CTD patients have similar clinical correlates, including psychiatric comorbidity and school, neuropsychological and psychosocial functions (Kidd *et al.* 1980, Pauls *et al.* 1981, Pauls *et al.* 1984, Spencer *et al.* 1995).

Using various population selection methods and case ascertainment strategies, prevalence studies report that the prevalence of TS ranges from 0.5 to 59 per 10 000, and the prevalence of tic disorders is 420 per 10 000 (Lucas *et al.* 1982, Burd *et al.* 1986, Caine *et al.* 1988, Comings *et al.* 1990, Apter *et al.* 1993, Costello *et al.* 1996). Not surprisingly, the prevalence using clinical samples is underestimated (0.5–0.7 per 10 000) compared to that using community samples (4.3–59.2 per 10 000). The male to female ratio also decreases from 4–9 : 1 to 1.3–1.6 : 1 when community cases are used to estimate the prevalence.

Several prevalence studies in TS have been conducted in particular populations. For example, TS appears to be relatively low in the African-American population (Shapiro *et al.* 1978, Erenberg *et al.* 1986). However, the recent community-based epidemiology study by Costello *et al.* found no difference in the prevalence of tic disorders or TS among African-American children and Caucasian children (Costello *et al.* 1996).

The age of onset of tic disorders is typically between 2 and 15 years, with a modal age of 5–7 years. Vocal tics occur as initial symptoms in fewer than 20% of cases and tend to have a slightly older age of onset than motor tics (Jagger *et al.* 1982, Shapiro *et al.* 1988, Bornstein *et al.* 1990). Onset of symptoms is typically marked by transient tic episodes followed by more persistent motor or vocal tics. However, in rare cases, TS may erupt with dozens of sudden, forceful tics occurring every minute. The most common initial symptoms are facial tics, particularly eye tics (Bornstein *et al.* 1990). As CTD and TS progress, new tic symptoms appear and previous ones may disappear. The original single tics may be augmented by movements of the limbs and body. Simple rapid tics may become complex, orchestrated movements involving one or many muscle groups. Noises may evolve into words and phrases. Coprolalia, once considered the pathognomic feature of TS, is observed in less than 10% of cases using current diagnostic criteria (R. A. King, personal communication, 1997). Each patient's tic repertoire is distinctive and sometimes reflects an array of unwanted movements and vocalizations, including rare self-mutilating tics. The overall severity of tics usually waxes and wanes in cycles lasting weeks or months. During sleep, frequency and forcefulness of tics diminish, but at least in some children, tics do not entirely disappear.

Initially, children may be unaware that they are having tic symptoms. Over the course of months, most children become aware of their tics. By age 10 or 11, most children recognize and report a faint premonitory sensation that precedes a tic and that is momentarily relieved by performance of the tic (Leckman *et al.* 1993). This sensory experience that typically consists of a feeling of tightness, increased sensitivity, or a mounting discomfort, located in specific body parts. Other patients report a more generalized bodily tension.

Usually of brief duration, individual tics rarely last more than a second. Tics tend to occur in bouts with brief inter-tic intervals (less than 1–2 s). It also appears that bouts of tics themselves occur in bouts and that this bout-like structure is maintained over longer intervals, producing the waxing and waning of symptoms so characteristic of this disorder. If confirmed, this pattern may be especially useful in explaining the natural course of TS across multiple temporal scales (seconds, hours, weeks, and months), and may provide a fundamental insight into some of the underlying neurobiological process.

Attention deficit hyperactivity disorder (ADHD) and obsessive–compulsive disorder (OCD) are the two most common psychiatric conditions that accompany TS. Better understanding of whether they are part of the TS spectrum disorders is crucial. It will sharpen the definition of the TS phenotype and in turn, lead to more accurate identification of study subjects. As early as 1945, Mahler *et al.* described restlessness, hyperkinesis and impulsivity as a pre-tic behavior disorder (Mahler *et al.* 1945). Since then, hyperactivity, inattentiveness, impulsivity, and difficulty in the regulation of activity, often with low frustration tolerance in TS patients, have been reported by many other investigators. These symptoms of ADHD may appear before the onset of tics, or may worsen with the onset of tics. Frequently, comorbid ADHD is a greater source of impairment than are the tics. They often cause more difficulties in peer and family relationships and academic achievement.

Furthermore, the severity of ADHD may be more predictive of impaired social adjustment, regardless of tic severity (Dykens *et al.* 1990, Stokes *et al.* 1991, Carter *et al.* 1994). In clinic cases of TS, 40–50% of children reportedly have comorbid ADHD, and in epidemiological studies, 8–27% comorbidity of ADHD has been reported (Caine *et al.* 1988, Apter *et al.* 1993). There has been an ongoing effort to understand whether ADHD is a phenotypic variant of TS, or whether high comorbidity of ADHD is just a reflection of selection bias caused by the use of clinic cases. The finding of 8% comorbidity of ADHD in the population-based study by Apter *et al.* (1993) supports the view that ascertainment bias may account for the high frequency of ADHD in clinic populations. A second approach to the study of comorbidity in TS is the use of family studies. Family genetic studies have found that relatives of probands with TS were at greater risk for ADHD than controls regardless of the presence of ADHD in the TS probands, but the rates of ADHD in relatives are much greater among relatives of the probands with TS and ADHD than those of the probands with TS alone. These findings suggest that there may be two types of individuals with TS and ADHD, those in which ADHD is independent of TS and those in which ADHD is secondary to the occurrence of TS (Pauls *et al.* 1986a, 1993).

OCD has been observed in 7–40% of TS cases in epidemiological samples (Caine *et al.* 1988, Apter *et al.* 1993), compared with 28–62% from clinics or membership rolls from the Tourette Syndrome Association (Pauls *et al.* 1986b, Grad *et al.* 1987, Pitman *et al.* 1987). Additionally, occurrence of TS and/or tics has been reported in 15–59% of patients with OCD (Swedo and Leonard 1994). Along with the high comorbidity rate of TS and OCD, systematic family studies suggest that some forms of OCD may be a phenotypic variant of TS. For example, the increased rate of OCD in first-degree relatives of TS probands has been noted regardless of the presence of OCD in the TS probands (Pauls *et al.* 1986b, 1991). Recent empirical studies have reported consistent and remarkable differences in these two putative types of OCD. In general, tic-related OCD has prepubertal onset, male predominance, a mix of aggressive and sexual obsessions, concerns of symmetry and exactness, tic-like compulsions, and a preceding 'just right' perception before performance of their compulsions. In contrast, non-tic-related OCD is characterized by a peri- or postpubertal onset, sex-equivalent vulnerability, predominant contamination worries and cleaning compulsions, and preceding obsessive worries and anxiety that are recognized as prompting other compulsive performance (George *et al.* 1993, Baer 1994, Holzer *et al.* 1994, Leckman *et al.* 1994, de Groot *et al.* 1995, Leckman *et al.* 1995).

Studies of natural history

Natural history studies provide information that is valuable because such studies guide clinical treatment decisions, and enable clinicians to counsel patients and their families concerning the course and prognosis of the disorder.

Most of the natural history studies available for tic disorders and TS have been conducted retrospectively, with varying numbers of study subjects ranging from 10 to 251 and varying duration of follow-up ranging from 0.5 to 38 years.

In general, these studies have found that tics occur in childhood and are at their worst in the first decade. For most patients, tic disorders and TS improve during late adolescence or early adulthood. Four early follow-up studies of tic disorders, which included transient tic disorders and chronic motor tic disorders as well as TS, reported on 15–220 subjects. The follow-up duration ranged from 1 to 18 years, and the subjects had an age range at follow-up from 6 to 29 (Zausmer 1954, Torup 1962, Lucas *et al.* 1967, Corbett *et al.* 1969). Based on the author's own criteria for remission and improvement of tics, these studies reported remission of tic symptoms in 33–50%, improvement in tics in 43–82% and no changes or worsening of tics in 6–24% of patients who were not treated with medication. One follow-up study of 58 children who were diagnosed with transient tic disorder at initial evaluation reported that the children whose initial symptoms were either both motor and vocal tics, or vocal tics alone, had higher risk for subsequent development of TS at follow-up evaluation (Bruun and Budman 1997). Follow-up studies of TS had duration of 0.5–38 years, with 15–251 subjects who ranged in age from 6 to 85 at follow-up (Mahler and Luke 1946, Bruun *et al.* 1976, Asam 1982, Mak *et al.* 1982, Erenberg *et al.* 1987a, Bruun 1988, Sandor *et al.* 1990, Park *et al.* 1993). These studies of

TS patients who were not treated with medication reported that 11–52% of patients experienced remission, 25–81% had improvement in tics and 28–100% had unchanged tic severity at follow-up.

However, interpretation and comparability of the findings from natural history studies of tic disorders are limited by the use of

- potential sampling bias because most of the subjects were recruited from clinics, not from communities

- retrospective study designs and consequent bias in recalling the natural course of the disease

- variable duration of the follow-up interval

- inconsistent and sometimes inadequate evaluation of tic severity at baseline and follow-up.

Intervention studies

Interventions for tic disorders and TS are divided into three categories: pharmacotherapy, behavioral therapy, and neurosurgical procedures.

Pharmacotherapy

Pharmacotherapeutic intervention is predominantly used for patients with tic disorders and TS. Various kinds of agents have been studied, based on empirical and theoretical considerations.

Antidopaminergic agents

Haloperidol is a central dopamine D_2 receptor antagonist and also has some adrenergic α_1 antagonistic activity. Case reports and uncontrolled studies which were conducted either retrospectively or prospectively have reported that haloperidol can effectively suppress tics in 45–80% of patients (Seignot 1961, Lucas *et al.* 1967, Shapiro and Shapiro 1968, Erenberg *et al.* 1987a). Double-blind randomized clinical trials (RCTs) have showed that haloperidol (mean dosage = 4.5 mg per day) is superior to placebo in suppressing tics (Ross and Moldofsky 1978, Shapiro *et al.* 1989). However, haloperidol can be associated with serious side-effects (such as sedation, acute dystonia, and akathisia), resulting in discontinuation in many patients despite beneficial effects on tics (Ross and Moldofsky 1978, Erenberg 1992, Silva *et al.* 1996). Fortunately, long-term complications of haloperidol therapy, such as tardive dyskinesia, are rare in TS patients. However, tic exacerbation and marked withdrawal dyskinesias frequently occur following discontinuation of haloperidol (Caine and Polinsky 1981, Riddle *et al.* 1987, Singh and Jankovic 1988).

Pimozide is a more specific central dopamine D_2 receptor antagonist with no anti-norepinephrine effect. As expected from its pharmacological characteristics, pimozide has been reported to have similar effectiveness in tic suppression to haloperidol, with fewer adverse effects, in both uncontrolled and controlled double-blind studies (Ross and

Moldofsky 1978, Shapiro *et al.* 1983a, Erenberg *et al.* 1987b, Shapiro *et al.* 1989, Sallee *et al.* 1997). Recently, one double-blind, placebo-controlled crossover study of haloperidol and pimozide in children and adolescents reported that pimozide was superior to haloperidol in relative efficacy (Sallee *et al.* 1997).

Tetrabenazine exerts its antidopaminergic effects by depleting presynaptic dopamine storage granules and blocking postsynaptic dopamine receptors. In uncontrolled, open-label studies, the beneficial effects of tetrabenazine have been reported (Jankovic *et al.* 1984, Jankovic and Orman 1988). More recently, dopamine agonists such as *pergolide* and *talipexole* have been used in the treatment of tics with inconsistent results (Goetz *et al.* 1994, Lipinski *et al.*, 1997). These agents are believed to exert modulatory effects on dopaminergic activity resulting in a decrease in tic symptoms.

Atypical antipsychotic agents

The pharmacological characteristics of atypical antipsychotic agents, such as preferential involvement of limbic and cortical dopaminergic circuits and relative sparing of the nigrostriatal dopaminergic system, provide the theoretical basis for examining their therapeutic effects in TS patients (Gerlach and Peacock 1995). Such agents include clozapine, risperidone, and sulpiride.

Clozapine is a potent serotonin 5-HT$_2$ receptor antagonist and a weak dopamine D$_2$ receptor antagonist. Successful treatment outcomes of tardive-TS, which is a variant of tardive dyskinesia, with clozapine have been reported in case reports (Kalian *et al.* 1993, Jaffe *et al.* 1995). However, a controlled, double-blind, crossover clinical trial of clozapine failed to demonstrate its tic-suppressing effect in TS subjects (Caine *et al.* 1979).

Risperidone is a potent antagonist at both the serotonin 5-HT$_2$ and dopamine D$_2$ sites. Three prospective open-label studies in a total of 56 TS subjects showed that risperidone reduced tics to 25–66% of their baseline severity (van der Linden *et al.* 1994, Lombroso *et al.* 1995, Bruun and Budman 1996).

Sulpiride has a highly selective dopamine D$_2$ receptor antagonist effect. One uncontrolled retrospective study showed that sulpiride had beneficial effects in 59% of treated TS patients (Robertson et al. 1990). Taken together, these findings suggest that D$_2$ receptor blockade is the essential pharmacological action for the neuroleptics.

α_2 Adrenergic agonist

Clonidine is a central α_2-adrenergic agonist. In an open-label study and a controlled single-blind study, clonidine was reported to be effective in reducing tics, especially vocal tics, and other behavioral problems such as attentional problems and low frustration tolerance, in 25–70% of TS subjects (Cohen *et al.* 1980, Shapiro *et al.* 1983b, Leckman *et al.* 1985). Further study findings in controlled clinical trials have been equivocal (Goetz *et al.* 1987, Leckman *et al.* 1991).

Guanfacine has similar pharmacological characteristics to clonidine, but also has several potential advantages. It is more selective in its receptor affinity profile, it has a longer half-life, and less sedative and hypotensive side-effects than clonidine. Two uncontrolled open-label studies showed that guanfacine improves symptoms of ADHD (Horrigan and Barnhill 1995, Hunt *et al.* 1995). A third study reported a modest beneficial effects on the reduction of tics (Chappell *et al.* 1995).

Hormonal agents

Exacerbation of tic symptoms in two TS subjects with the use of an *anabolic steroid* was reported in a case report (Leckman and Scahill 1990). A controlled double-blind crossover study of *flutamide,* an androgenic receptor blocker, showed that it has modest tic suppressing effects, primarily on motor tics (Peterson *et al.* 1994).

A variety of other pharmacological and other interventions have been tried in TS, but sufficient data are not available to judge their merits.

Behavioral therapy

The types of behavioural therapy that have been used for tic disorders and TS include massed negative practice, contingency management, relaxation training, self-monitoring, and habit reversal. Mostly, single-subject experimental designs have reported beneficial effects of behavioral therapies on tic disorders and TS. Only habit reversal, which uses a competing response to prevent the occurrence of tics, has been studied in randomized controlled studies of subjects with chronic tic disorders and TS. Habit reversal was reported to be superior in reducing tics compared to massed practice and no treatment (Azrin *et al.* 1980).

Neurosurgical treatments

Neurosurgery has been performed primarily on patients who suffered from disabling tic disorders and comorbid conditions and has targeted frontal cortical, cingulate cortical, thalamic, or cerebellar brain areas. The findings of case reports are inconclusive (Chappell *et al.* 1997).

Short-term and long-term outcome

Tic severity outcomes with pharmacotherapy

Two early studies of tic disorders examined tic outcomes of the patients who had pharmacological intervention at follow-up (Torup 1962, Lucas *et al.* 1967). These studies were conducted in a retrospective way with 15–220 study subjects and duration of follow-up ranging from 2 to 16 years. They reported remission of tics in 10%, improvement of tics in 64–70% and unchanged or worsening of tic severity in 20% of patients at follow-up. Six studies that have been conducted retrospectively, with the number of study subjects ranging from 15 to 78 and duration of follow-up ranging from 0.5 to 20 years, reported tic outcomes in TS patients who were treated with medications, mainly haloperidol and pimozide (Bruun *et al.* 1976, Shapiro *et al.* 1978, Asam 1982, Mak *et al.* 1982, Erenberg *et al.* 1987a, Sandor *et al.* 1990). In these studies, tic severity at follow-up was rated as remission in 14–33%, improvement in 33–100% and no change or worsening of tics in 3–36% of the patients.

Psychosocial outcomes

In early studies of tic disorders, psychosocial outcomes at follow-up showed fair to good social adjustment in 66% of patients and achievement of high school or university education in 33%

of patients (Lucas *et al.* 1967). Of the TS patients, 25–98% achieved more than a high school education, 13–54% got married, and 61–90% were employed, with 35% of the jobs classified as professional in one study (Mahler and Luke 1946, Asam 1982, Mak *et al.* 1982, Erenberg *et al.* 1987a, Bruun 1988, Goetz *et al.* 1992). However, some studies reported a failure on the part of TS patients to achieve parental social class due to restricted educational and vocational opportunities (Asam 1982, Sandor *et al.* 1990). Family functioning, independent of parental psychopathology was reported to be associated with ADHD and anxiety disorder, decreased adaptive behavior, and increased maladaptive behaviors and lower self-esteem, but not in tic severity outcome or learning disorders (Carter *et al.* 1994).

Continuity versus discontinuity

It is generally accepted that the onset of tic disorders and TS occurs in the first decade of life and that symptoms for a majority of cases are markedly reduced in late adolescence and early adulthood (Leckman *et al.* 1998). Burd *et al.* (1986) reported a disparity in the prevalence of TS among children and adults of 5.2 per 10 000 versus 0.5 per 10 000 in his prevalence study of TS in North Dakota, and attributed this disparity to the quiescence of tic symptoms in adulthood and the underdiagnosis of TS in adults (Burd *et al.* 1986).

However, given the ascertainment bias and these other limitations, caution is warranted in interpreting this data. This disparity does not necessarily represent the reduction of symptoms in early adulthood. For example, there may be important birth cohort variations in health status produced by unique environmental and social factors across these different birth cohorts. Also, there may be fundamental difference in healthcare services such that child cases are more readily identified in the current era.

Risk and prognostic factors

Risk factors

Risk factors are defined as factors that contribute to the persistence of tic disorders at follow-up and that are associated with a poor outcome.

There is little information available in this area. Risk factors that are known to be influential on the course of Tourette's syndrome include chronic intermittent psychosocial stresses such as being teased or severely criticized for having tic symptoms, exposure to cocaine or other CNS stimulants, and thermal stress in a few well-documented cases (for review, see Leckman *et al.* 1997).

Prognostic factors

Prognostic factors are defined as factors that are present at the beginning of the disorders and are either positively or negatively associated with outcomes. The natural course of a disease varies considerably from patient to patient; it is therefore important to predict which patients will do well and which ones will not. Low IQ and poor school performance were related to downward drift of social class and poor social adjustment (Mak *et al.* 1982). In early studies in patients with tic disorders, female gender, onset age between 6–8, longer duration of follow-up and sleep disorder at initial evaluation were associated with a good prognosis, whereas patients whose parents had persistent tics in adulthood, who had conflicts in the home, body tics or vocal tics (especially coprolalia), comorbid affective disorders, and obsessionality at initial evaluation were found to have a poor prognosis (Zausmer 1954, Torup 1962, Corbett *et al.* 1969). In TS patients, remission was found more frequently in patients from a high social class who also tended to have milder tics (Shapiro *et al.* 1978). Additionally, patients who had mild tics at their worst ever period, at mid or late-youth or throughout youth, tended to have mild adult tics (Goetz *et al.* 1992). Also, Mahler and Luke (1946) observed that organized outdoor physical activity appeared to help their patients develop a more integrative personality and to recover from TS or to have improved symptoms. They attributed this more favorable outcome to tension-reducing influence of physical activity (Mahler and Luke 1946). Patients who had moderate to severe tic severity in late youth tended to have more severe adult tics (Goetz *et al.* 1992). Interestingly, medication, response of tics to medication, childhood tic severity, and coprolalia did not seem to have prognostic value in TS patients in later studies (Erenberg *et al.* 1987a, Sandor *et al.* 1990, Goetz *et al.* 1992, Leckman *et al.*, in press). Severity of maternal stress during pregnancy, male gender of the patient, and severe nausea and/or vomiting during the first trimester of pregnancy were reported to be significantly associated with tic severity at follow-up (Leckman *et al.* 1990).

Conclusion

Tic disorders are childhood onset neuropsychiatric condition that emerge as the result of the effects of genetic, neurobiological, and environmental factors operating during development. Systematic research paradigms have been developed to understand these disorders that emphasize multidisciplinary approaches. Advances in genetics will permit the identification of disease genes, which in turn, will allow a more accurate diagnosis of the disorders and more effective identification of environmental risk and protective factors. Knowledge of the specific vulnerability genes and risk factors will permit the development of the animal models and the ability to monitor the expression and function of the gene products over the course of normal development. Such animal models can be used to test the role of various risk and protective factors and to speed the development of the interventions aimed at preventing severe outcomes. Advances in developmental neuroscience will widen our understanding of the role of specific neurobiological pathways in these disorders, which will enable us to use accurate animal models of the disorders to maximum advantage. Based on the rapid progress of the past decade, we anticipate major advances in the understanding of the pathogenesis of tic disorders in the near future.

To achieve this goal, a prospective birth cohort design to evaluate the study subjects selected by a valid diagnostic criteria and assessed at multiple points of time with various standardized assessment tools would be most desirable to minimize information bias and maximize measurement reliability. Inclusion of community cases and valid comparison groups in such studies will enable generalization of future study findings.

Acknowledgment

The authors thank Drs Patricia Feineigle and Lawrence Scahill for their generous help with the preparation of this chapter.

References

APA (1994). In *Diagnostic and Statistical Manual of Mental Disorders*, 4th edn, pp. 78–85, 100–105, 417–423. American Psychiatric Association, Washington, DC.

Apter, A., Pauls, D.L., Bleich, A., Zohar, A.H., Kron, S., Ratzoni, G., Dycian, A., Kotler, M., Weizman, A., Gadot, N., and Cohen, D.J. (1993). An epidemiological study of Gilles de la Tourette's syndrome in Israel. *Archives of General Psychiatry*, **50**, 734–738.

Asam, U. (1982). A follow-up study of Tourette syndrome. In *Advances in neurology*, Vol. 35., ed. A.J.,Friedhoff and T.N. Chase, pp. 285–286. Raven Press, New York.

Azrin, N.H., Nunn, R.G., and Frantz, S.E. (1980). Habit reversal vs. negative practice treatment of nervous tics. *Behavioral Therapy*, **11**, 169–178.

Baer, L. (1994). Factor analysis of symptom subtypes of obsessive compulsive disorder and their relation to personality and tic disorders. *Journal of Clinical Psychiatry*, **55**, 18–22.

Bornstein, R.A., Stefl, M.E., and Hammond, L. (1990). A survey of Tourette syndrome patients and their families : the 1987 Ohio Tourette survey. *Journal of Neuropsychiatry and Clinical Neuroscience*, **2**, 275–281.

Bruun, R.D. (1988). The natural history of Tourette's syndrome. In *Tourette's syndrome and tic disorders : Clinical understanding and treatment*, ed. D.J. Cohen, R.D. Bruun, and J.F. Leckman, pp. 21–39. Wiley, New York.

Bruun, R.D. and Budman, C.L. (1996). Risperidone as a treatment for Tourette's syndrome. *Journal of Clinical Psychiatry*, **57**, 29–31.

Bruun, R.D. and Budman, C.L. (1997). The course and prognosis of Tourette syndrome. In *Tourette syndrome*, ed. J. Jankovic, pp. 291–198. Neurologic Clinics Vol. 15, W.B. Saunders, Philadelphia.

Bruun, R.D., Shapiro, A.K., and Shapiro, E. (1976). A follow up of eighty patients with Tourette's syndrome. *Psychopharmacology Bulletin*, **12**, 15–17.

Burd, L., Kerbeshian, J., Wikenheiser, M., and Fisher, W. (1986). A prevalence study of Gilles de la Tourette syndrome in North Dakota school-age children. *Journal of American Academy of Child Psychiatry*, **25**, 552–553.

Caine, E.D., McBride, M.C., Chiverton, P., Bamford, K.A., Rediess, S., and Shiao, J. (1988). Tourette's syndrome in Monroe County school children. *Neurology*, **38**, 472–475.

Caine, E.D. and Polinsky, R.J. (1981). Tardive dyskinesia in persons with Gilles de la Tourette's disease. *Archives of Neurology*, **38**, 471–472.

Caine, E.D., Polinsky, R.J., Kartzinel, R., and Ebert, M.H. (1979). The trial use of clozapine for abnormal involuntary movement disorders. *American Journal of Psychiatry*, **136**, 317–320.

Carter, A.S., Pauls, D.L., Leckman, J.F., and Cohen, D.J. (1994). A prospective longitudinal study of Gilles de la Tourette's syndrome. *Journal of the American Academy of Child and Adolescent Psychiatry*, **33**, 377–385.

Chappell, P.B., Riddle, M.A., Scahill, L.D., Lynch, K.A., Schultz, R., Arnsten, A., Leckman, J.F., and Cohen, J.F. (1995). Guanfacine treatment of comorbid attention-deficit hyperactivity disorder and Tourette's syndrome: Preliminary clinical experience. *Journal of the American Academy of Child and Adolescent Psychiatry*, **34**, 1140–1146.

Chappell, P.B., Scahill, L.D., and Leckman, J.F. (1997). Future therapies of Tourette syndrome. In *Tourette syndrome*, ed. J. Jankovic, pp. 429–450. Neurologic Clinics Vol. 15, W.B. Saunders, Philadelphia.

Cohen, D.J., Detlor, J., Young, J.G., and Shaywitz, B.A. (1980). Clonidine ameliorates Gilles de la Tourette syndrome. *Archives of General Psychiatry*, **37**, 1350–1357.

Comings, D.E., Himes, J.A., and Comings, B.G. (1990). An epidemiologic study of Tourette's syndrome in a single school district. *Journal of Clinical Psychiatry*, **51**, 463–469.

Corbett, J.A., Mathews, A.M., Connell, P.H., and Shapiro, D.A. (1969). Tics and Gilles de la Tourette's syndrome: a follow-up study and critical review. *British Journal of Psychiatry*, **115**, 1229–1241.

Costello, E.J., Angold, A., Burns, B.J., Stangl, D.K., Tweed, D.L., Erkanli, A., and Worthman, C.M. (1996). The Great Smoky Mountains study of youth—goals, design, methods, and the prevalence of DSM III-R disorders. *Archives of General Psychiatry*, **53**, 1129–1136.

de Groot, C.M., Bornstein, R.A., Janus, M.D., and Mavissakalian, M.R. (1995). Patterns of obsessive compulsive symptoms in Tourette subjects are independent of severity. *Anxiety*, **1**, 268–274.

Dykens, E.M., Leckman, J.F., Riddle, M.A., Hardin, M.T., Schwartz, S., and Cohen, D.J. (1990). Intellectual, academic, and adaptive functioning of Tourette syndrome children with and without attention deficit disorder. *Journal of Abnormal Child Psychology*, **18**, 607–614.

Erenberg, G. (1992). Treatment of Tourette's syndrome with neuroleptic drugs. In *Tourette Syndrome: Genetics, neurobiology and treatment*, ed. T.N. Chase, A.J. Friedhoff, and D.J. Cohen, pp. 241–243. Advances in Neurology Vol. 58, Raven Press, New York.

Erenberg, G., Cruse, R.P., and Rothner, A.D. (1986). Tourette syndrome : an analysis of 200 pediatric and adolescent cases. *Cleveland Clinic Quarterly*, **53**, 127–131.

Erenberg, G., Cruse, R.P., and Rothner, A.D. (1987a). The natural history of Tourette Syndrome: a follow-up study. *Annals of Neurology*, **22**, 383–385.

Erenberg, G., Cruse, R.P., and Rothner, A.D. (1987b). The use of pimozide in young children with Tourette's syndrome. *Annals of Neurology*, **22**, 435.

George, M.S., Trimble, M.R., Ring, H.A., Sallee, F.R., and Robertson, M.M. (1993). Obsessions in obsessive-compulsive disorder with and without Gilles de la Tourette's syndrome. *American Journal of Psychiatry*, **150**, 93–97.

Gerlach, J. and Peacock, L. (1995). New antipsychotics: the present status. *International Clinical Psychopharmacology*, **10** (Suppl. 3), 39–48.

Gilles de la Tourette, G. (1885). Etude sur une affection nerveuse caracterisée par de l'incoordination motrice accompagnée d'écholalie et de copralalie. *Archives of Neurology*, **9**, 19–42, 158–200.

Goetz, C.G., Stebbins, G.T., and Thelen, J.A. (1994). Talipexole and adult Gilles de la Tourettes syndrome: double-blind, placebo-controlled clinical trial. *Movement Disorder*, **9**, 315–317.

Goetz, C.G., Tanner, C.M., Stebbins, G.T., Leipzig, G., and Carr, W.C. (1992). Adults' tics in Gilles de la Tourette's syndrome: description and risk factors. *Neurology*, **42**, 784–788.

Goetz, C.G., Tanner, C.M., Wilson, R.S., Carroll, V.S., Como, P.G., and Shannon, K.M. (1987). Clonidine and Gilles de la Tourette's syndrome: double-blind study using objective rating methods. *Annals of Neurology*, **21**, 307–310.

Grad, L.R., Pelcovitz, D., Olson, M., Matthews, M., and Grad, G.J. (1987). Obsessive-compulsive symptomatology in children with Tourette's syndrome. *Journal of the American Academy of Child and Adolescent Psychiatry*, **26**, 69–73.

Holzer, J., Goodman, W.K., Price, L.H., Baer, L., Leckman, J.F., and Heninger, G.R. (1994). Obsessive compulsive disorder with and without a chronic tic disorder : a comparison of symptoms in 70 patients. *British Journal of Psychiatry*, **164**, 469–473.

Horrigan, J.P. and Barnhill, L.J. (1995). Guanfacine for treatment of attention-deficit hyperactivity disorder in boys. *Journal of Child and Adolescent Psychopharmacology*, **5**, 215–223.

Hunt, R.D., Arnsten, A.F.T., and Asbell, M.D. (1995). An open trial of guanfacine in the treatment of attention-deficit hyperactivity disorder. *Journal of the American Academy of Child and Adolescent Psychiatry*, **34**, 50–54.

Jaffe, E., Tremeau, F., Sharif, Z., and Reider, R. (1995). Clozapine in tardive Tourette syndrome. *Biological Psychiatry*, **38**, 196–197.

Jagger, J., Prusoff, B.A., Cohen, D.J., Kidd, K.K., Carbonari, C.M., and John, K. (1982). The epidemiology of Tourette syndrome: a pilot study. *Schizophrenia Bulletin*, **8**, 267–278.

Jankovic, J. and Orman, J. (1988). Tetranbenzaine therapy of dystonia, chorea, tics, and other dyskinesias. *Neurology*, **38**, 391–394.

Jankovic, J., Glaze, D.G., and Frost, J.D., Jr. (1984). Effects of tetrabenazine on tics and sleep of Gilles de la Tourette's syndrome. *Neurology*, **34**, 688–692.

Kalian, M., Lerner, V., and Glodman, M. (1993). Atypical variants of tardive dyskinesia, treated by a combination of clozapine with propranolol and clozapine with tetrabenazine. *Journal of Nervous and Mental Disorder*, **181**, 649–651.

Kidd, K.K., Prusoff, B.A., and Cohen, D.J. (1980). The familial pattern of Tourette syndrome. *Archives of General Psychiatry*, **37**, 1336–1339.

Leckman, J.F. and Scahill, L. (1990b). Possible exacerbation of tics by androgenic steroids. *New England Journal of Medicine*, **322**, 1674.

Leckman, J.F., Detlor, J., Harcherik, D.F., Ort, S., Shaywitz, B.A., and Cohen, D.J. (1985). Short- and long-term treatment of Tourettes syndrome with clonidine: a clinical perspective. *Neurology*, **35**, 343–351.

Leckman, J.F., Dolnansky, E.S., Hardin, M.T., Clubb, M., Walkup, J.T., Stevenson, J., and Pauls, D. (1990). Perinatal factors in the expression of Tourettes Syndrome: an exploratory study. *Journal of the American Academy of Child and Adolescent Psychiatry*, **29**, 220–226.

Leckman, J.F., Hardin, M.T., Riddle, M.A., Stevenson, J., Ort, S.I., and Cohen, D.J. (1991). Clonidine treatment of Gilles de la Tourettes syndrome. *Archives of General Psychiatry*, **48**, 1168–1176.

Leckman, J.F., Walker, D.E., and Cohen, D.J. (1993). Premonitory urges in Tourettes Syndrome. American Journal of Psychiatry, 150, 98–102.

Leckman, J.F., Walker, D.E., Goodman, W.K., Pauls, D.L., and Cohen, D.J. (1994). Just

Right perception associated with compulsive behavior in Tourettes Syndrome. *American Journal of Psychiatry*, 151, 675–680.

Leckman, J.F., Grice, D.E., Barr, L.C., deVries, A.L.C., Martin, C., Cohen, D.J., Goodman, W.K., and Rasmussen, S.A. (1995). Tic-related vs. non-tic related obsessive compulsive disorder. *Anxiety*, **1**, 208–215.

Leckman, J.F., Peterson, B.S., Anderson, G.M., Arnsten, A.F.T., Pauls, D.L., and Cohen, D.J. (1997). Pathogenesis of Tourette's syndrome. *Journal of Child Psychology and Psychiatry*, **38**, 119–142.

Leckman, J.F., Zhang, H., Vitale, A., Lahnin, F., Lynch, K., Bondi, C., Kim, Y., and Peterson, B.S. (1998). Course of tic severity; the first two decades. *Pediatrics*, **102**, 14–19.

Lipinski, J.F., Salle, F.R., and Jackson, C. (1997). Dopamine agonist treatment of Tourette disorder in children: results of an open-label trial of pergolide. *Movement Disorder*, **12**, 402–407.

Lombroso, P.J., Scahill, L., King, R.A., Lynch, K.A., Challell, P.B., Peterson, B.S., McDougle, C.J., and Leckman, J.F. (1995). Risperidone treatment of children and adolescents with chronic tic disorders: a preliminary report. *Journal of the American Academy of Child and Adolescent Psychiatry*, **34**, 1147–1152.

Lucas, A.R., Auffman, P.E., and Morris, E.M. (1967). Gilles de la Tourettes disease: a clinical study of fifteen cases. *Journal of the American Academy of Child Psychiatry*, **6**, 700–722.

Lucas, A.R., Beard, C.M., Rajput, A.H., and Kurland, L.T. (1982). Tourette syndrome in Rochester, Minnesota, 1968–1979. In *Advances in Neurology*, Vol. 35, ed. A.J. Friedhoff and T.N. Chase, pp. 267–269. Raven Press, New York.

Mahler, M.S. and Luke, J.A. (1946). Outcome of the tic syndrome. *Journal of Nervous and Mental Disease*, **103**, 433–445.

Mahler, M.S., Luke, J.A., and Daltroff, W. (1945). Clinical and follow-up study of the tic syndrome in children. *American Journal of Orthopsychiatry*, **15**, 631–647.

Mak, F.L., Chung, S.Y., Lee, P., and Chen, S. (1982). Tourette syndrome in the Chinese: a follow-up of 15 cases. In *Advances in Neurology*, Vol. 35, ed. A.J. Friedhoff, and T.N. Chase, pp. 281–283. Raven Press, New York.

Park, S., Como, P.G., Cui, L., and Kurlan, R. (1993). The early course of the Tourette's syndrome clinical spectrum. *Neurology*, **43**, 1712–1715.

Pauls, D.L., Cohen, D.J., Heimbuch, R., Detlor, J., and Kidd, K.K. (1981). Familial pattern and transmission of Gilles de la Tourette syndrome and multiple tics. *Archives of General Psychiatry*, **38**, 1091–1093.

Pauls, D.L., Kruger, S.D., Leckman, J.F., Cohen, D.J., and Kidd, K.K. (1984). The risk of Tourette's syndrome and chronic multiple tics among relatives of Tourette's syndrome patients obtained by direct interview. *Journal of the American Academy of Child Psychiatry*, **23**, 134–137.

Pauls, D.L., Hurst, C.R., Kruger, S.D., Leckman, J.F., Kidd, K.K., and Cohen, D.J. (1986a). Gilles de la Tourette's syndrome and attention deficit with hyperactivity. *Archives of General Psychiatry*, **43**, 1177–1179.

Pauls, D.L., Towbin, K.E., Leckman, J.F., Zahner, G.E.P., and Cohen, D.J. (1986b). Gilles de la Tourette's syndrome and obsessive compulsive disorder. *Archives of General Psychiatry*, **43**, 1180–1182.

Pauls, D.L., Raymond, C.L., Stevenson, J.M., and Leckman, J.F. (1991). A family study of Gilles de la Tourette syndrome. *American Journal of Human Genetics*, **48**, 154–163.

Pauls, D.L., Leckman, J.F., and Cohen, D.J. (1993). Familial relationship between Gilles de la Tourette's syndrome, attention deficit disorder, learning disabilities, speech disorders, and stuttering. *Journal of the American Academy of Child and Adolescent Psychiatry*, **32**, 1044–1050.

Peterson, B.S., Leckman, J.F., Scahill, L., Naftolin, F., Keefe, D., Charest, N.J., King, R.A., Hardin, M.T., and Cohen, D.J. (1994). Steroid hormones and Tourette's syndrome: early experience with antiandrogen therapy. *Journal of Clinical Pharmacology*, **14**, 131–135.

Pitman, R.K., Green, R.C., Jenike, M.A., and Mesulam, M.M. (1987). Clinical comparison of Tourette's disorder and obsessive-compulsive disorder. *American Journal of Psychiatry*, **144**, 1166–1171.

Riddle, M.A., Hardin, M.T., Towbin, K.E., Leckman, J.F., and Cohen, D.J. (1987). Tardive dyskinesia following haloperidol treatment in Tourette's syndrome. *Archives of General Psychiatry*, **44**, 98–99.

Robertson, M.M., Schnieden, V., and Lees, A.J. (1990). Management of Gilles de la Tourette syndrome using sulpiride. *Clinical Neuropharmacology*, **13**, 229–235.

Ross, M.S. and Moldofsky, H. (1978). A comparison of pimozide and haloperidol in the treatment of Gilles de la Tourette's syndrome. *American Journal of Psychiatry*, **135**, 585–587.

Sallee, F.R., Nesbitt, L., Jackson, C., Sine, L., and Sethuraman, G. (1997). Relative efficacy of haloperidol and pimozide in children and adolescents with Tourette's disorder. *American Journal of Psychiatry*, **154**, 1057–1062.

Sandor, P., Musisi, S., Moldofsky, H., and Lang, A. (1990). Tourette syndrome =: a follow-up study. *Journal of Clinical Psychopharmacology*, **10**, 197–199.

Seignot, M.J.N. (1961). A case of Gilles de la Tourette cured by R1625. *Annals of Medico-psychology*, **119**, 578–579.

Shapiro, A.K. and Shapiro, E. (1968). Treatment of Gilles de la Tourette's syndrome with haloperidol. *British Journal of Psychiatry*, **114**, 345–350.

Shapiro, A.K., Shapiro, E., Bruun, R.D., and Sweet, R.D. (1978). In *Gilles de la Tourette Syndrome*. Raven Press, New York.

Shapiro, A.K., Shapiro, E., and Eisenkraft, G.J. (1983a). Treatment of Gilles de la Tourette syndrome with pimozide. *American Journal of Psychiatry*, **140**, 1183–1186.

Shapiro, A.K., Shapiro, E., and Eisenkraft, G.J. (1983b). Treatment of Gilles de la Tourette's syndrome with clonidine and neuroleptics. *Archives of General Psychiatry*, **40**, 1235–1240.

Shapiro, A.K., Shapiro, E.S., Young, J.G., and Feinberg, T.E. (1988). In *Gilles de la Tourette Syndrome*, pp. 90–91 Raven Press, New York.

Shapiro, E.S., Shapiro, A.K., Fulop, G., Hubbard, M., Mandeli, J., Nordlie, J., and Phillips, R.A. (1989). Controlled study of haloperidol, pimozide and placebo for the treatment of Gilles de la Tourette's syndrome. *Archives of General Psychiatry*, **46**, 722–730.

Silva, R.R., Munoz, D.M., Daniel, W., Barickman, J., and Friedhoff, A.J. (1996). Causes of haloperidol discontinuation in patients with Tourette's disorder: Management and alternatives. *Journal of Clinical Psychiatry*, **57**, 129–135.

Singh, S.K. and Jankovic, J. (1988). Tardive dyskinesia in patients with Tourette's syndrome. *Movement Disorder*, **3**, 274–280.

Spencer, T., Biederman, J., Harding, M., Wilens, T., and Faraone, S. (1995). The relationship between tic disorders and Tourettes Syndrome revisited. *Journal of the American Academy of Child and Adolescent Psychiatry*, **34**, 1133–1139.

Stokes, A., Bawden, H.N., Camfield, P.R., Backman, J.E., and Dooley, J.M. (1991). Peer problems in Tourette's disorder. *Pediatrics*, **87**, 36–42.

Swedo, S.E. and Leonard, H.L. (1994). Childhood movement disorders and obsessive compulsive disorder. *Journal of Clinical Psychiatry* **55**, 32–37.

Torup, E. (1962). A follow-up study of children with tics. *Acta Paediatrica* **51**, 261–268.

van der Linden, C., Bruggeman, R., and van Woerkom, T.A.M. (1994). Serotonin-dopamine antagonist and Gilles de la Tourette's syndrome: an open pilot dose-titration study with risperidone. *Movement Disorder*, **9**, 687–688.

WHO (1992). In *ICD-10 Classification of Mental and Behavioral Disorders; Clinical descriptions and diagnostic guidelines*, pp. 282–284. World Health Organization, Geneva.

Zausmer, D.M. (1954). The treatment of tics in childhood—a review and a follow-up study. *Archives of Disease in Childhood* **29**, 537–542.

18 Variants of gender differentiation

Heino F.L. Meyer-Bahlburg

Of the three main diagnostic categories in the Sexual and Gender Identity Disorders section of DSM-IV, only one, gender identity disorder (GID), is applied to children below teenage (APA 1994, pp. 532–8). No diagnostic category of sexual behavior disorder has been defined for children; sexual dysfunctions and paraphilias are diagnosed only in adolescents and adults. Although quite a few preteenage children need help with sexual behavior problems, especially following sexual abuse, these problems are either not diagnostically categorized at all or understood as a component of another diagnostic category such as conduct disorder or post-traumatic stress disorder. Therefore, this chapter is limited to variants of gender development such as GID in childhood as defined in DSM-IV and the gender identity problems of individuals born with somatic intersexuality or other forms of genital ambiguity (in DSM-IV classified as GID Not Otherwise Specified [GID NOS]). Because of space limitations we do not address the current debate on whether GID and gender problems should be removed from the DSM or otherwise 'depathologized'; the developmental research questions would largely remain the same.

Clinical picture

GID in genitally normal, non-intersex individuals is defined by strong and persistent identification with the other sex in combination with persistent gender dysphoria, i.e. discomfort about one's assigned sex or a sense of inappropiateness in the gender role of that sex (APA 1994, pp. 532–3). Children with GID may say that they wish to be or indeed are the other sex and show marked preoccupation with cross-gender activities. For instance, boys with GID like to dress up in girls' or women's outfits, take female roles in pretend games, prefer girls' toys and game activities, have a strong preference for girls as playmates, tend to avoid rough-and-tumble play and male-typical sports and other activities, and may reject their own genitalia. Girls with GID show the corresponding reverse behaviors.

Gender problems in children and adolescents with intersexuality or other forms of genital ambiguity are diverse and range in severity from parental concerns about slightly gender-atypical behavior through the child's doubts of his/her assigned gender to gender dysphoria, a clinical picture similar to GID, and gender change. The problems vary with the intersex syndrome, the genital status, the prenatal and postnatal sex-hormone milieu, the quality of medical management, age, the psychosocial history, especially of the home situation, and cultural context. The more severe problems such as patient-initiated gender change tend to take place during adolescence and even adulthood rather than in childhood (Meyer-Bahlburg

1994, Meyer-Bahlburg *et al.* 1996). Because of the great variety of medical intersex conditions, their rarity, the phenotypic variability of each, and the limited behavioral data available, the empirical evidence concerning the distribution of gender-behavioral patterns and problems can only be considered preliminary for most syndromes.

To date, none of the few existing studies on the prevalence of child psychiatric diagnoses in the general population has included an assessment of GID. Crude upper-bound estimates of the prevalence of GID can be derived from epidemiological data on the prevalence of parent-based reports of cross-gender wishes and behavior in their children (Meyer-Bahlburg 1985), but probably only a small percentage of such children would meet DSM-IV criteria for GID. A lower-bound estimate might be provided by the prevalence of adults with GID ('transsexuals' prior to DSM-IV) in the general population which—based on clinical referrals—are estimated to range around 1 : 30 000 men and 1 : 100 000 women in western industrialized countries (Meyer-Bahlburg 1985) except for the Netherlands, where the prevalence of adults with GID has recently been estimated as 1 : 11 000 men and 1 : 30 400 women (Bakker *et al.* 1993). As only a small fraction of children with GID will carry the syndrome forward into adolescence and go on to hormonal and surgical sex reassignment in adulthood, the prevalence of adulthood transsexualism constitutes a major underestimate of the frequency of childhood GID. Reported rates for males are usually higher than for females. The gender difference is even more pronounced for clinical referrals: at the largest known clinic specialized on such children the Male:Female ratio is approximately 6 : 1 (Zucker and Bradley 1995, p. 32).

Solid epidemiological figures for the prevalence or incidence of intersex syndromes are difficult to obtain. For the most frequent syndrome in 46,XX individuals, early onset (classical) congenital adrenal hyperplasia (CAH), estimates for the prevalence among live female newborns in North America cluster around 1 : 12 000 (New *et al.* 1989), but there are marked differences between ethnic groups. Estimates of the prevalence of intersex patients in general depend on which syndromes are included; generally accepted figures do not exist, especially not for the incidence of newborns with genital ambiguity significant enough to raise questions about the appropriate gender assignment.

Even more difficult is the establishment of the prevalence or incidence of gender problems among the various categories of intersex patients, owing to the lack of standard definitions of gender problems and the absence of any epidemiological data in this regard. Some of the existing data suggest an enormous variability in the rate of gender problems among syndromes and/or cultural settings. For instance, of 46,XX individuals with classical CAH in the US who are prenatally exposed to high levels of androgens, but raised female when correctly diagnosed in infancy, very few appear to change gender voluntarily in their lifetime (Meyer-Bahlburg *et al.* 1996). By contrast, of 46,XY individuals with 5-α-reductase deficiency (5α-RD) in a remote rural area of the Dominican Republic who at birth look very much like ordinary females and are raised as females, the majority change gender during the adolescent and young adult years when they undergo marked spontaneous somatic virilization (Imperato-McGinley *et al.* 1979). Thus, statements regarding the prevalence of gender problems among intersex individuals across syndromes and cultures may be very misleading. As to the gender ratio, the available data suggest more frequent patient-initiated gender change from female-raised to male than the other way around (Meyer-Bahlburg 1994).

Natural course studies

GID in childhood

The majority of children with GID are referred to clinical services between about 4 and 6 years of age, but referrals occur—at a lower rate—at any later age of childhood and adolescence. In reviewing the child's history at the initial evaluation, most parents report an onset of marked cross-gender behavior between the ages of 2 and 4 years. Initially, both parents and professionals such as family pediatricians and nursery school teachers tend to see the behavior as a transient phase, but if it persists into kindergarten age, parents and professionals gradually become concerned and look for help. (Whether there are 2–4 year old children who develop full GID for a brief transient period has not been studied systematically.)

Data on what happens subsequently are very limited. There are only a few clinical follow-up reports on very small samples of male patients with GID (Bailey and Zucker 1995) and one systematic controlled prospective follow-up study (Green 1987) of boys initially recruited at 4–12 years of age. The results suggest that most boys with early-identified GID do not carry the syndrome over into adolescence and adulthood. Six clinical follow-up studies with a total of 55 boys yielded the following breakdown:

- 5 transsexual (with a homosexual orientation)

- 1 heterosexual transvestite

- 15 heterosexual

- 21 homosexual

- 13 not GID and not classifiable as to sexual orientation (Zucker and Bradley 1995, p. 285).

At the last reported follow-up (age 14–24 years) of Green's (1987) sample, only one man was seriously considering medical sex reassignment, about 20–25% were heterosexual, and the remainder homosexual. As most of the boys in the prospective studies underwent some kind of psychological therapy, we do not have systematic data on the natural history of GID in childhood without professional intervention. All available evidence suggests, however, that in males the long-term outcome of adult homosexuality is relatively common and of adult GID relatively uncommon, i.e. in most cases the GID appears to fade during the years of middle childhood.

Retrospective data from adolescent patients with GID (Zucker and Bradley 1995, pp. 302–18; Cohen-Kettenis and van Goozen 1997) also indicate early onset of the condition. The same applies to adult women with GID (Bailey and Zucker 1995). Adult men with GID, by contrast, appear to represent one of two different pathways (Blanchard 1990): either early onset GID combined with androphilia (erotic attraction to men) in adolescence and adulthood, or adult onset of GID (following a history of transvestic fetishism around the time of puberty) usually associated with gynecophilia (erotic attraction to women) or autogynephilia (sexual arousal in men produced by the sound or image of themselves as women). Most adults with GID who undergo hormonal and surgical sex reassignment to the desired gender function socially and psychiatrically at least as well as before or better (Petersen and Dickey 1995).

Gender problems in intersexuality

In the majority of persons with intersexuality, the gender identity develops in agreement with the gender assigned in infancy, although there can be considerable variability in the degree of behavioral or psychological femininity/masculinity. In interpreting this observation, one has to keep in mind, however, that gender is not assigned on a random basis. In recent decades, 46,XX individuals with intersexuality whose internal reproductive system is (predominantly) female have usually been assigned to the female gender, no matter how large their clitoropenis is. 46,XY individuals with a micropenis, i.e. a penis size of 2 ½ SD or more below the male norm, have frequently been assigned to the female gender, no matter how much they were masculinized otherwise. Thus, both categories include individuals who were raised as females despite histories of—relative to normal females—increased prenatal androgen exposure that presumably affected the developing brain and is the most likely explanation for the frequently observed partial behavioral masculinization. Nevertheless, only a minority of intersex patients appear to develop marked gender identity problems. Since different intersex syndromes seem to vary greatly in regard to gender development, a syndrome-specific analysis is necessary. For illustration, we briefly compare the life trajectory of three syndromes: complete androgen insensitivity (CAIS), classical CAH, and the pubertal change syndrome of 5α-RD (for medical details, see Grumbach and Conte 1998).

Complete androgen insensitivity (CAIS)

46,XY individuals with CAIS have functioning testes and at least normal testosterone levels but lack functioning androgen receptors. At birth, the external genitalia appear female, but the vagina is typically short and the other internal female structures are absent because of the action of the mullerian inhibiting factor of the testes. Because of the female appearance, these children are raised as females. The diagnosis may be made at birth if by that time the testes have descended into the labia majora. Many of these patients, however, are diagnosed not before adolescence when little or no pubic and axillary hair develops and menarche fails to occur. Owing to the normal testicular production of estrogens which, in this syndrome, is unopposed by androgen effects, these women develop breasts. The testes are usually removed before age 20 because of an increased risk of testicular malignancy, and exogenous estrogens are prescribed from then on. Frequently, the vagina needs lengthening by surgery or dilatation. There is only a very limited number of published psychological studies, all with small sample sizes. CAIS women as a group do not differ from control women in overall gender-role behavior, gender identity, and erotic attraction to males, although they may experience varying degrees of emotional difficulties related to the issue of infertility, to medical procedures, and to the way they are informed about the diagnosis. To my knowledge, the literature does not contain a single case report of a 46,XY CAIS individual raised female who later has voluntarily changed gender to male.

Congenital adrenal hyperplasia (CAH)

In classical CAH, 46,XX individuals are exposed to varying degrees of excess androgens produced in the adrenal secondary to a genetic defect in adrenal glucocorticoid synthesis. As a consequence, at birth, their external genitalia are variably masculinized, although the internal reproductive system is female. For some the genital masculinization is so extreme that the nature of their condition is not recognized and they are assigned to the male gender. If finally, around pubertal age, the correct endocrine diagnosis is made, the majority of such male-reared patients apparently decides to remain male, undergo surgery to remove the internal female reproductive organs, and begin testosterone replacement therapy.

When correctly diagnosed in infancy, 46,XX children with CAH are assigned and raised as girls, usually treated chronically with glucocorticoid replacement, which also largely normalizes the adrenal androgen production, and if necessary with mineralocorticoid replacement. Early genital surgery—particularly clitoral surgery of various forms—is mostly directed at feminizing the appearance of the external genitalia, followed often by vaginal surgery in childhood or adolescence to permit peno-vaginal intercourse. If glucocorticoid replacement is well managed, these women will experience menstruation and are fertile.

For girls with classical CAH, shifts of childhood gender-role behavior from stereotypically feminine in the direction of male-typical ('tomboyish') have been documented in a number of studies (Meyer-Bahlburg *et al.* 1996). By analogy to findings in non-human mammals, the organizational effects of excess prenatal androgens on the brain are the most plausible biological explanation of the behavioral masculinization. Adolescent and adult women with classical CAH show an increased rate of bisexual and homosexual erotic imagery and—to a lesser extent—behavior (Zucker *et al.* 1996). Yet most of the affected 46,XX individuals appear to maintain a female gender identity even if exposed to additional virilization in adolescence and adulthood. Relatively few 46,XX cases raised female have been reported to experience significant problems with their gender and, when presented with the choice, elected to change their gender to male, usually during the adolescent or adult years. If gender change occurs, it typically takes place in individuals with a history of prolonged genital ambiguity due to delay or absence of feminizing genital surgery, and/or a history of prolonged virilization due to poor or absent glucocorticoid replacement therapy (Meyer-Bahlburg *et al.* 1996).

5-α-reductase deficiency (5α-RD)

As a consequence of their enzyme deficiency, individuals with 5α-RD (Wilson *et al.* 1993) cannot convert testosterone into dihydrotestosterone, which is the essential androgen for the formation of external male genitalia, and are born with female-appearing external genitalia, but male internal genitalia. These patients begin to masculinize markedly with the onset of puberty, their testes descend into the labia majora, their clitoris develops into a relatively short hypospadiac penis of about average diameter, and their entire body virilizes markedly. In a remote rural area of the Dominican Republic where, owing to inbreeding, a sizeable number of such individuals could be identified, most of these individuals appeared to have developed a sexual attraction to females and assumed a male gender identity and role some time in later adolescence or young adulthood (Imperato-McGinley *et al.* 1979).

Interventions

GID in childhood

The literature concerning the treatment of childhood GID (Zucker and Bradley 1995, pp.265–82) is typically limited to case reports, and most descriptions of treatment regimens refer to one of three categories:

- intense psychodynamically oriented or psychoanalytic treatment of the child that appears to focus on child–parent relationships and conflicts (e.g. Coates and Wolfe 1995, Meyer and Dupkin 1985)

- intense behavior therapy utilizing mostly techniques of positive reinforcement of overt gender-typical behaviors by the therapist and the parents, and/or their self-monitoring by the child (Rekers 1985, Rekers *et al.* 1990)

- eclectic approaches involving, for instance, psychotherapy of the child and parental counseling (e.g. Green *et al.* 1972), or a parent- and peer-based treatment protocol emphasizing change of the psychosocial milieu at home without direct child–therapist contact (Meyer-Bahlburg, submitted).

There are also a few individual reports on group therapy with GID boys using differential reinforcement of gender-role behavior (Green and Fuller 1973), reinforcement of masculine behavior and social skills training (Bates *et al.* 1975), or group counseling sessions with the parents of GID boys (Pleak and Anderson 1993). With regard to girls with GID, the therapy research is even more limited and confined to a few case reports with similar therapeutic approaches. In conclusion, no well-established standard treatment regimens for childhood GID are currently available, neither psychological nor pharmacological.

Gender problems in intersexuality

Because of the defining genital ambiguity, the management questions concerning intersex patients are more complex than those concerning non-intersex children with GID. In regard to gender, the first issue to be decided in intersex children is the assignment of gender at birth. A second issue is the reassignment of gender in children, adolescents, or adults for whom the correct medical diagnosis is only made after the initial assignment of gender. A third question is how to manage the child, adolescent, or adult with intersexuality who develops a gender problem.

With regard to gender assignment and reassignment, there are basically three policies (Meyer-Bahlburg 1998b):

- the traditional *true sex policy* with a diagnostic focus on the indicators of biological sex

- the *optimal gender policy* with a primary emphasis on expectations for future functioning and, for reassignment decisions after infancy, on the child's gendered self-concept and behavioral development (Money *et al.* 1955, Money 1994)

- a *'third gender' policy* emerging implicitly or explicitly from the critical examination of prevailing medical policies by such consumer organizations as the Intersex Society of North America (ISNA, 1995) and the transgender movement.

Associated with any policy on gender assignment and reassignment are specific decisions regarding the surgical treatment of the genitalia and sex-hormone treatment in adolescence, both designed—in the case of the optimal gender policy—to render the somatic appearance of the person with intersexuality maximally compatible with the assigned gender. Unfortunately, some medical procedures may have significant negative implications for the patients' psychosocial development and sexual functioning, but because of space limitations the details of medical management of intersexuality cannot be dealt with here.

Medical and psychosocial interventions have to address a multitude of issues (Meyer-Bahlburg 1993, Money 1994) owing to the great variability in patient presentation depending on the type of syndrome, its severity, the chosen gender of assignment, the child's age, and his/her medical management history. The number of intersex syndromes is large, their prevalence low, and the prevalence of individuals with a specific intersex syndrome and significant gender problems even lower. Therefore, systematic studies of intervention approaches to gender problems in intersex patients have not yet been conducted and will require major interinstitutional collaboration, if reasonable sample sizes are to be obtained.

Short-term and long-term outcomes

GID in childhood

Treatment success in terms of reduction of cross-gender behavior has been reported for each of the three major categories of individual therapy, but the literature is limited to case reports. Our own new parent- and peer-based treatment approach has so far only been examined by way of a chart-review study of 11 consecutive cases of boys including 8 with GID and 3 with marked GID NOS; the treatment was successful in 10 (Meyer-Bahlburg, submitted). Obviously, the lack of controlled clinical trials of children with GID does not permit any statements regarding the comparative efficacy of the treatment approaches. Such statements are further complicated by the enormous variability in treatment intensity ranging from a total of a few weekly sessions to years of several sessions per week. Zucker *et al.* (1985), in a survey of treatment cases covering diverse treatment approaches, concluded that the 'degree of [gender-related] behavioral change at follow-up correlated positively with number of therapy sessions and the child therapists' emphasis on gender-identity issues'. The case reports involving dynamic treatment approaches have the added disadvantage that they leave very unclear which of the many therapeutic activities and techniques employed over the years of treatment actually account for symptomatic change, or whether the multi-year treatment added anything beyond the long-term process of fading of the cross-gender identity.

Clinicians working in this area generally assume that successful GID therapy, at the very least, reduces the duration of the marked expression of cross-gender behavior in most children and thereby lessens the risk of negative side-effects of GID in terms of negative reactions from the peer group and others. Yet, it remains to be systematically demonstrated that this is indeed the case. It is even less clear whether the long-term outcome in terms of sexual orientation or adult gender identity is affected by any treatment approach. In Green's study (1987, p. 318), 12 boys with GID were treated with his (eclectic) treatment program; 9 of the 12 emerged as bisexual or homosexual, a percentage not statistically different from the entire sample of GID boys. At this stage of the research, we have no reason to assume that treatment of GID during childhood affects at all the long-term outcome in terms of sexual orientation or adult GID.

Gender problems in intersexuality

For reasons discussed earlier, no standardized psychosocial intervention approaches have been formulated for the psychosocial management of intersexuality, and therefore no systematic clinical trials have been conducted. Given the long-term implications, it seems doubtful that 'placebo'-controlled intervention trials of gender assignment and reassignment will ever be conducted, and systematic trials of other psychosocial procedures face considerable logistic difficulties. Thus, beyond the illustrative data on the developmental course of specific intersex syndromes in specific environments such as those presented earlier, systematic data on short-term and long-term outcomes of specific intervention approaches are not yet available.

Continuity versus discontinuity

GID in childhood

As mentioned earlier, the very limited evidence available indicates that continuation of childhood GID into adolescence and adulthood occurs only rarely. The data available do not permit any predictions of a transsexual outcome. Green's (1987) data suggest that a homosexual outcome (as compared to a heterosexual one) might be related to the child's degree of female role-taking and to variables indicating low availability of the father. Yet, to this author, the findings also appear compatible with the interpretation that the overall severity of the GID correlates with later homosexuality. In any case, much larger samples would be needed for firmer conclusions.

Gender problems in intersexuality

The variability of gender problems in intersexuality is too great and the empirical evidence too limited to permit satisfactory statements on continuity and discontinuity.

Risks and prognostic factors

GID in childhood

Early speculations about the origin of GID focused on biological explanations related to intersexuality. Yet abnormalities of sex chromosomes, postpubertal sex-hormone production, and neuroendocrine indications of prenatal hormone abnormalities could not be reliably found in males with GID, whereas a significant minority of adult females with GID tended to show some minor increases in adult androgens to levels characteristic of women with hirsutism (Bosinski *et al.* 1997). Although modest associations of androgen levels and various aspects of gender-role behavior have been described in women, GID is seen rarely among women with marked degrees of hirsutism. Zhou *et al.* (1995) were the first authors—and so far the only ones—to report on a structural brain difference between adult individuals with and without GID, namely in the central subdivision of the bed nucleus of the stria terminalis, which is known to be involved in the regulation of sexual behavior in non-human mammals. In the small sample of male-to-female transsexual men, its volume was female-sized, i.e. smaller than in both heterosexual and homosexual men without GID. Given the recent difficulties in establishing any replicable finding on sex differences in specific human brain structures, independent confirmation is needed.

Are there temperamental features that predispose a child to the development of GID under specific environmental conditions? In treating boys with GID, one is often impressed by the persistence of a temperamental syndrome that includes low interest in rough-and-tumble play and sports, low aggressiveness with other boys, aesthetic sensibility, and high emotionality, even after successful therapy of the GID itself. Coates and Wolfe (1995) have provided some preliminary systematic small-sample data based on retrospective maternal report showing that approximately 60% of untreated GID boys met the criteria of the inhibited child syndrome. About the same percentage showed increased sensory sensibility, which may be the basis for the often observed increased aesthetic and artistic talents of such individuals. Coates and Person (1985) found a high rate of separation anxiety in their boy sample as well as depressive features. Bradley and Zucker (1997) quote unpublished data by A. Birkenfeld-Adams indicating that boys with GID have 'largely insecure attachments'. These small-sample data certainly do not permit any conclusions about the age at onset of the behavioral features relative to the age at onset of GID, but are of great interest for future research on predisposing factors.

Even if these predisposing factors should be confirmed, however, additional factors are needed to explain the development of GID itself, when one considers the fact that the prevalence of children with the inhibited child syndrome or with anxiety disorders seems to be much higher than that of children with GID. In this regard, the psychosocial mechanisms involved in normal gender development (Ruble and Martin 1997) are of primary interest. With regard to reinforcement patterns, Green (1987) reported lack of parental discouragement of cross-gender behavior, and Mitchell (1991) showed that mothers of boys with GID showed increased reinforcement of feminine behavior and less reinforcement of masculine behavior. Occasionally, not only parental tolerance of cross-dressing, but repeated active cross-dressing of a boy by a family member, appears to be associated with the development of GID. The motivations underlying the particular parental reinforcement patterns are probably highly variable and may include, for instance, strong and persistent disappointment about having given birth to a boy when a girl was desired (Zucker and Bradley 1995, p. 213), disdain for aggressive behavior—perceived as male-typical—or of males altogether related to a mother's own history of physical abuse, or a strong ideology favoring androgynous rearing (Meyer-Bahlburg, unpublished clinical observations; for similar examples, see Zucker and Bradley 1995, p. 224–5). Reinforcement patterns are also linked to parental psychopathology. For instance, Zucker and Bradley (1995, pp. 237–9) showed that a composite measure of maternal psychopathology, as assessed by a complex index, was most closely related to the tolerance or encouragement of feminine behavior in boys with GID and (negatively) to the reinforcement of masculine behavior. Perhaps even the reported increased physical attractiveness, especially of facial features, of boys with GID—or decreased physical attractiveness of girls with GID—may enhance parental propensity for reinforcement patterns that foster cross-gender behavior (Zucker and Bradley 1995, p. 193–7). However, these data come from cross-sectional—although well-controlled—studies and do not permit a distinction between pre-GID appearance and the influence of GID itself on facial and related physical features.

Whereas the data on reinforcement patterns experienced by boys with GID are compatible with what one would predict from the role of reinforcement in normative gender development, data on cognitive-developmental factors in the development of GID are very limited. A detailed assessment of gender schemas—both of others and of self—for children with GID is yet to be done. Clinically, many boys with GID appear to display rather extreme degrees of femininity (as also observed in many adult male transsexuals). It well exceeds the degree of femininity or cross-gender behavior that one typically sees in the more extreme forms of intersexed children (Meyer-Bahlburg, unpublished data) and the discrepancy between boys with GID and controls on standardized gender scales surpasses the sex difference between normal males and females. Differences in gender-role behavior between boys with and without intersexuality and between boys and girls are likely to reflect, in part, sex-related biological differences that are larger than those between boys with GID and control boys. Therefore it seems more plausible that the extreme cross-gender behavior of GID children reflects cognitive variables including self-socialization rather than biological factors, but this remains to be tested.

The various psychosocial factors involved in the development of GID are not limited to the family, but include the entire social milieu, particularly the peer group whose strong influence on many facets of child socialization including gendered behavior is well documented (Parker *et al.* 1995).

Gender problems in intersexuality

The many diverse forms of intersexuality originate in abnormalities of the sex chromosomes or genes that participate in the sex-determining processes and in marked deviations from the norm of the prenatal sex-hormone milieu (including the function of sex-hormone receptors), due to either endogenous factors, e.g. genetically based enzyme abnormalities, or to exogenous factors, e.g. sex hormone administration during pregnancy (Grumbach and Conte 1998). Postnatally, we assume that the same psychosocial mechanisms (Ruble and Martin 1997) operate in the gender development of intersex children as in others, and that it is a combination of these psychosocial mechanisms that overrule the conflicting biological factors in cases where the gender assignment is successful.

The very limited evidence available indicates that under the prevailing management policies in the US only a minority of individuals with intersexuality will develop significant gender problems, and even fewer seek gender-reassignment in adolescence or later. Yet, the rate at which significant gender problems occur appears to be greater than expected by random cooccurrence of intersexuality and GID (Meyer-Bahlburg 1994, Meyer-Bahlburg *et al.* 1996). A number of biological and psychosocial factors may be involved. The most plausible biological factor is the sex-hormone based organization of the brain during sex-hormone-sensitive developmental periods. However, we are not yet certain which of the three major models of mammalian sex-hormone effects on the sex-dimorphic organization of brain and behavior applies to humans:

- the androgen-only model which focuses on prenatal or perinatal sensitive periods (Money and Ehrhardt 1972, Dörner 1976)
- the two-pathway theory involving both pre/perinatal androgens and estrogens in the masculinization and defeminization of brain and behavior (Meyer-Bahlburg 1997)
- the newly proposed model by Fitch and Denenberg (1998; Meyer-Bahlburg, 1998a) which adds to the two-pathway model processes of feminization and demasculinization that depend on low-dose estrogen during later (postnatal) sensitive periods.

To what extent the pre- and perinatal hormonal milieu determines gender identity is currently under intense debate. Recently, individual cases have been described where 46,XY individuals with a presumably normal prenatal hormonal milieu but non-hormonal penile underdevelopment or loss were assigned or reassigned and raised as females, but had themselves re-reassigned to male in adolescence (e.g. ablatio penis: Diamond and Sigmundson 1997, cloacal bladder exstrophy: Reiner and Meyer-Bahlburg 1995), and it has been argued that the sex-hormone-induced brain predisposition was the cause of the re-reassignment. However, Bradley *et al.* (1998) have presented the follow-up evaluation of a second case of ablatio penis followed by sex reassignment to female in infancy at a considerably earlier age than the other case; this woman was bisexual, but without gender dysphoria. Also, the majority of the 46,XY individuals born with cloacal exstrophy of the bladder and raised female who have been studied to date have not changed gender (Reiner and Meyer-Bahlburg 1995, Meyer-Bahlburg, unpublished data), although their relatively young age does not preclude gender change at a later age. These observations indicate that the presumptive predisposition by prenatal hormones does not in itself dictate the development of gender identity, and that other mechanisms participate. Much evidence from human studies does support an association of prenatal androgenization with the later development of masculinized gender-role behavior (e.g. Money and Ehrhardt 1972, Hines and Collaer 1993), but a gender identity as male or female can apparently be developed and maintained by individuals who vary widely in behavioral masculinity/femininity.

Perhaps it takes the combination of prenatal and pubertal androgenization of the brain to determine a male gender identity, as Imperato-McGinley *et al.* (1979) have argued on the basis of their data on 46,XY individuals with 5α-RD in the Dominican Republic. Yet, the data show that, when these female-raised children began to develop severe virilization in adolescence, gender change took many years and some never changed their gender (Meyer-Bahlburg 1982). Also late-treated CAH women who were born with ambiguous genitalia and experienced progressive virilization from early on, before glucocorticoid treatment became available, rarely changed their gender to male (Ehrhardt *et al.* 1968, Meyer-Bahlburg *et al.* 1996). Finally, simple determination of gender identity by prenatal and pubertal androgens combined does not appear to explain the occurrence of GID (transsexualism) in non-intersex men.

The concept of a 'sensitive period' of brain development was applied by Money and the Hampsons (Money *et al.* 1957) to the contribution of psychosocial factors on gender development, in analogy to the development of speech. This was prompted by their finding that adjustment problems or psychopathology in intersex patients were increased the more, the later—after the age of 18 months—a gender change was instituted by physicians without consideration of the child's behavioral development. Such early sensitive periods for psychosocial effects may be important for psychosexual differentiation in both intersex and GID patients and has much clinical plausibility, but still awaits systematic empirical validation.

Even if we assume that both hormonal and psychosocial factors contribute to gender development, it remains a major problem for the clinician, who is faced with the gender assignment decision of how to determine at birth the strength of the hormonal and social influences that will affect the child born with genital ambiguity. On the one hand, genital appearance (degree of genital masculinization in 46,XX infants or of genital undermasculinization in 46,XY infants) and gender-behavior outcome are only poorly correlated (e.g.

Dittmann *et al.* 1990). On the other hand, we have no good way of predicting future gender-typing behavior of the parents. There are a few exceptions. We are reasonably confident (based on the collective clinical experience of people in the field—partly documented in form of case reports) that consistency of rearing in one or the other gender role by both parents and other family members is more difficult to achieve

- if the professional team does not agree on the course of action to take
- if the parents and other family members are not sure of the appropriateness of the gender decision
- if there is a long period of uncertainty about the decision
- if the child continues to look genitally ambiguous or, later, develops strong secondary sex characteristics of the other sex.

The last point is supported by some systematic empirical evidence, namely data on modest-sized samples of intersexed individuals that link such persistent somatic ambiguities to increased rates of gender transpositions, i.e. gender change and/or homosexual orientation (Money *et al.* 1986, Money and Norman 1987, Money 1991, see also Meyer-Bahlburg *et al.* 1996).

Conclusions

The continuing public nature/nurture debate of psychosexual differentiation by largely unifactorially oriented representatives of biology or the social sciences appears to be increasingly out of step with the status of the research in this area. Even on the genetic level of the differentiation of gonads and genitalia, it has become apparent that sexual differentiation is a complex process involving multiple genes, and recent animal research has made it likely that some of the sex-dimorphic features of CNS function and behavior are directly related to the effects of genes without sex-hormone mediation (Pilgrim and Reisert 1992). The endocrine aspect of sexual differentiation has also gained in complexity and involves multiple hormones and metabolites that are active during subsystem-specific hormone-sensitive periods of development, although we do not yet know which of the major hormonal models is the most appropriate one for human psychosexual differentiation. The very existence of the phenomenon of GID in non-intersex individuals suggests that psychosocial 'nurture' during the early preschool years—presumably in conjunction with temperamental factors whose developmental basis needs further elaboration—can override hormonal predispositions. Psychosocial 'nurture' itself is comprised of a number of discrete mechanisms of social learning. In addition, cognitive-developmental factors play a major role and may derive their strong affective fuel from problems in early attachment development, although the initial findings in this area are in urgent need of confirmation. Nothing in the limited research available on the relatively uncommon variants of gender development such as GID in childhood and gender problems in intersexuality suggests that their development is any less complex than the normative development of gender whose complexity we have gradually come to understand (Ruble and Martin 1997). A comprehensive model of psychosexual differentiation will require detailed empirical grounding of the interactive aspects of multiple biological, social, and psychological factors and of their transactional relationships where applicable.

References

APA (1994). *Diagnostic and statistical manual of mental disorders*, 4th edn. American Psychiatric Association, Washington, DC.

Bailey, J.M. and Zucker, K.J. (1995). Childhood sex-typed behavior and sexual orientation: A conceptual analysis and quantitative review. *Developmental Psychology*, **31**, 43–55.

Bakker, A., van Kesteren, P.J. M., Gooren, L.J. G., and Bezemer, P.D. (1993). The prevalence of transsexualism in the Netherlands. *Acta Psychiatrica Scandinavica*, **87**, 237–238.

Bates, J.E., Skilbeck, W.M., Smith, K.V.R., and Bentler, P.M. (1975). Intervention with families of gender-disturbed boys. *American Journal of Orthopsychiatry*, **45**, 150–157.

Blanchard, R. (1990). Gender identity disorders in adult men. In *Clinical management of gender identity disorders in children and adults*, ed. R. Blanchard and B.W. Steiner, pp. 47–76. American Psychiatric Press, Washington, DC.

Bosinski, H.A.G., Peter, M., Bonatz, G., Arndt, R., Heidenreich, M., Sippell, W.G., and Wille, R. (1997). A higher rate of hyperandrogenic disorders in female-to-male transsexuals. *Psychoneuroendocrinology*, **22**, 361–380.

Bradley, S.J., Oliver, G.D., Chernick, A.B., and Zucker, K.J. (1998). Experiment of nurture: Ablatio penis at 2 months, sex- reassignment at 7 months, and a psychosexual follow-up in young adulthood. *Pediatrics*, **102**, http://www.pediatrics.org/cgi/content/full/102/1/e9.

Bradley, S.J. and Zucker, K.J. (1997). Gender identity disorder: A review of the past 10 years. *Journal of the American Academy of Child and Adolescent Psychiatry*, **36**, 872–880.

Coates, S. and Person, E.S. (1985). Extreme boyhood femininity: Isolated behavior or pervasive disorder? *Journal of the American Academy of Child Psychiatry*, **24**, 702–709.

Coates, S.W. and Wolfe, S.M. (1995). Gender identity disorder in boys: The interface of constitution and early experience. *Psychoanalytic Inquiry*, **15**, 6–38.

Cohen-Kettenis, P.T. and van Goozen, S.H.M. (1997). Sex reassignment of adolescent transsexuals: A follow-up study. *Journal of the American Academy of Child and Adolescent Psychiatry*, **36**, 263–271.

Diamond, M. and Sigmundson, H.K. (1997). Sex reassignment at birth. Long-term review and clinical implications. *Archives of Pediatrics and Adolescent Medicine*, **151**, 298–304.

Dittmann, R.W., Kappes, M.H., Kappes, M.E., Börger, D., Stegner, H., Willig, R.H., and Wallis, H. (1990). Congenital adrenal hyperplasia: I. Gender-related behavior and attitudes in female patients and sisters. *Psychoneuroendocrinology*, **15**, 401–420.

Dörner, G. (1976). *Hormones and brain differentiation*. Elsevier, Amsterdam.

Ehrhardt, A.A., Evers, K., and Money, J. (1968). Influence of androgen and some aspects of sexually dimorphic behavior in women with the late-treated adrenogenital syndrome. *Johns Hopkins Medical Journal*, **123**, 115–122.

Fitch, R.H. and Denenberg, V.H. (1998). A role for ovarian hormones in sexual differentiation of the brain. *Behavioral and Brain Sciences*, **21**, 311–352.

Green, R. (1987). *The sissy boy syndrome and the development of human sexuality*. Yale University Press, New Haven, CT.

Green, R. and Fuller, M. (1973). Group therapy with feminine boys and their parents. *International Journal of Group Psychotherapy*, **23**, 54–68.

Green, R., Newman, L.E., and Stoller, R.J. (1972). Treatment of boyhood transsexualism: An interim report of four years experience. *Archives of General Psychiatry*, **26**, 213–217.

Grumbach, M.M. and Conte, F.A. (1998). Disorders of sex differentiation. In *Williams' Textbook of Endocrinology*, 9th edn, eds. J.D. Wilson, D.W. Foster, H.M. Kronenberg, and P.R. Larsen, pp. 1303–1425. W.B. Saunders, Philadelphia.

Hines, M. and Collaer, M.L. (1993). Gonadal hormones and sexual differentiation of human behavior: Developments from research on endocrine syndromes and studies of brain structure. *Annual Review of Sex Research*, 4, 1–48.

Imperato-McGinley, J., Peterson, R.E., Gautier, T., and Sturla, E. (1979). Androgens and the evolution of male-gender identity among male pseudohermaphrodites with 5α-reductase deficiency. *New England Journal of Medicine*, **300**, 1233–1237.

ISNA (1995). *Recommendations for treatment: intersex infants and children.* Pamphlet available from Intersex Society of North America, PO Box 31791, San Francisco, CA 94131, USA.

Meyer, J.K. and Dupkin, C. (1985). Gender disturbance in children: An interim clinical report. *Bulletin of the Menninger Clinic*, **49**, 236–269.

Meyer-Bahlburg, H.F.L. (1982). Hormones and psychosexual differentiation: Implications for the management of intersexuality, homosexuality, and transsexuality. *Clinics in Endocrinology and Metabolism*, **11**, 681–701.

Meyer-Bahlburg, H.F.L. (1985). Gender identity disorder of childhood. Introduction. *Journal of the American Academy of Child Psychiatry*, **24**, 681–683.

Meyer-Bahlburg, H.F.L. (1993). Gender identity development in intersex patients. *Child and Adolescent Psychiatric Clinics of North America*, **2**, 501–512.

Meyer-Bahlburg, H.F.L. (1994). Intersexuality and the diagnosis of gender identity disorder. *Archives of Sexual Behavior*, **23**, 21–40.

Meyer-Bahlburg, H.F.L. (1995). Psychoneuroendocrinology and sexual pleasure. The aspect of sexual orientation. In *Sexual nature, sexual culture*, ed. P.R. Abramson and S.D. Pinkerton, pp. 135–153. University of Chicago Press, Chicago.

Meyer-Bahlburg, H.F.L. (1997). The role of prenatal estrogens in sexual orientation. In *Sexual orientation: toward biological understanding*, ed. L. Ellis and L.Ebertz, pp. 41–51. Praeger, Westport, CT.

Meyer-Bahlburg, H.F.L. (1998a). Estrogens in human psychosexual differentiation. *Behavioral and Brain Sciences*, **21**, 336–337.

Meyer-Bahlburg, H.F.L. (1998b). Gender assignment in intersexuality. *Journal of Psychology and Human Sexuality*, **10**, 1–21.

Meyer-Bahlburg, H.F.L. (submitted). Gender identity disorder in young boys: A parent-and peer-based treatment protocol.

Meyer-Bahlburg, H.F.L., Gruen, R.S., New, M.I., Bell, J.J., Morishima, A., Shimshi, M., Bueno, Y., Vargas, I., and Baker, S.W. (1996). Gender change from female to male in classical CAH. *Hormones and Behavior*, **30**, 319–332.

Mitchell, J.N. (1991). Maternal influences on gender identity disorder in boys: Searching for specificity. Unpublished doctoral dissertation, York University, Downsview, Ontario.

Money, J. (1991). *Biographies of gender and hermaphroditism in paired comparisons.* Elsevier, Amsterdam.

Money, J. (1994). *Sex errors of the body and related syndromes. A guide to counseling children, adolescents, and their families*, 2nd edn. Paul H. Brookes, Baltimore, MD.

Money, J. and Ehrhardt, A.A. (1972). *Man and woman—boy and girl. Differentiation and dimorphism of gender identity from conception to maturity*, pp. 117–125 and 146–166. Johns

Hopkins University Press, Baltimore, MD.

Money, J. and Norman, B.F. (1987). Gender identity and gender transposition: Longitudinal outcome study of 24 male hermaphrodites assigned as boys. *Journal of Sex and Marital Therapy*, **13**, 75–92.

Money, J., Hampson, J.G., and Hampson, J.L. (1955). Hermaphroditism: Recommendations concerning assignment of sex, change of sex, and psychologic management. *Bulletin of the Johns Hopkins Hospital*, **97**, 284–300.

Money, J., Hampson, J.G., and Hampson, J.L. (1957). Imprinting and the establishment of gender role. *Archives of Neurology and Psychiatry*, **77**, 333–336.

Money, J., Devore, H., and Norman, B.F. (1986). Gender identity and gender transposition: Longitudinal outcome study of 32 male hermaphrodites assigned as girls. *Journal of Sex and Marital Therapy*, **12**, 165–181.

New, M.I., White, P.C., Pang, S., Dupont, B., and Speiser, P.W. (1989). The adrenal hyperplasias. In *The metabolic basis of inherited disease*, 6th edn, ed. C.R. Scriver, A.L. Beudet, W.S. Sly, and D.Valle, pp. 1881–1917. McGraw-Hill, New York

Parker, J.G., Rubin, K.H., Price, J.M., and DeRosier, M.E. (1995). Peer relationships, child development, and adjustment: A developmental psychopathology perspective. In *Developmental psychopathology*, Vol.2. *Risk, disorder and adaptation*, ed. D. Cicchetti and D.J. Cohen, pp. 96–161. Wiley, New York.

Petersen, M.E. and Dickey, R. (1995). Surgical sex reassignment: A comparative survey of international centers. *Archives of Sexual Behavior*, **24**, 135–156.

Pilgrim, C. and Reisert, I. (1992). Differences between male and female brains—developmental mechanisms and implications. *Hormone and Metabolic Research*, **24**, 353–359.

Pleak, R.R. and Anderson, D.A. (1993). Group psychotherapy for parents of boys with gender identity disorder of childhood. (Poster) International Academy of Sex Research, June meeting, Pacific Grove, CA.

Reiner, W.G. and Meyer-Bahlburg, H.F.L. (1995). Psychosexual implications of gender reassignment at birth. (Poster). American Academy of Child and Adolescent Psychiatry, 42nd Annual Meeting, New Orleans, LA., 17–22 October. *Scientific Proceedings of the Annual Meeting*, p. 115 (NR-102).

Rekers, G.A. (1985). Gender identity problems. In *Handbook of clinical behavior therapy with children*, ed. P.A. Bornstein and A.E. Kazdin, pp. 658–699. Dorsey Press, Homewood, IL.

Rekers, G.A., Kilgus, M., and Rosen, A.C. (1990). Long-term effects of treatment for gender identity disorder of childhood. *Journal of Psychology and Human Sexuality*, **3**, 121–153.

Ruble, D.N. and Martin, C.L. (1997). Gender development. In *Handbook of child psychology*, 5th edn, ed. W. Damon, Vol. 3: *Social, emotional, and personality development*, ed. N. Eisenberg, pp. 933–1016, Wiley, New York.

Wilson, J.D., Griffin, J.E., and Russell, D.W. (1993). Steroid 5α-reductase 2 deficiency. *Endocrine Reviews*, **14**, 577–593.

Zhou, J.N., Hofman, M.A., Gooren, L.J., and Swaab, D.F. (1995). A sex difference in the human brain and its relation to transsexuality. *Nature*, **378**(6552), 68–70.

Zucker, K.J. and Bradley, S.J. (1995). *Gender identity disorder and psychosexual problems in children and adolescents*. Guilford, New York.

Zucker, K.J., Bradley, S.J., Doering, R.W., and Lozinski, J.A. (1985). Sex-typed behavior in cross-gender-identified children: Stability and change at a one-year follow-up. *Journal of the*

American Academy of Child Psychiatry, **24**, 710–719.

Zucker, K.J., Bradley, S.J., Oliver, G., Blake, J., Fleming, S., and Hood, J. (1996). Psychosexual assessment of women with congenital adrenal hyperplasia. *Hormones and Behavior*, **30**, 300–318.

19 Child maltreatment

Michelle New and David Skuse

Clinical picture

Since the first published studies in child abuse and neglect (Kempe *et al.* 1962), there has been a dramatic growth in professional interest in the subject (Knutson and DeVet 1995). The US National Research Council's Panel on Research on Child Abuse and Neglect considered over 2000 articles (NRC 1993). We aim to provide a partial overview of research on risks and outcomes, from a developmental perspective. Definitions of child abuse inevitably vary according to the uses for which they have been devised. Differences of emphasis occur between definitions for legal, clinical diagnostic, and research purposes. Developmental considerations need to be taken into account in defining abuse, as do cultural and other contextual factors (Cicchetti and Toth 1995). Behaviors which are construed as abusive or neglectful in infancy differ from those that indicate maltreatment of an adolescent (Finkelhor 1995). Medical and social definitions differ from legal definitions in their focus on parental adjustment and parental actions (Cicchetti and Toth 1995).

Research on risks and outcomes of child abuse and neglect has suffered from a lack of adequate sampling and appropriate control groups. A theoretical foundation for sample selection should be guided by the purposes of the study (Kinard 1994) but in practice the sample chosen is usually one of convenience. Many studies contain samples of mixed gender (Green 1993) but equivalent abusive experiences may affect boys and girls differently (Kendall-Tackett *et al.* 1993, Wolfe and McGee 1994). Generalization of results is limited by the source of subjects studied. For example, sexual abuse victims recruited from hospitals and emergency rooms are likely to be younger and more severely abused than those referred from social services and child protection services. Non-abused comparisons are essential so as to remove from subsequent analysis, so far as possible, variables that are irrelevant to the hypothesis or hypotheses being tested, but which may independently influence the outcome (Kendall-Tackett *et al.* 1993, Kinard 1994, Knutson and De Vet 1995). For example, pre-existing or concurrent traumatic events unrelated directly to the abuse (e.g. family breakdown) may influence outcomes too.

Intervention studies

Mental health treatment following child abuse is now well established, but is variable in its theoretical rationale. Few interventions have been rigorously evaluated due to sampling problems and a lack of comparison groups (see Finkelhor and Berliner 1995, Briere 1996,

Saunders and Williams 1996). Because the consequences of abuse are likely to be confounded by other concurrent stressors, whose impact follows disclosure, both intervention and treatment outcome appraisal are exceptionally difficult (Berliner and Saunders 1996). Evaluations of treatment effectiveness should use standardized assessments (Berliner and Saunders 1996). Focused cognitive-behavioral interventions may be effective (Cohen and Mannarino 1996, Deblinger and Heflin 1996, Deblinger *et al.* 1996). Although we can now be confident that abused children can improve during a course of treatment, more empirical studies are needed to determine the nature of variables influencing treatment outcome.

Short-term and long-term effects

General effects

Maltreatment during early childhood may have both physical and psychological sequelae (Skuse and Bentovim 1994). The psychological consequences are often the most profound and enduring (Garbarino and Vondra 1987, Claussen and Crittenden 1991). In recent years parallels have been drawn between the impact of abusive and aversive childhood events and the symptoms associated with post-traumatic stress disorder (PTSD) (e.g. McLeer *et al.* 1992). If it could be shown convincingly that the consequences for emotional and behavioral adjustment of child maltreatment, whether sexual, physical, or emotional, were similar, the conventional subdivision of abusive experiences might require revision. Recent studies and reviews suggest that a integrated approach may serve our understanding better (Briere 1992, Cicchetti and Toth 1995, Finkelhor and Berliner 1995, Mullen *et al.* 1996). However, there is no consensus view on the matter. We shall consider first the general impact of abuse and neglect upon child development before going on to discuss in detail the impact of sexual, physical, and emotional abuse separately.

The dominant area of concern regarding emotional development during infancy and early childhood is the quality of the relationship between parent and child. Attachment theory suggests that children's expectations of adult availability and responsiveness are generalizations, developed during infancy and toddlerhood through interaction with their primary attachment figures (Crittenden and Ainsworth 1989). Relationships with novel adults, encountered in childcare settings and schools, are linked to children's expectations about adult availability and responsiveness which influence both the construction of new relationships and the ability to explore and cope with the demands of new and stressful situations (Sroufe and Fleeson 1986). Early insecure, especially disorganized or disorientated, attachments are associated with neglect and abuse (Carlson *et al.* 1989). Subsequently the child's relationships with unfamiliar adults outside the home can be impaired, leading to abnormal patterns of social interaction. Abused preschoolers may avoid people who make friendly overtures toward them and may be unpleasant or even aggressive toward same-age peers (Klimes-Dougan and Kistner 1990). They may fail to respond with concern, empathy, and sadness to peer distress (Main and George 1985).

The socioemotional adjustment of school-age children may also be adversely affected. Regardless of the abuse they have suffered, self esteem is likely to be depressed, behavior is likely to be withdrawn or aggressive, and peer relations are impaired (Kaufman and Cicchetti

1989). Until the past few years little was known about the effects of early maltreatment upon children's social perceptions, upon the way in which they construct, interpret, and structure their social world, what understanding they have of other's emotions, what attributions they ascribe to the behavior of others, how they justify their own behavior, and how their moral judgments compare with those of non-maltreated children (Smetana and Kelly 1989). Abused children may be significantly less able to identify and label the emotional states of others, less able to describe social and interpersonal causes of specific emotions, and less able to understand social roles than non-abused children.

The detrimental impact of abuse and neglect upon cognitive development is also well recognized. Maltreated children usually score lower than expected on cognitive tests and have poorer school achievements than demographically matched peers (Hoffman-Plotkin and Twentyman 1984). Older maltreated children show a relatively high incidence of language delay and deviation (e.g. Vondra *et al.* 1990). Compared to normative data, or to non-abused children of similar intelligence, they score significantly less well on standardized language tests and also on the verbal scales of intelligence tests (e.g. Gibbons *et al.* 1995). Intellectual impairments might result from a variety of sources. For example, many maltreated children are raised in social environments that are typified by a low degree of reciprocity, low rates of verbal interaction, limited playful exchanges, and a lack of harmony. Occasionally adverse outcomes may result from neurological damage due to head injury or from inadequate nutrition, but perinatal stress and maternal mental illness can also influence intellectual development. Factors associated with social deprivation may confound the direct effects of abuse and neglect. Socially deprived subjects are in general unduly cautious and inhibited in the presence of unfamiliar adults, thereby compromising their ability to learn at school. Individual characteristics may be important too. Many abused and neglected children lack motivation during testing and consequently underperform (Aber and Allen 1987).

Interpersonal processes that lead to disorders of behavioral adjustment are rather better understood, due in large measure to the careful work of Patterson and his colleagues (e.g. Patterson *et al.* 1989). Their home observation methodology provided convincing evidence that parenting styles characterized by explosiveness, irritability, and threats tend to train children in the use of aggressive behavior. Children generalize this aggressive interpersonal style to interactions with peers and teachers at school (e.g. Simons *et al.* 1991).

Sexual abuse

Sexual abuse is defined as 'any sexual contact between an adult and a sexually immature child for the purposes of the adult's sexual gratification; or any sexual contact to a child made by the use of force, threat, or deceit to secure the child's participation; or sexual contact to which a child is incapable of consenting by virtue of age or power differentials and the nature of the relationship with the adult' (Finkelhor and Korbin 1988). The National Center on Child Abuse and Neglect (NCCAN) in the US recorded that approximately 1.9 per 1000 children are sexually abused each year (Office of Human Development Services 1988). In the UK, 0.26 per 1000 children are sexually abused each year according to official records (Home Office, London 1994). Such prevalence figures are compiled from interviews with adults about their childhood experiences, and from statistics of children placed on child protection registers and statistics for convictions of sexual offenses (Gulbenkian Foundation 1995).

The impact of sexual abuse on development takes many forms. Emotional and behavioral consequences can last well into adulthood (Browne and Finkelhor 1986, Beitchman *et al.* 1991, Finkelhor 1995, Mullen *et al.* 1996). Clinical research using subjects referred from child protection or criminal justice departments (Berliner and Elliott 1996) has found higher rates of psychological disturbance than among non-abused clinical samples (e.g. Kendall-Tackett *et al.* 1993, Boney-McCoy and Finkelhor 1995). Fears, post-traumatic stress symptoms, and sexualized behavior occur more frequently in sexually abused children than non-abused children (McLeer *et al.* 1992, Kendall-Tackett *et al.* 1993, Berliner and Elliott 1996, Deblinger and Heflin 1996). No single symptom or cluster of symptoms seems to be typical but there may be a developmental pattern. Preschool age children are more likely to show anxiety, nightmares, internalizing, externalizing and inappropriate sexual behaviors than older children (Kendall-Tackett *et al.* 1993). Those of school age are more likely to show fear, aggression, nightmares, school problems, and hyperactivity. Adolescents are more likely to show depression, withdrawn, suicidal or self-injurious behaviors, somatic complaints, delinquent activity, running away, and substance abuse.

In their community survey of adult women abused as children, Mullen *et al.* (1996) found that the similarities in outcome between physical, emotional, and sexual abuse in terms of their association with adult psychopathology are greater than their differences. Sexual abuse was, however, specifically associated with sexual problems. Although many poor adult outcomes were apparently influenced by a broad 'matrix of childhood disadvantage', Mullen *et al.* (1996) suggest the severity of the abusive experience in terms of degree of intimacy, and the nature of the perpetrator–victim relationship, have important moderating influences upon outcome. One further important consequence of child sexual abuse is the risk of revictimization. A recent review suggested that women who were sexually abused as children were at risk of experiencing physical and/or sexual abuse as adults (Messman and Long 1996).

Physical abuse

In the US at least 4.3 per 1000 children are victims of child physical abuse (Office of Human Development Services 1988). UK figures indicate that 1 child per 1000 is a victim of child physical abuse each year (Gulbenkian Foundation 1995). Injury is usual, and a distinction is made between accidental and non-accidental injuries to children.

- Non-accidental injury is more likely, but not invariable, if there has been a delay in seeking or failure to seek medical help.

- An account of the 'accident' which is vague, lacking in detail, and varies with each telling, is suspicious; innocent incidents are related in vivid ways that ring true.

- An account of the incident which is not compatible with the injury observed is also suspicious.

- Parental affect which is abnormal and does not reflect the degree of concern and anxiety one would expect in circumstances following a genuine accident also arouses suspicion. Abusing parents tend to be preoccupied with their own problems.

- Other aspects of the parents' demeanor may give cause for concern, including hostility, the rebuttal of accusations that have not explicitly been made, or attempts to leave (with or without the injured child) before medical investigations are complete.

- An appearance of the child and the interaction with the parents may also give cause for concern; many abused children look sad, withdrawn, and frightened. In some cases they show 'frozen watchfulness'.

- Finally, the child may say something to arouse suspicion (Speight 1997).

Children who have been subjected to the most severe physical maltreatment, or have experienced a combination of neglect, emotional, and physical abuse, suffer the greatest detriment to their socioemotional development. They experience problems with self- esteem, ego control, and ego resiliency (Egeland *et al.* 1983, Cicchetti and Olsen 1991). A recent 10 year follow-up of formerly physically abused children has recently been completed in the UK (Gibbons *et al.* 1995). Children were seen at a mean age of 11 years. Both teachers and parents regarded the formerly abused children as showing greater evidence of behavioral and emotional maladjustment than age-matched controls. Other studies have found an excess of depressive disorders before puberty (Kaufman 1991).

Relatively little has been written about the impact of physical abuse and neglect upon adolescents (Power *et al.* 1988, Garbarino 1989). Yet a national study of incidence of child abuse in the US (US Department of Health and Human Services 1988) reported that adolescents accounted for 47% of alleged cases, the great majority of which were substantiated upon investigation. Adolescent abuse is less likely to be reported to the protective services than are cases of abuse involving other age groups. The incidence of adolescent maltreatment equals or exceeds the incidence of maltreatment of younger children; psychological and sexual abuse predominate. Girls are at greater risk at this age than are boys (e.g. Power and Eckenrode 1990). Unlike the majority of families known to abuse younger children, those who maltreat their adolescent offspring are not predominantly socioeconomically disadvantaged (Garbarino *et al.* 1986, Vondra 1986). Families containing step-parents are more likely to maltreat them than families in which both parents are biologically related to their children (Farber and Joseph 1985). A survey among runaway and homeless youths in New York State during 1986–87 found that the majority were girls 15–16 years of age, of whom 60% claimed to have been physically abused by their families, 42% to have suffered emotional abuse, 48% neglect, and 21% sexual abuse (Power and Eckenrode 1990). Biological mothers were the usual perpetrators of maltreatment (63%), followed next in frequency by biological fathers (45%). The consequences of abuse upon adolescent adjustment may be severe, and a causal relationship between abuse and attempted or completed suicide has been hypothesized (e.g. Silverman *et al.* 1996, Yang and Clum 1996, Wagner 1997).

Emotional abuse and neglect

Emotional abuse and neglect of children may take many forms, from a lack of care for their physical needs, through a failure to provide consistent love and nurture, to overt hostility and rejection. Emotional abuse is rarely the sole reason for seeking child protection through legal action, yet evidence is accumulating that its long-term consequences upon social, emotional, cognitive, and behavioral development may be far-reaching and profound. Characteristic features include the habitual verbal harassment of a child by disparagement, criticism, threat, and ridicule and the inversion of love; by verbal and non-verbal means, rejection and withdrawal are substituted.

Neglect comprises both a lack of physical care-giving and supervision, and a failure to fulfill the developmental needs of the child in terms of cognitive stimulation. Although direct observations of parenting may raise suspicions about the presence of emotional abuse or neglect, the situation is usually suggested by its consequences for the child in terms of emotional and behavioral adjustment. All abuse entails some emotional ill treatment. There is often accompanying physical or sexual abuse. However, even without signs of physical or sexual maltreatment and disclosure of specific abusive activities, it is sometimes still possible to recognize characteristic groups of features that demand further investigation (see Skuse 1993).

Current knowledge on emotional abuse and neglect does not yet allow us causally to link specific patterns of maltreatment to particular delays and disorders. The symptoms we regard as suspicious may not invariably be indicative of abuse and neglect. Nevertheless, it is import- ant to recognize that the cessation of emotional abuse and its substitution by sensitive care, often in an alternative family, is usually followed by rapid and dramatic improvement in dev- elopmental attainments, behavior, and socioemotional adjustment (Skuse 1988, 1992). In this sense, the diagnosis can be validated in retrospect. There may also be evidence of a deterioration over time in cognitive abilities whilst the child is living in the abusive home. Motor development will in general be less affected than skills based on language such as practical reasoning. Serial testing every 6 months or so with a standardized instrument such as the Denver scales (Frankenburg 1975) can yield valuable information. Scores should be calculated as a percentage, with the quotient of mental age divided by chronological age used to view trends.

One specific consequence of long-term abuse and neglect is lack of physical growth in the absence of any organic disorder. Failure to recognize the etiology of psychosocial short stature may imperil not only the children's future physical development but also their intelligence, their social adjustment, and their emotional well-being. Skuse *et al.* (1996a,b) have identified two forms of this physical consequence of abuse. The first is referred to as *hyperphagic short stature* because of the associated insatiable appetite for food and drink. It may be distinguished from other cases of growth failure associated with abuse in which affected children lose their appetite. We have called the latter variant the *anorexic subtype*, which should not be confused with anorexia nervosa for affected children are not usually preoccupied with their body image (Skuse and Gilmour 1997).

Hyperphagic short stature (Skuse *et al.* 1996a,b) is not yet recognized as a distinct entity within the International Classification of Diseases (WHO 1992), a deficiency which hampers clinical recognition, inhibits epidemiological investigations into prevalence, and limits research into its etiology and management. Children with hyperphagic short stature are not only exceptionally small for their age, they have a range of distinctive behavioral symptoms. The diagnosis is based on a combination of current and historical features. It is not normally made before 2–3 years of age, probably because the neuropsychological and neurophysiolo- gical mechanisms mediating the characteristic features require a certain maturation of the central nervous system to become evident. Symptoms include disorders of sleep and appetite, together with disturbed patterns of defecation or urination in many instances. The key etiological factor is severe and prolonged stress, which is usually but not exclusively associated with emotional abuse. Most children living in stressful environments, however, do not display the characteristics of hyperphagic short stature, which may indicate a genetic predisposition. Siblings in a family with an affected child who share both biological parents are at about a 40% risk of developing the condition. Half-siblings and step-siblings do not appear to be at risk. All children in a family with an affected sibling must be examined and a full history taken. Cases have poor attention, often a hyperkinetic disorder, and associated learning difficulties. Poor receptive and expressive language skills are usual, in combination with relatively less impaired non-verbal abilities. Affected children may be receiving special education on the grounds of mild to moderate learning difficulties; their mean IQ is at least 1 SD below the population mean (Gilmour 1996, Skuse *et al.* 1996a).

Impaired linear growth may also follow failure to thrive in infancy; recent prospective longitudinal studies have shown that many affected children remain significantly shorter than their peers at least until puberty (Dowdney *et al.* 1997). Failure to thrive is rarely due to overt abuse or neglect (Skuse *et al.* 1995a). The usual cause is probably chronic malnutrition, which may be due as much to the individual characteristics of the child as to the parenting that child is receiving (Skuse *et al.* 1995b). For example, over a third of so-called non-organic cases of failure to thrive have dysfunctional oromotor skills that render it difficult for them to feed efficiently (Reilly *et al.* 1997), thus placing additional demands upon their care-givers to monitor nutritional intake.

Continuities versus discontinuities

Both professional child care workers, and indeed the general public, tend to assume that harsh parenting styles are transmitted across generations, but several researchers have noted significant limitations in the data cited in support of that relationship (Kaufman and Zigler 1987, Burgess and Youngblade 1988). Research during the 1960s and early 1970s suggested a strong association between engaging in abusive parenting and having been a victim of maltreatment (e.g. Kempe *et al.* 1962, Green *et al.* 1974). Recent studies, using greater methodological rigor, have found only a modest association between a history of harsh and abusive parenting and current parenting practices in the next generation (Egeland *et al.* 1987, Rutter 1989). Speculation about the processes that mediate intergenerational effects are often couched in terms of social learning theory (e.g. Burgess and Youngblade 1988). Researchers sharing this perspective believe that harsh parenting influences the next generation through a process of modeling and reinforcement. However, opinions are diverse about what exactly is learned. Severe coercive measures could simply be part of normal parenting (Straus *et al.* 1980). Those who have experienced such parenting could therefore use harsh parenting methods with their own children in an unthinking way (Simons *et al.* 1991). Alternatively, an abused individual could consciously apply set of rules or normative beliefs about the desirability, or perhaps the necessity, of strict physical discipline in child rearing. Patterson and his colleagues (Patterson 1982, Patterson *et al.* 1989) have provided convincing evidence that parenting style characterized by explosiveness and irritability and threats tends to train a child in the use of aggressive behavior and an aggressive approach to social interactions in general could be transmitted across generations (Burgess and Youngblade 1988) as a result of hostile parenting practices (see Elder *et al.* 1986, Caspi and Elder 1988, Simons *et al.* 1991,).

Risks and prognostic factors

In recent years there have been increasingly sophisticated attempts to combine environmental, social, and personal components that are known to contribute to child abuse into theoretical frameworks that summarize the processes, so that later adjustment in cases of abuse can be predicted. Belsky (1980) and Finkelhor (1995) present frameworks for understanding the way in which being the victim of abuse at various points throughout childhood and adolescence could affect adversely later emotional, behavioral, cognitive, and physical development. Abuse can disrupt a infant's attachment to the primary care-giver (e.g. Bowlby 1982). In later childhood the consequences differ according to the specific cognitive abilities of the child, which can influence their appraisal and subsequent coping of abusive experiences.

There have been many attempts to identify influences that could increase the risk of parents abusing their children. In recent years the contribution made by the parent's attributional processes has become a matter of increasing interest. By attributions we mean parent's beliefs about the causes of their child's behaviors and of the child's response to their attempts to control undesirable behaviors (Rosenberg and Reppucci 1983, Bugental *et al.* 1989). Larrance and Twentyman (1983) noted that abusive mothers tended to adopt rigid, categorical ideas about their child's personality (Sameroff and Feil 1985), and assumed their child possessed enduring unattractive attributes, such as stubbornness and irritability. Attributions for common behaviors, such as crying confirmed the parent's negative view of the child (e.g. 'he is doing it just to upset me'). Interventions need to take into account the tendency abusive parents have to perceive that they themselves have very little power to control their child's behavior. In contrast, they regard their children as having a great deal of power.

The association between parental depression and child abuse is complex. Although a depressed parent may be at greater risk of abusing their child, adults who were abused as children may be at greater risk of developing a depressive disorder (Burbach and Borduin 1986, Downey and Coyne 1990, Rutter 1990). Maladjusted children may exacerbate their parent's mental disorder. Hence difficulties may beget difficulties, with irritable and negative exchanges being initiated by both parties, and child maladjustment may be compounded (e.g. Radke-Yarrow *et al.* 1991). The same interpersonal factors, such as marital discord that induce depression in mothers, could lead to both parenting and child problems (Belsky and Vondra 1989). Other risk factors include individual child characteristics, including perinatal factors such as low birthweight and prematurity (Lynch and Roberts 1982, Benedict and White 1985), which may be associated with an excess of difficult temperamental qualities. An aversive cry, especially if related to neurological disorders, is often a source of parental stress (Donovan and Leavitt 1985). Coercive and oppositional behavior in older abused children may put them at increased risk of being abused (e.g. Wolfe and Mosk 1983, Lahey *et al.* 1984) although it is often hard to determine the direction of cause and effect (Lorber *et al.* 1984, Dowdney and Pickles 1991).

Socioeconomic circumstances are relevant too. Abuse occurs more frequently among families of lower socioeconomic status (e.g. Straus and Gelles 1986) especially those with a lack of social supports, such as extended families (e.g. Gaudin and Polansky 1986). It is associated with high levels of intrafamilial stress (eg, Browne 1986), and recent adverse life events (Justice *et al.* 1985). Abuse within families of lower socioeconomic status has been associated with a greater use of authoritarian punishment, lower parental involvement and heightened conflict, and a lack of emphasis on independence together with disciplinary techniques that exert undue control and are punitive (e.g. Trickett and Kuczynski 1986). Although having been abused as a child is not a necessary or sufficient cause of becoming an abusive parent, the way in which adults conceptualize their childhood contributes significantly to the way in which they view and practice child rearing (Egeland *et al.* 1987, Kaufman and Zigler 1987).

Conclusions

In summary, the major determinants of parenting behavior are the personality and psychological wellbeing of that individual, his or her own experience of parenting practices, the characteristics of the child, socioeconomic influences, and contextual sources of stress and support. The role played by broader societal influences has not yet been established. Parental competence is multiply determined and consequently is buffered against threats from any single source of influence. A breakdown in parental coping that results in physical or emotional abuse of a child is engendered by a whole range of circumstances acting in concert, rather than one key event or predisposition (Belsky and Vondra 1989). The predisposition to engage in sexual abuse is similarly complex, although there is substantial evidence that it is overwhelmingly men who are responsible—whether the victims are boys or girls (Skuse *et al.* 1997).

Society's own attitude to the abuse of children may well be relevant to the risks of such behavior. When Sweden introduced legislation prohibiting parents from physically punishing their children, the aim was not primarily to institute a series of prosecutions for a common parenting practice but to change the climate of opinion toward corporal punishment so as to make it less acceptable to society at large (Commission on Children's Rights 1978). Perhaps societal attitudes towards violence and societal expectations about what is appropriate discipline at home and at school are of considerable importance (Zigler and Hall 1989). So long as violence is portrayed by the media for its entertainment value (e.g. Friedrich-Cofer and Huston 1986), and corporal punishment within the home is the rule rather than the exception (e.g. Straus *et al.* 1980) the use of physical force as either a method of behavioral control or as an expression of anger and frustration may seem to be condoned by society (for review see Widom 1989). Both direct services to children and families and research programs on child abuse are likely to be influenced by prevailing public policy (e.g. Knutson and DeVet 1995, Berliner and Elliott 1996).

References

Aber, J.L. and Allen, J.P. (1987). The effects of maltreatment on young childrens socioemotional development: an attachment theory perspective. *Developmental Psychology*, **23**, 406–414.

Beitchman, J.H., Zucker, K.J., Hood, J.E., daCosta, G.A., and Akman, D. (1991). A review of the short-term effects of child sexual abuse. *Child Abuse and Neglect*, **15**, 537–556.

Belsky, J. (1980). Child maltreatment: an ecological integration. *American Psychologist*, **35**, 320–335.

Belsky, J. and Vondra, J. (1989). Lessons from child abuse: the determinants of parenting. In *Child maltreatment. Theory and research on the causes and consequences of child abuse and neglect*, ed. D. Cicchetti and V. Carlson, pp. 153–202. Cambridge University Press, New York.

Benedict, M.L. and White, R.B. (1985). Selected perinatal factors and child abuse. *American Journal of Public Health*, **75**, 780–781.

Berliner, L. and Elliott, D.M. (1996). Sexual abuse of children. In *The APSAC handbook on child maltreatment*, ed. J. Briere, L. Berliner, J.A. Bulkley, C. Jenny, and T. Reid. Sage, Thousand Oaks, CA.

Berliner, L. and Saunders, B.E. (1996). Treating fear and anxiety in sexually abused children: Results of a controlled 2-year follow-up study. *Child Maltreatment*, **1**, 294–309.

Boney-McCoy, S. and Finkelhor, D. (1995). The psychosocial sequelae of violent victimization in a national youth sample. *Journal of Consulting and Clinical Psychology*, **63**, 726—736.

Bowlby, J. (1982). *Attachment and loss: attachment*. Basic Books, New York.

Briere, J. (1992). *Child abuse trauma: theory and treatment of the lasting effects*. Sage, Newbury Park, CA.

Briere, J. (1996). Treatment outcome research with abused children: Methodological considerations in three studies. *Child Maltreatment*, 1, 348–352.

Browne, D.H. (1986). The role of stress in the commission of subsequent acts of child abuse and neglect. *Journal of Family Violence*, **1**, 289–297.

Browne, A. and Finkelhor, D. (1986). Impact of child sexual abuse: A review of the research. *Psychological Bulletin*, **99**, 66–77.

Bugental, D.B., Blue, J., and Cruzcosa, M. (1989). Perceived control over caregiving outcomes: implications for child abuse. *Developmental Psychology*, **25**, 532–539.

Burbach, D. and Borduin, C. (1986). Parent-child relations and the etiology of depression: a review of methods and findings. *Clinical Psychology Review*, **6**, 133–153.

Burgess, R. and Youngblade, L. (1988). The intergenerational transmission of abusive parental practices: a social interactional analysis. In *New directions in family violence research*, ed. R. Gelles, G. Hotaling, D. Finkelhor, and M. Straus. Sage, Beverly Hills, CA.

Carlson, V., Cicchetti, D., Barnett, D., and Braunwald, K. (1989). Disorganized/disoriented attachment relationships in maltreated infants. *Developmental Psychology*, **25**, 525–531.

Caspi, A. and Elder, G.H. Jr. (1988). Emergent family patterns: the intergenerational construction of problem behavior and relationships. In *Relationships within families: mutual influences*, ed. R.A. Hinde and J. Stevenson-Hinde, pp. 218–240.Oxford University Press, New York.

Cicchetti, D. and Olsen, K. (1991). The developmental psychopathology of child maltreatment. In *Handbook of developmental psychopathology*, ed. M. Lewis and S. Miller, pp. 261–279. Plenum, New York.

Cicchetti, D. and Toth, S.L. (1995). A developmental psychopathology perspective on child abuse and neglect. *Journal of the American Academy of Child and Adolescent Psychiatry*, **34**, 541—565.

Claussen, A.H. and Crittenden, P.M. (1991). Physical and psychological maltreatment: relations among types of maltreatment. *Child Abuse and Neglect*, **15**, 5–18.

Cohen, J.A. and Mannarino, A.P. (1996). A treatment outcome study for sexually abused preschool children: Initial findings. *Journal of the American Academy of Child and Adolescent Psychiatry*, **35**, 42—50.

Commission on Children's Rights (1978). *Barnesratt: On forbud not aga.* Swedish Department of Justice, Stockholm. (In Swedish).

Crittenden, P.M. and Ainsworth, M.D.S. (1989). Child maltreatment and attachment theory. In *Child maltreatment. theory and research on the causes and consequences of child abuse and neglect*, ed. D. Cicchetti and V. Carlson, Cambridge University Press, New York, pp. 432–463.

Deblinger, E. and Heflin, A. (1996). *Treating sexually abused children and their nonoffending parents: a cognitive-behavioral approach.* Sage, Thousand Oaks, CA.

Deblinger, E., Lippman, J., and Steer, R. (1996). Sexually abused children suffering posttraumatic stress symptoms: Initial treatment outcome findings. *Child Maltreatment*, **1**, 310–321.

Donovan, W.L. and Leavitt, L.A. (1985). Physiologic assessment of mother–infant attachment. *Journal of the American Academy of Child Psychiatry*, **24**, 65–70.

Dowdney, L. and Pickles, A. (1991). Expression of negative affect within disciplinary encounters: is there dyadic reciprocity? *Developmental Psychology*, **27**, 606–617.

Dowdney, L., Skuse, D., Morris, K., and Pickles, A. (1998). Short normal children and environmental disadvantage: a longitudinal study of growth and cognitive development from 4 to 11 years. *Journal of Child Psychology and Psychiatry*, **39**, 1017–1029.

Downey, G. and Coyne, J.C. (1990). Children of depressed parents: an integrative review. *Psychological Bulletin*, **108**, 50–76.

Egeland, B., Sroufe, L.A., and Erickson, M.F. (1983). Developmental consequences of different patterns of maltreatment. *Child Abuse and Neglect*, **7**, 459–469.

Egeland, B., Jacobvitz, D., and Papatola, K. (1987). Intergenerational continuity of abuse. In *Child abuse and neglect: biosocial dimensions*, ed. R.J. Gelles and J.B. Lancaster, pp. 255–276. Aldine de Gruyter, New York.

Elder, G.H., Caspi, A., and Downey, G. (1986). Problem behavior and family relationships: life course and intergenerational themes. In *Human Development and the life course: multidisciplinary perspectives*, ed. A. Sorensen, F. Weinert, and L. Sherrod, pp. 293–340. Erlbaum, Hillsdale, NJ.

Farber, E. and Joseph, J. (1985). The maltreated adolescent: patterns of physical abuse. *Child Abuse and Neglect*, **9**, 201–206.

Finkelhor, D. (1995). The victimization of children: A developmental perspective. *American Journal of Orthopsychiatry*, **65**, 177–193.

Finkelhor, D. and Berliner, L. (1995). Research on the treatment of sexually abused children: A review and recommendations. *Journal of the American Academy of Child and Adolescent Psychiatry*, **34**, 1408–1423.

Finkelhor, D. and Korbin, J. (1988). Child abuse as an international issue. *Child Abuse and Neglect*, **12**, 3—23.

Frankenburg, W.K. (1975). Revised Denver Developmental Screening Test. *Journal of Pediatrics*, **87**, 125–128.

Friedrich-Cofer, L. and Huston, A.C. (1986). Television violence and aggression: the debate continues. *Psychological Bulletin*, **100**, 364–371.

Garbarino, J. (1989). Troubled youth, troubled families: the dynamics of adolescent maltreatment. In *Child maltreatment. theory and research on the causes and consequences of child abuse and neglect*, ed. D. Cicchetti, and V. Carlson, pp. 685–706. Cambridge University Press, New York.

Garbarino, J. and Vondra, J. (1987). Psychological maltreatment: issues and perspectives. In *Psychological maltreatment of children and youth*, ed. M. Brassard, B. Germain, and S. Hart. Pergamon, New York.

Garbarino, J., Guttman, E., and Seeley, J.W. (1986). *The psychologically battered child*. Jossey-Bass, San Francisco.

Gaudin, J.M. and Polansky, N.A. (1986). Social distancing of neglectful families. *Children and Youth Services Review*, **8**, 1–12.

Gibbons, J., Gallagher, B., Bell, C., and Gordon, D. (1995). *Development after physical abuse in early childhood*. Department of Health Studies in Child Protection, HMSO, London.

Gilmour, J.D. (1996). The genetic influences of hyperphagic short stature. Unpublished PhD thesis, University of London.

Green, A.H. (1993). Child sexual abuse: Immediate and long-term effects and intervention. *Journal of the American Academy of Child and Adolescent Psychiatry*, **32**, 890–902.

Green, A.H., Gaines, R.W., and Sandgrund, A. (1974). Child abuse: a pathological syndrome of family interaction. *American Journal of Psychiatry*, **131**, 882–886.

Gulbenkian Foundation (1995). *Report on the Commission on Children and Violence*. Calouste Gulbenkian Foundation, London.

Hoffman-Plotkin, D. and Twentyman, C.T. (1984). A multimodal assessment of behavioral and cognitive deficits in abused and neglected preschoolers. *Child Development*, **55**, 794–802.

Home Office (1994). *Criminal Statistics England and Wales, 1993*. HMSO, London.

Justice, B., Calvert, A., and Justice, R. (1985). Factors mediating child abuse as a response to stress. *Child Abuse and Neglect*, **9**, 365–372.

Kaufman, J. (1991). Depressive disorders in maltreated children. *Journal of the American Academy of Child and Adolescent Psychiatry*, **30**, 257–265.

Kaufman, J. and Cicchetti, D. (1989). Effects of maltreatment on schoolage childrens socioemotional development: assessments in a day-camp setting. *Developmental Psychology*, **25**, 516–524.

Kaufman, J. and Zigler, E. (1987). Do abused children become abusive parents? *American Journal of Orthopsychiatry*, **57**, 186–191.

Kempe, C.H., Silverman, F.N., Steele, B.F., Droegemueller, W., and Silver, H.K. (1962). The battered child syndrome. *Journal of the American Medical Association*, **181**, 17–24.

Kendall-Tackett, K.A., Willimas, L.M., and Finkelhor, D. (1993). Impact of sexual abuse on children: A review and synthesis of recent empirical studies. *Psychological Bulletin*, **113**, 164–180.

Kinard, E.M. (1994). Methodological issues and practical problems in conducting research on maltreated children. *Child Abuse and Neglect*, **18**, 645–656.

Klimes-Dougan, B. and Kistner, J. (1990). Physically abused preschoolers responses to peers' distress. *Developmental Psychology*, **26**, 599–602.

Knutson, J.F. and De Vet, K.A. (1995). Physical abuse, sexual abuse, and neglect. In *Handbook of pediatric psychology*, ed. M.C. Roberts. Guildford, New York.

Lahey, B.B., Conger, R.D., Atkeson, B.M., and Treiber, F.A. (1984). Parenting behavior and emotional status of physically abusive mothers. *Journal of Consulting and Clinical Psychology*, **52**, 1062–1071.

Larrance, D.T. and Twentyman, C.T. (1983). Maternal attributions and child abuse. *Journal of Abnormal Psychology*, **92**, 449–457.

Lorber, R., Felton, D.K., and Reid, J.B. (1984). A social learning approach to the reduction of coercive processes in child abusive families: a molecular analysis. *Advances in Behavior Research and Therapy*, **6**, 29–45.

Lynch, M.A. and Roberts, J. (1982). *Consequences of child abuse*. Academic Press, London.

Main, M. and George, C. (1985). Responses of abused and disadvantaged toddlers to distress in age mates: a study in the day care setting. *Developmental Psychology*, **21**, 407–412.

McLeer, S.V., Deblinger, E., Henry, D., and Orvaschel, H. (1992). Sexually abused children at high risk for post-traumatic stress disorder. *Journal of the American Academy of Child and Adolescent Psychiatry*, **31**, 875–879.

Messman, T.L. and Long, P.J. (1996). Child abuse and its relationship to revictimization in adult women: A review. *Clinical Psychology Review*, **16**, 397–420.

Mullen, P., Martin, J.L., Anderson, J.C., Romans, S.E., and Herbison, G.P. (1996). The long-term impact of the physical, emotional and sexual abuse of children: A community study. *Child Abuse and Neglect*, **20**, 7–21.

NRC (1993). *Understanding Child Abuse and Neglect.* Panel on Research on Child Abuse and Neglect, Commission on Behavioral and Social Sciences and Education, National Research Council.

Office of Human Development Services (1988). *Study findings: Study of national incidence and prevalence of child abuse and neglect, 1988.* U.S. Government Printing Office, Washington, DC.

Patterson, G.R. (1982). *Coercive family process*. Castalia, Eugene, OR.

Patterson, G.R., DeBaryshe, B.D., and Ramsay, E. (1989). A developmental perspective on antisocial behavior. *American Psychologist*, **44**, 329–335.

Power, J.L. and Eckenrode, J. (1990). Maltreatment among runaway and homeless youths. *Child Abuse and Neglect*, **14**, 87–98.

Power, J.L., Eckenrode, J., and Jaklitsch, B. (1988). The maltreatment of adolescents. *Child Abuse and Neglect*, **1**, 189–199.

Radke-Yarrow, M., Richters, J., and Wilson, W.E. (1991). Child development in a network of relationships. In *Individuals in a network of relationships*. ed. R. Hinde and J. Stevenson-Hinde. Cambridge University Press, Cambridge.

Reilly, S., Skuse, D., Wolke, D., and Stevenson, J. (1998). Oral motor dysfunction in children who fail to thrive: Organic or non-organic? *Developmental Medicine Child Neurology*, in press.

Rosenberg, M.C. and Reppucci, N.D. (1983). Abusive mothers: perceptions of their own and their children's behavior. *Consulting Psychology*, **51**, 674–682.

Rutter, M. (1989). Intergenerational continuities and discontinuities. In *Child maltreatment: theory and research on the causes and consequences of child abuse and neglect*, ed. D. Cicchetti and V. Carlson, pp. 317–348. Cambridge University Press, New York.

Rutter, M. (1990). Commentary: some focus and process considerations regarding effects of parental depression on children. *Developmental Psychology*, **26**, 60–67.

Sameroff, A.J. and Feil, L.A. (1985). Parental concepts of development. In *Parental belief systems: the psychological consequences for children*, ed. I.E. Sigel. Erlbaum, NJ. Mahwah.

Saunders, B.E. and Williams, L.M. (1996). Introduction. focus section on treatment outcome research. *Child Maltreatment*, **1**, 293.

Silverman, A.B., Reinherz, H.Z., and Giaconia, R.M. (1996). The long-term sequelae of child and adolescent abuse—a longitidunal community study. *Child Abuse and Neglect*, **20**, 709–723.

Simons, R.L., Whitbeck, L.B., Conger, R.D., and Chyi-In, W. (1991). Intergenerational transmission of harsh parenting. *Developmental Psychology*, **27**, 159–171.

Skuse, D. (1988). Extreme deprivation in early childhood. In *Language development in exceptional circumstances*, ed. K. Mogford and D. Bishop, pp. 29–46. Churchill Livingstone, London.

Skuse, D. (1992). The relationship between deprivation, physical growth and the impaired development of language. In *Specific speech and language disorders in children: correlates, characteristics and outcomes*, ed. P. Fletcher and D. Hall, pp. 29–50. Whurr, London.

Skuse, D. (1993). Epidemiological and definitional issues in failure to thrive. In *Child and Adolescent Psychiatric Clinics of North America*, ed. J. Woolston, pp. 37–59. W.B. Saunders, Philadelphia.

Skuse, D. and Bentovim, A. (1994). Physical and emotional maltreatment. In *Child and adolescent psychiatry: modern approaches*, ed. M. Rutter, E. Taylor, and L.Hersov, pp. 209–229. Blackwell Scientific, Oxford.

Skuse, D. and Gilmour, J. (1997). Psychological disorders associated with short stature. In *Growth disorders: pathophysiology and treatment*, ed. C. Kelnar, H. Stirling, M. Savage, and P. Saenger. Chapman and Hall, London.

Skuse, D., Gill, D., Reilly, S., Wolke, D., and Lynch, M. (1995a). Failure to thrive and the risk of child abuse: a prospective population survey. *Journal of Medical Screening*, **2**, 145–150.

Skuse, D., Wolke, D., Reilly, S., and Chan, I. (1995b). Failure to thrive in human infants: the significance of maternal well-being and behaviour. In *Motherhood in human and nonhuman primates: biosocial determinants*, ed. C.R. Pryce, R.D. Martin, and D. Skuse, pp 162–170. Karger, Basel.

Skuse, D., Albanese, A., Stanhope, R., Gilmour, J., and Voss, L. (1996a). A new stress-related syndrome of growth failure and hyperphagia in children, associated with reversibility of growth hormone insufficiency. *Lancet*, **348**, 353–8.

Skuse, D., Gilmour, J., Stanhope, R., Albanese, A., and Voss, L. (1996b). Stress-related growth failure. *Lancet*, **348**, 1104–5.

Skuse, D., Stevenson, J., Hodges, J., Bentovim, A., New, M., Williams, B., Andreou, C., Lanyado, M., McMillan, D. (1997). *The influence of early experience of sexual abuse on the formation of sexual preferences during adolescence*. Final Report to the Department of Health. Behavioural Sciences Unit, London.

Smetana, J.G. and Kelly, M. (1989). Social cognition in maltreated children. In *Child maltreatment: theory and research on the causes and consequences of child abuse and neglect*, ed. D. Cicchetti and V. Carlson, pp. 620–646. Cambridge University Press, New York.

Speight, N. (1997). Non-accidental injury. In *ABC of child abuse*, 3rd edn, ed. R. Meadow, pp. 5–8. BMJ Publishing, London.

Sroufe, L.A. and Fleeson, J. (1986). Attachment and the construction of relationships. In *Relationships and development*, ed. W. Hartup and Z. Rubin, pp. 51–71. Cambridge University Press, New York.

Straus, M.A. and Gelles, R.J. (1986). Change in family violence from 1975–1985. *Journal of*

Marriage and the Family, **48**, 465–479.

Straus, M., Gelles, R., and Steinmetz, S. (1980). *Behind closed doors: violence in the American family*. AnchorBooks/Doubleday, Garden City, NY.

Trickett, P.K. and Kuczynski, L. (1986). Childrens misbehaviors and parental discipline strategies in abusive and nonabusive families. *Developmental Psychology*, **22**, 115–123.

US Department of Health and Human Services (1988). *Study Findings: Study of the National Incidence and Prevalence of Child Abuse and Neglect*, pp. 5–8. US Department of Health and Human Services, Washington, D.C.,

Vondra, J. (1986). The socioeconomic context of parenting. Unpublished Master's thesis, Pennsylvania State University.

Vondra, J., Barnett, D., and Cicchetti, D. (1990). Self-concept, motivation and competence among preschoolers from maltreating and comparison families. *Child Abuse and Neglect*, **14**, 525–540.

Wagner, B.M. (1997). Family risk factors for child and adolescent suicidal behavior. *Psychological Bulletin*, **121**, 246–298.

WHO (1992). *International Statistical Classification of Diseases and Related Health Problems (ICD-10)*. World Health Organization. Geneva.

Widom, C.S. (1989). Child abuse, neglect and adult behavior: Research design and findings on criminality, violence, and child abuse. *American Journal of Orthopsychiatry*, **59**, 355–367.

Wolfe, D.A. and McGee, R. (1994). Dimensions of child maltreatment and their relationship to adolescent adjustment. *Development and Psychopathology*, **6**, 165–181.

Wolfe, D.A. and Mosk, M.D. (1983). Behavioural comparisons of children from abusive and distressed families. *Journal of Consulting and Clinical Psychology*, **51**, 702–708.

Yang, B. and Clum, G.A. (1996). Effects of early negative life experiences on cognitive-functioning and risk for suicide : A review. *Clinical Psychology Review*, **16**, 177–195.

Zigler, E. and Hall, N.W. (1989). Physical child abuse in America: past, present, and future. In *Child maltreatment: theory and research on the causes and consequences of child abuse and neglect*, ed. D. Cicchetti and V. Carlson, pp. 38–75. Cambridge University Press: New York.

Index